Preanesthetic Assessment 2

Preanesthetic Assessment 2

Edited by
Elizabeth A.M. Frost

B

Birkhäuser
Boston · Basel · Berlin

Elizabeth A.M. Frost, M.D.
Department of Anesthesiology
Albert Einstein College of Medicine
  of Yeshiva University
Montefiore Medical Center
Bronx, NY 10461
U.S.A.

Printed on acid-free paper.

The chapters in this volume are revised and updated articles that originally appeared in consecutive issues of *Anesthesiology News* from 1987 to 1989. They appear here as a service to the medical-anesthesiology community with the cooperation and kind permission of McMahon Publishing Company, New York.

ISBN-13: 978-0-8176-3430-8   e-ISBN-13: 978-1-4684-6765-9
DOI: 10.1007/978-1-4684-6765-9

Typeset by Bi-Comp, Inc., York, Pennsylvania.

9 8 7 6 5 4 3 2 1

*Dedicated to Dr. Paul Goldiner, our Chairman,
for his enthusiastic support and unending devotion
to education in Anesthesiology*

Foreword

The primary mission of the medical school is to create new doctors. Once the medical student has received his or her doctorate, the medical school's interest in, and acceptance of, responsibility for the continued professional development of the physician ceases almost entirely.

Yet, with scientific advances in medicine increasing exponentially and the inevitable erosion of memory with time, teachings from our schools of medicine become increasingly irrelevant, forgotten, or both. To maintain competence, the physician must continuously re-educate him- or herself. CME—Continuing Medical Education—will probably never attain the status of the medical school's degree-granting undergraduate program, but medical schools and their faculties must recognize their responsibility, not only for *creating* competent physicians but also for *maintaining* that competence.

With these words I introduced the first volume of *Preanesthetic Assessment* in 1986. The series was a product of a Continuing Medical Education program initiated by the Department of Anesthesiology, Albert Einstein College of Medicine/Montefiore Medical Center. Controversy continues to exist over the lasting educational value of conferences that bring physicians together. Moreover, because of time or financial constraints, only a small number of anesthesiologists are able to attend seminars on a frequent basis. By producing a monthly, current, clinical series in conjunction with *Anesthesiology News* over these 4 years, we have been able to make state-of-the-art analyses available to all anesthesiologists.

Since the inception of this program in 1985, the Albert Einstein College of Medicine Office of Continuing Medical Education has received over 4,000 completed post-tests and requests for CME credit. Formal evaluations conducted by the office of Continuing Medical Education and *Anesthesiology News* have continued to underscore the enthusiasm with which the series has been accepted and its inherent usefulness. With the publication of the first 26 lessons in book form, anesthesiologists in

Europe and South America became familiar with the program and encouraged its continuation.

Although it is vital to verify and record the continuing educational endeavors of each practitioner, the highest form of education is pursued for its own sake—because of its own intrinsic value to the physician apart from credentialing and licensing requirements. The *Preanesthetic Assessment* program has proven its value to anesthesiologists. In Volume 2, the 24 lessons published in the second two years of the program have been assembled and updated to provide a convenient reference, not only for anesthesiologists preparing for Oral Board examinations, but also for clinicians confronted daily by routine and sometimes not-so-routine cases in the operating room.

VICTOR B. MARROW, M.A.

Director, Continuing Medical Education,
Assistant Professor of Bioethics,
Albert Einstein College of Medicine,
Montefiore Medical Center, Bronx, New York

Contents

Contributors

MICHAEL S. ACKERMAN, M.D.
Chief Resident in Anesthesiology, Albert Einstein College of Medicine, Montefiore Medical Center, Bronx, New York, USA.

RAGHUBAR P. BADOLA, M.D., F.F.A.R.C.S.
Assistant Professor of Anesthesiology, Albert Einstein College of Medicine, Montefiore Medical Center, Bronx, New York, USA.

SVETLANA BONNER, M.D.
Fellow in Neuroanesthesia, Department of Anesthesiology, Albert Einstein College of Medicine, Bronx, New York, USA.

ALRICK BROOKS, M.D.
Staff Anesthesiologist, Georgia Medical Center, Macon, Georgia, USA.

JONATHAN S. DAITCH, M.D.
Captain, U.S.A.F., U.S.A.F. Medical Center, Wright Patterson Air Force Base, Beavercreek, Ohio, USA.

JAN M. DAVIES, M.D.
Associate Professor, Foothills Hospital, University of Calgary, Calgary, Alberta, Canada.

ANIL DE SILVA, M.D.
Fellow in Neuroanesthesia, Albert Einstein College of Medicine, Montefiore Medical Center, Bronx, New York, USA.

C.J. EAGLE, M.D.
Assistant Professor, Foothills Hospital, University of Calgary, Calgary, Alberta, Canada.

WILLIAM T. GENTRY, M.D.
Resident in Anesthesiology, Albert Einstein College of Medicine, Montefiore Medical Center, Bronx, New York, USA.

GARY HARTSTEIN, M.D.
Instructor in Anesthesiology, Albert Einstein College of Medicine, Bronx, New York, USA.

ROSS A. MALLEY, M.D.
Fellow in Neuroanesthesiology, Albert Einstein College of Medicine, Bronx, New York, USA.

SYLVIA McMULLAN, M.D.
Staff Anesthesiologist, Phelps Memorial, Tarrytown, New York, USA.

EFREM MILLER, M.D.
Staff Anesthesiologist, Desert Samaritan Hospital & Health Center, Mesa, Arizona, USA.

IRENE OSBORN, M.D.
Assistant Professor of Anesthesiology, Albert Einstein College of Medicine, Montefiore Medical Center, Bronx, New York, USA.

WERNER PFISTERER, M.D., M.S. ED.
Assistant Professor of Anesthesiology, Albert Einstein College of Medicine, Bronx, New York, USA.

ROBERT ROSENLUND, M.D.
Staff Anesthesiologist, Wadsworth V.A. Medical Center, Los Angeles, California, USA.

SALVATORE C. SCALAFANI, M.D.
Department of Anesthesiology, St. Joseph's Hospital and Medical Center, Paterson, New Jersey, USA.

GERALD SCHEINMAN, M.D.
Staff Anesthesiologist, Prince George Hospital, Lanham, Maryland, USA.

CATHY WALL THOMAS, M.D.
Department of Anesthesiology, University of North Carolina, North Carolina Memorial Hospital, Chapel Hill, North Carolina, USA.

CHARLES W. WHITTEN, M.D.
Staff Anesthesiologist, University of Texas, Dallas, Texas, USA.

RANDALL D. WILHOIT, M.D.
Instructor, Department of Anesthesiology, Bowman Gray School of Medicine, Wake Forest University Medical Center, Winston-Salem, North Carolina, USA.

Introduction

Now almost 5 years have passed since the first meeting with Mr. Ward Byrne, the editor of *Anesthesiology News,* when we discussed the development of an educational series for clinical anesthesiologists. The articles, although complete in themselves, were to be bound by the common theme of Preanesthetic Assessment. In the beginning, I had many doubts that we would be able to complete enough articles on time for even one year. However, we passed that first hurdle. Practitioners across the United States expressed interest both by writing to *Anesthesiology News* and by registering with our office of Continuing Medical Education to receive credit for completing the lessons.

We soon had enough material to present in book form. Volume 1 contained the first 26 lessons. It was enthusiastically received both in this country and abroad as a convenient, practical reference source and as an aid in studying for Board examinations. Almost immediately, we received inquiries as to when Volume 2 would be ready and if we could establish a biannual project. The next 24 articles, each one reviewing a different topic, are now assembled and while we are proud to present Volume 2, our confidence does not yet extend to an affirmative reply on the second request.

As with the early lessons, I have continued to involve our residents and junior faculty as much as possible. I am delighted that anesthesiologists from other programs have also asked to contribute. Few of these young physicians have realized at the outset how much research and hard work are involved before a lesson is completed. There have been many discussions, some quite heated, before a manuscript has been finally sent to press. But I am proud to share their joy in their achievements and I am delighted at the understanding and awareness that has continued to grow between the residents and the attending physicians who have acted as reviewers. As the series has become more widely known, some of our authors have even found placement interviews much easier.

As was done in Volume 1, attempts have been made to update each article, although the material is essentially the same as that published in

Anesthesiology News. The questions have been included at the end as a self-assessment test.

Again, I express my gratitude to the staff of *Anesthesiology News,* Ward Byrne, Elizabeth Douglas, and Tatiana Chillrud for their willing cooperation and continued support. I thank the staff of Birkhäuser for confidence in this project, and most of all my sincere appreciation to the residents and staff who have helped me make the deadlines on time.

ELIZABETH A.M. FROST, M.D.

CHAPTER 1

The Patient with Abdominal Aortic Aneurysm*

Raghubar P. Badola

Case History. *An 86-year-old man presented in the Emergency Room with a chief complaint of dull abdominal pain radiating to both flanks. He had been treated for hypertension for 25 years and at the time of admission he was taking propranolol 40 mg twice daily, hydrochlorothiazide 25 mg on alternate days, and alphamethyldopa 250 mg daily.*

The patient reported chest pain on climbing one flight of stairs, relieved promptly by sublingual nitroglycerin. Although the patient had been informed that he had hyperglycemia, he was not on any medication to control his blood sugar. He had been admitted to the hospital 6 months earlier with a transient ischemic attack that resolved without evidence of neurologic deficit.

Blood pressure was 160/100 mmHg, pulse 86/min and regular laboratory findings were as follows: hematocrit 31%, hemoglobin 10.2 gm, white blood cell count 9700/mm³; serum electrolytes—potassium 3.0 mEq/l, sodium 135 mEq/l, chloride 101/mEq/l; blood glucose 225 mg/dl, BUN 50 mg, creatinine, 2.0 mg. The electrocardiogram showed normal sinus rhythm, with evidence of an old inferior wall infarct. Chest x-ray showed evidence of bilateral basal congestion and mild congestive heart failure.

A diagnosis of abdominal aortic aneurysm was confirmed by ultrasound and CT scan. The patient was scheduled for repair of the aneurysm on a semiemergent basis.

Introduction

When an abdominal aortic aneurysm (AAA) was first resected more than a quarter of a century ago, the operation was considered a prohibitively risky undertaking. Now, surgery of the aorta and its major branches is a common procedure because of improved surgical techniques, advances in

---

* Reviewed by Dr. Kurt Weingerter, Fellow in Vascular Surgery, Department of Surgery, Montefiore Medical Center.

monitoring, better anesthetic agents and adjuvants, and greater under-standing of normal and pathologic vascular physiology.[1] Risk of aneu-rysm rupture is an ever-present danger as the aneurysm gradually increases in size over time. The larger the aneurysm, the greater the chances of rupture: With an aneurysm of 5 cm diameter, the chance of rupture is 10% per year, increasing to 40% per year for aneurysms of 7 cm diameter.[2] Elective repair should be undertaken as soon as possible because the mortality is much higher if rupture has occurred. Mortality rate with elective surgery is about 3.9%.[3]

Signs and Symptoms

Most AAAs are asymptomatic, although on occasion some patients may experience bounding abdominal pulsations in the upper abdomen. Lum-bar or lower back pain is a grave sign, suggesting rupture or impending rupture. More frequently, the diagnosis is made during a routine physical examination or the aneurysm is found incidentally on gastrointestinal or genitourinary tract x-ray studies, or CT scan or ultrasound examinations performed for other complaints.

Age as a Risk Factor

Patients with AAAs are usually in the sixth to ninth decade of life and are likely to have other significant impairments. Physiologic functions decline with age, with a decrease in reserve that manifests most often at times of stress. Perioperative morbidity and mortality increase with age. One analysis showed that death within 7 days of surgery occurred in 1.5% of all surgical patients from 21–50 years of age, in 4.4% of those patients 61–70 years of age, and in 8.2% of those patients over the age of 80.[4]

TABLE 1.1. Prevalence (%) of coexisting disease in patients with abdominal aortic aneurysm, 1984–1986*.

	%
Hypertension	45
Angina	8
Congestive heart failure	5
Previous myocardial infarction	15
Presence of arrhythmias	2
Renal failure	4
Chronic obstructive pulmonary disease	5

* Data provided by S. Gupta, MD, Division of Vascular Surgery, Montefiore Medical Center, Bronx, N.Y.

Older patients frequently suffer multisystem involvement and concomitant diseases. Degenerative arterial disease is a generalized process and vascular pathology in the aorta suggests similar pathologic changes in other parts of the arterial tree. Coronary, cerebral, or renal vessels may be affected, at different rates in different areas, with consequent impairment of the respective organ. Concomitant systemic diseases are more common in the elderly. One review of patients admitted to a special geriatric unit gave the average number of diseases per patients as 6.[5] The high prevalence of coexisting coronary artery disease, hypertension, renal disease, diabetes, and chronic obstructive pulmonary disease in patients with acquired vascular disease is well documented.[3] (See Table 1.1.)

Preoperative Assessment

Myocardial infarction is the most common cause of death following intact aortic aneurysm repair—40–60% of perioperative deaths, and 3–9% of immediate deaths (intraoperatively or first 48 hours postoperatively).[36] Nearly 35% of patients undergoing abdominal aortic surgery develop congestive heart failure in the postoperative period, either as a consequence of myocardial infarction or exposure of the myocardium to excessive work load, eg, persistent hypertension, aortic stenosis, or regurgitation.[7] A thorough evaluation of the patient's current cardiac status is therefore essential, with a return to the best physiologic and psychological balance possible before surgery.

Cardiovascular System

Between 50 and 70% of patients presenting for vascular surgery have clinical manifestations of coronary artery disease; 40–50% have had previous myocardial infarction; 10–20% have angina[6]; 30–60% of asymptomatic patients may have severe coronary disease with greater than 70% stenosis of one or more vessels.[8]

Of patients presenting for major vascular surgery, 10–15% have congestive heart failure. If time permits, it should be treated over the course of a few days with bed rest, salt restriction, diuretics (furosemide), potassium supplementation, and when necessary, with digoxin or other inotropic support. Vasodilators such as nitroglycerin will reduce the work load of the failing ventricle.

Surgery of abdominal aortic aneurysms is associated with a high incidence of perioperative infarction even in patients without severe coronary artery disease, related to the patient's age, stress, long duration of surgery, and large fluid shifts. Patients with obvious coronary artery disease who are candidates for coronary artery bypass grafting should have that done before elective aneurysm repair. In rare, desperate situations, both procedures may have to be performed simultaneously if the patient has a tender expanding symptomatic aneurysm in danger of rupture, coexisting with severe coronary artery disease.

In the patient with dysrhythmias, the cause should be sought and treated preoperatively, if at all possible. Dysrhythmias may be caused by diseases of the myocardium and conducting tissue, electrolyte abnormalities, and hypertension.

Supraventricular dysrhythmias, including premature atrial contractions, do not require therapy if they occur fewer than 3–5/min and vital signs are stable. Paroxysmal atrial tachycardia is best treated with verapamil. Digoxin I.V. and propranolol are second-line therapy. Atrial flutter responds best to verapamil and electrocountershock of 10–20 watt-seconds, especially if the dysrhythmia is of recent onset. In long-standing cases, digitalis is effective in slowing the ventricular rate.

Ventricular dysrhythmias, if they occur more often than 6/min, are multifocal, or appear 3 or more in a row (ventricular tachycardia), should be treated with procainamide 20 mg/min I.V. to a loading dose of 1 gm. If there is enough time for oral control, the drug may be given orally 250–500 mg four times daily.

Ischemic heart disease should be treated preoperatively. If there is a history of recent myocardial infarction, surgery should be avoided if at all possible. Three different studies have shown increased risk of infarction (37%, 27%, and 5.8%, respectively) in the first 3 months after surgery. Between 3 and 6 months, the respective risk decreased to 16%, 11%, and 2.3%. After 6 months, the risk was 6%, 5%, and 1.7%, respectively.[9–11]

Hypertension should be well controlled in the preoperative period, with antihypertensive medication continued up to the day of surgery and resumed as soon as possible postoperatively. Clonidine presents problems when used in this setting. It is generally available only as an oral preparation and has a short half-life. Decreased intestinal function postoperatively may make its absorption unpredictable, with the possibility of rebound hypertension. Also, naloxone may antagonize the antihypertensive effects of clonidine. If possible, one of the other antihypertensive medications (eg, labetalol, verapamil) should be used for preoperative stabilization.

Electrolyte abnormalities should be corrected. If serum potassium is less than 3mEq/l, potassium should be replaced orally over 3–4 days until the serum level returns to normal. If oral replacement is not feasible, potassium should be given I.V. over 24–48 hours at a rate of 20 mEq/hr, with not more than 240 mEq in a 24-hour period.

Myocardial Performance Curve

Construction of a myocardial performance curve may improve patient evaluation and care. The pulmonary artery wedge pressure (PAWP) is elevated by infusing salt-poor albumin and lactated Ringer's solution. At each incremental elevation of PAWP, cardiac index (CI) is determined in triplicate by thermodilution. Plotting CI versus PAWP gives the slope of the Starling-type myocardial performance curve.[3] (See Figure 1.1.)

Three types of myocardial performance curves are shown in the figure. During volume infusion in patients with good myocardial reserve (patient "A"), cardiac output increases for each increment in PAWP. Patients with a poorer myocardium (eg, patient "B") have a peak in cardiac performance and with further increases in PAWP, the cardiac output decreases. The third type (eg, patient "C") demonstrates a steady decline in cardiac performance. Volume therapy is designed to raise the PAWP to the point at which cardiac performance peaks or, if this does not occur, to a maximum of 10–12 mmHg with a CI exceeding 2.5.

Left ventricular stroke work index can be used instead of CI.[12] The cardiac performance curve may move up or down depending upon various sympatho-mimetic stimulations caused by surgery or depression caused by some inhalational anesthetic agents and intravenous barbiturates. The curve also changes markedly during crossclamping and unclamping of the aorta. The PAWP level that gives optimal performance preoperatively also gives optimal cardiac performance intraoperatively. In the type "C" patient, cardiac contractility must be increased by use of dopamine or dobutamine, thereby reducing the PAWP.

Once the pulmonary artery catheter is in place, the balloon is deflated and a mixed venous sample is obtained. Measurements of mixed venous oxygen tension are very sensitive indicators of adequacy of cardiac output for total body metabolic needs.[13] If the mixed venous saturation is much lower than normal (40 mmHg), oxygen transport is inadequate. Even a small decline in cardiac output can be serious.

Respiratory System

Patients with AAAs commonly have a long history of heavy smoking. Longstanding congestive cardiac failure adds to pulmonary insufficiency. Thus, these patients frequently have borderline respiratory failure. Preanesthetic assessment includes chest x-ray, bedside pulmonary function tests, and arterial blood gas analyses. If the patient is

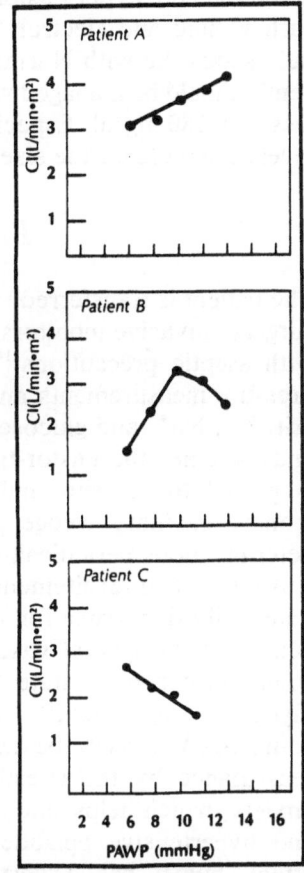

FIGURE 1.1. Myocardial Performance Curves.

still an active smoker, he should be encouraged to stop immediately as the carboxyhemoglobin-level decrease seen in 24 hours will help to increase O_2 carrying capacity in critical situations. Bronchodilators (aminophyll-ine, B2 receptor stimulators) may be beneficial. If there is evidence of infection, sputum for culture should be taken and appropriate antibiotic therapy started. Consultation with a respiratory therapist is useful. Although little immediate improvement in structural lung function may be obtained, familiarization with respiratory equipment preoperatively makes for greater efficiency in effect after the surgery.

Other Systems

Chronic renal failure is a frequent complication in patients with aortic aneurysms, especially if the aneurysm is at the level of the origin of the renal artery. Also, injection of radiopaque contrast for diagnostic radio-logic procedures may impair kidney function. Chronic hypovolemia, diabetes, and hypertension are further contributory factors. As noted earlier, fluid and electrolyte balance should be corrected. Replacement fluid should be with Normosol® or lactated Ringer's solution. Hypergly-cemia should be managed with regular insulin until the blood sugar level is less than 180 mg/dl. Especially during periods of stress, high blood sugar levels can increase the size of a cerebral infarct during an hypoxic event.

Preanesthetic Plan

The patient is transferred to the intensive care unit on the evening before surgery. Invasive monitors should be inserted under local anesthesia and with aseptic precautions.[14] The radial artery is cannulated for arterial pressure measurements and analysis of blood pH, PO_2, PCO_2, hemato-crit, K^+, Na^+, and glucose. The right internal jugular vein is cannulated and a 4-lumen thermistor-tipped, flow-directed pulmonary artery catheter is placed to measure pulmonary artery pressures continuously, pul-monary capillary wedge pressures intermittently, and cardiac output determinations periodically.

Anxiety and excitement in the immediate preoperative period are potentially dangerous for AAA patients. Hypertension and increases in heart rate, peripheral vascular resistance, and myocardial oxygen con-sumption can precipitate an angina attack, cardiac dysrhythmias, and myocardial infarction.[14,15] It is important, therefore, that patients under-going AAA surgery be adequately sedated. A preoperative visit and reassurance by the anesthesiologist establish good rapport and allay anxiety, which helps smooth induction of anesthesia without excitement and hypertensive episodes. Diazepam has an excellent tranquilizing effect, but it has a very long half-life (16–18 hours) and is quite unpredictable in duration of effect in the elderly. If it is used, the dosage should be reduced to 2.5–5 mg. Alternative drugs include hydroxyzine

25–50 mg or a small dose (approximately 25 mg) of diphenhydramine. Reduced dosages of premedication drugs should be used in patients with low cardiac output states. Elderly patients in shock or patients in whom the aneurysm has ruptured should not be sedated before the airway has been established and cardiovascular support has been instituted.

Anesthetic Plan

Monitoring

Adequate monitoring is essential, including continuous display of ECG and direct continuous arterial blood pressure recording. Sudden hypertension on crossclamping of the aorta or severe blood loss during unclamping are not uncommon, and continuous arterial pressure monitoring is essential to determine rational therapy. The pulmonary artery catheter is invaluable in managing the rapid shifts in preload and afterload and estimating myocardial performance (see Table 1.2.). An esophageal stethoscope with temperature probe and an indwelling urinary catheter are other essential monitors. Pulse oximetry, capnography, and frequent arterial blood gas analyses are now standards of care in all major vascular cases.

In some centers, monitoring during aortic surgery includes somatosensory evoked potential (SSEP) recordings. Repeated small stimuli are applied to the posterior tibial nerves and the evoked responses monitored

TABLE 1.2. Normal volumes for various parameters monitored during anesthesia for AAA resection.

Formula	Units	Normal Value
$SV = \dfrac{CO}{HR} \times 1000$	ml/beat	60-90
$SI = \dfrac{SV}{BSA}$	ml/beat/m^2	40-60
$LVSWI = \dfrac{1.36(MAP - PCWP)}{100} \times SI$	gram-meters/m^2	45-60
$RVSWI = \dfrac{1.36(PAP - PCWP)}{100} \times SI$	gram-meters/m^2	5-10
$SVR = \dfrac{MAP - CVP}{CO} \times 80$	dynes-sec/cm^{-5}	900-1500
$PVR = \dfrac{PAP - PCWP}{CO} \times 80$	dynes-sec/cm^{-5}	50-150

Key: PVR = Peripheral vascular resistance; MAP = mean arterial pressure; PCWP = pulmonary capillary wedge pressure; CVP = central venous pressure; SV = stroke volume; SI = stroke index; BSA = body surface area; LVSWI = left ventricular stroke work index; CO = cardiac output; HR = heart rate; RVSWI = right ventricular stroke work index; PAP = pulmonary artery pressure.

over the spine and cortex. Deleterious surgical manipulation or cardio-vascular changes causing hypoxic or ischemic events in the cord are recognized by increase in poststimuli latencies and decrease in amplitude of the waves. Appropriate therapy can then be instituted immediately.

Induction

Induction of anesthesia should be smooth, excitement free, and with minimal change in heart rate and blood pressure. Coughing, laryngo-spasm, hypertension, and tachycardia during induction may break the barrier of a dissecting or expanding AAA with diastrous results.

The trachea should be intubated only after adequate surgical anesthesia has been established. This may be achieved by administering adequate concentrations of inhalational anesthetic. MAC for endotracheal intuba-tion is about $1.3 \times$ MAC for surgical anesthesia.[15] In patients with poor ventricular function, a better choice of anesthetic technique would be to titrate the anesthetic depth with fentanyl or sufentanil, with muscle relaxation provided by vecuronium or atracurium.

Choice of anesthetic agents will be influenced by the condition of the individual patient and can be varied as long as the goals of smooth induction of anesthesia are met. Propranolol 1 mg or labetalol 5–10 mg helps to alleviate the hypertensive response to intubation. However, since a synergistic effect with nondepolarizing muscle relaxants may occur, the dose of these latter drugs should be decreased. Lidocaine 1 mg/kg I.V. has also been used as an adjunct to intubation.

Crossclamping

As part of the operative management, the aorta is crossclamped. Infrare-nal aortic crossclamping invariably increases vascular resistance about 40% and decreases stroke volume and cardiac output by 15–35%.[16–18] Arterial blood pressure is elevated but a dramatic rise is not a consistent finding. PCWP is increased and venous return to the heart is decreased as the pressure gradient in the vascular bed distal to the clamp from the capillaries to the venous system is zero. Patients with diminished cardiac reserve secondary to previous infarction or multivessel atherosclerotic heart disease frequently develop signs of cardiac decompensation and impending failure after infrarenal aortic crossclamping. This is character-ized by a sharp rise in PCWP, and a fall in cardiac output. There may be associated dysrhythmias and ECG evidence of subendocardial ischemia.

In patients without ischemic heart disease, on crossclamping there may be a decrease or no change in PCWP. Contractility of the ventricles increases to match the rise in the peripheral resistance.

With the release of the infrarenal aortic clamp, the artificially increased resistance is dissipated and afterload of the left ventricle is reduced. Cardiac output increases but this increase depends entirely upon the left ventricular filling pressure. The venous return is reduced due to ischemic vasodilation and vasomotor paralysis in the legs and pelvis during clamping. On unclamping, a large quantity of blood is pooled in this dilated and hyperemic vascular bed, diverting blood flow into the lower extremities and causing an internal steal.

Cardiac output falls if venous return does not match ventricular end-diastolic pressure (PCWP), and can result in severe hypotension and poor organ perfusion. This deleterious sequence of events is preventable—the PCWP should be raised to the value of maximum cardiac performance (Figure 1.1.) or 4–5 mm Hg above the control value by volume replacement before the clamp is released. When this is done, unclamping is associated with a smaller decrease in the cardiac output and less significant fall in blood pressure.

A rise in PCWP of 3 mmHg or more following aortic crossclamping is a sign of early cardiac decompensation. During crossclamping cardiac dysfunction worsens with time. There is an increase in the oxygen requirement of the heart and the cardiac output decreases. A continuous infusion of nitroglycerin 0.25 μg/kg/min during the period of crossclamping prevents the rise in the peripheral resistance and fall in cardiac output and restores myocardial contractility toward normal.[19]

Infrarenal aortic crossclamping is accompanied by a 75% increase in renal vascular resistance and a 38% decrease in renal blood flow.[18] Plasma levels of renin and angiotensin are elevated postoperatively. Renal hemodynamic deterioration persists for at least one hour after release of the aortic clamp. The mechanism of the renal changes is not clear. Prophylactic I.V. administration of mannitol (12.5—25 gm) before the clamp is applied seems to reverse or prevent the decrease in renal cortical blood flow.

Rarely, ischemic damage of the spinal cord can occur secondary to aortic crossclamping caused by interruption of blood flow through the low thoracic or high lumbar radicular artery supplying the spinal cord. Monitoring of SSEPs will, hopefully, provide early warning against such a disaster.

Fluid Management

Large amounts of fluid and blood are lost during AAA surgery due to tissue trauma, dissection, exposure of the abdominal cavity, and retroperitoneal edema. Blood loss is variable and depends on the technical problems involved during surgery, eg, poor vascular integrity, inadequate hemostasis, and anticoagulation. The aim of fluid therapy should be to maintain adequate blood volume (as determined by PCWP), adequate urine output (1 ml/kg/hour), and hematocrit of 30% or above. If urine output falls below 40 ml/hr in the presence of normal PCWP, therapy with mannitol and/or furosemide should be used.

All fluid and blood replacements must be warmed to prevent or minimize a fall in body temperature. Operating rooms should be warmed to 21°F, and inspired gases humidified. A warming mattress and radiant heat lamps can be used. Autotransfusion and the cell saver should be used to conserve blood loss and reduce the amount of bank blood required.

Emergency Aortic Surgery

If the patient presents with an aneurysm already dissecting or ruptured, he must be moved to the operating room as soon as possible. The anesthesiologist should call for as much help as possible to assist with resuscitation and establishment of intravenous access routes. Anesthesia is induced when the patient is prepared and draped and the surgical team is ready. Ketamine in small doses (25 mg increments), a large dose of muscle relaxant for endotracheal intubation, and controlled ventilation with 100% oxygen is one of the safer techniques in this setting.

A blood sample should be crossmatched with 12 units of blood and 4–5 units of O negative or type-specific blood should be at hand immediately. Six units of albumin 5% and adequate electrolyte solution must also be available, as well as several drugs including sodium bicarbonate, epinephrine, lidocaine, dopamine infusion, and nitroglycerin infusion.

Arterial cannulation should be accomplished and a central venous pressure catheter inserted as soon as possible. Blood gases should be examined frequently and oxygenation, ventilation, pH, electrolyte, and hematocrit corrected rapidly. If there is sudden loss of blood pressure when the abdomen is opened, the aorta should be clamped as early as possible while fluid and blood are replaced.

Acidosis can be corrected by the slow I.V. administration of sodium bicarbonate according to the formula:

Sodium bicarbonate (mEq) = .0.3 × body weight (kg) × base deficit/2

All patients must be observed in the intensive care unit for at least 24 hours after surgery.

References

1. Clark NJ, Stanley TH: Anesthesia for Vascular Surgery. In Miller RD (ed), Anesthesia, 2nd ed. New York: Churchill-Livingstone, 1986, pp 1519–61.
2. Rutherford RB: Infrarenal Aortic Aneurysms. In Rutherford RB (ed), Vascular Surgery. Philadelphia: W.B. Saunders, 1984. pp 755–71.
3. Whittemore AD, Clowes AW, Hechtman HB, et al: Aortic aneurysm repair—reduced operative mortality associated with maintenance of optimal cardiac performance. Ann Surg 1980;192:414–21.
4. Marx GF, Mateo CV, Orkin L: Computer analysis of postanesthetic deaths. Anesthesiology 1973;39:54–8.
5. Wilson LA, Lawson R, Porass W: Multiple disorders in the elderly. Lancet 1962;2:841–3.

6. Diehl JT, Cali RF, Hertzer NR, et al: Complications of abdominal aortic reconstruction—an analysis of perioperative risk factors in 557 patients. Ann Surg 1983; 197:49–6.
7. Young AE, Sandberg GW, Couch NP: The reduction of mortality of abdominal aortic aneurysm resection. Am J Surg 1977; 134:585–90.
8. Hertzer NR, Young JR, Kramer JR, et al: Routine coronary angiography prior to elective aortic reconstruction: results of selective myocardial revascularization in patients with peripheral vascular disease. Arch Surg 1979; 114: 1336–44.
9. Tarhan S, Moffit EA, Taylor WF, et al: Myocardial infarction after general anesthesia. JAMA 1972;220:1451–54.
10. Steen PA, Tinker JH, Tarhan S. Myocardial reinfarction after anesthesia and surgery. JAMA 1978;239:2566–70.
11. Rao TLK, Jacobs KH, Adel AI: Reinfarction following anesthesia in patients with myocardial infarction. Anesthesiology 1983;59:499–505.
12. Jeffrey CC, Kunsman J, Cullen DJ, et al: A prospective evaluation of cardiac risk index. Anesthesiology 1983;58:462–64.
13. Roy WL, Edelist G, Gilbert B: Myocardial ischemia during non-cardiac surgical procedures in patients with coronary artery disease. Anesthesiology 1979;51:393–97.
14. Lynn J, Stanley TH, Bidwai, AV, et al: Arterial blood pressure and pulse rate responses to pulmonary and radial artery catheterization prior to cardiac and major vascular surgery. Anesthesiology 1979;51:265–69.
15. Ykaitis RW, Blitt, CD, Angrillo JP: End-tidal halothane concentration for endotracheal intubation. Anesthesiology 1977;47:386–88.
16. Meloche R, Pottecher T, Audet J, et al: Haemodynamic changes due to clamping of the abdominal aorta. Can Anaesth Soc J 1977;24:20–34.
17. Attia RR, Murphy JD, Snider M, et al: Myocardial ischemia due to infrarenal aortic crossclamping during surgery in patients with severe coronary artery disease. Circulation 1976;53:961–65.
18. Gamulin Z, Forster A, Morel D, et al: Effects of infrarenal aortic cross-clamping on renal hemodynamics in humans. Anesthesiology 1984;61:394–9.
19. Zaidan JR, Guffin AV, Perdue G, et al: Hemodynamics of intravenous nitroglycerin during aortic clamping. Arch Surg 1982;117:1285–88.

The Patient with Pituitary Disease*

Irene Osborn

Case History. *A 41-year-old woman with the diagnosis of a suprasellar lesion was admitted for transsphenoidal hypophysectomy. The patient reported a 1-2 year history of headaches, with decreasing vision in the left eye. She also noted postmenopausal bleeding for 3 years. She denied other neurologic or physical problems at the time of admission.*

She had previously had a pilonidal cyst excision under general anesthesia without problems. Medical history was negative for hypertension, diabetes mellitus, cardiac symptoms, respiratory disease, or allergies, and the patient was not taking any medications. She smoked one pack of cigarettes a day but denied alcohol or drug use.

Physical examination revealed an obese woman (245 lb), who was alert, oriented, and cooperative. Vital signs were within normal limits. Head and neck examination revealed 4 missing upper teeth, but no other abnormalities were found. Chest examination was negative with lungs clear, and no cardiac murmurs. On neurological examination, the patient demonstrated intact cranial nerves but had a deficit in the left lateral visual field. No abnormalities were found on motor and sensory examinations.

Laboratory data included: hematocrit 32.4%, hemoglobin 10.7 gm, potassium 5.0 mEq/l, sodium 140 mEq/l. Endocrine evaluation was negative except for a serum prolactin level of 59 ng/ml (normal level, 5–10 ng/ml). Computed tomography scan showed a suprasellar lesion with extension into the left parasellar region. Angiography revealed a nonvascular pituitary lesion extending above the sella turcia. The patient was scheduled for transsphenoidal surgery.

---

* Reviewed by Dr. Alan Hirschfeld, Assistant Professor of Neurological Surgery, Albert Einstein College of Medicine, and Director of Neurological Surgery at the Bronx Municipal Hospital Center.

The Pituitary Gland

The pituitary is often called the "master gland" because its hormonal secretions affect many target organs within the body. Pituitary abnormalities are usually manifested by increased or decreased hormone secretion. Tumors of the pituitary may also expand to produce symptoms of headache, blindness, or obstructive hydrocephalus.

Location and Structure

The pituitary lies protected within the sella turcica of the sphenoid bone at the base of the skull. It is divided into an anterior lobe (adenohypophysis) that makes up 75% of the gland, and a posterior lobe (neurohypophysis). The pituitary stalk connects the posterior lobe to the hypothalamus (see Figure 2.1.), and a vascular trunk provides a connection for the anterior lobe.

The lateral walls of the sella are in direct proximity to the cavernous sinuses and thus to associated portions of the internal carotid artery and the oculomotor (III), trochlear (IV), trigeminal (V), and abducens (VI) nerves. The optic chiasma lies directly above the diaphragma sellae in

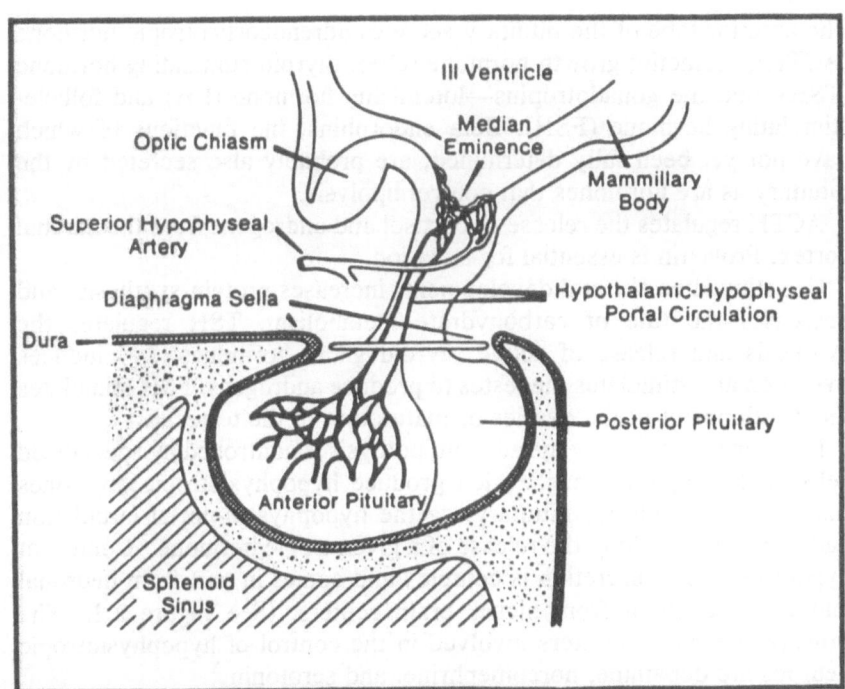

FIGURE 2.1. The pituitary and surrounding structures.

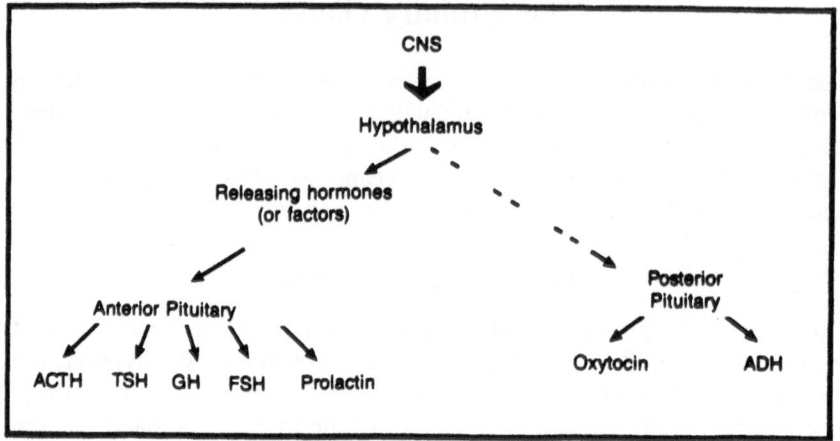

FIGURE 2.2. Hormones of the anterior and posterior pituitary.

front of the pituitary stalk. The hypothalamus controls the functions of the anterior pituitary by means of vascular connections and the posterior pituitary via nerve fibers.

Pituitary Hormones and Their Functions

The anterior lobe of the pituitary secretes adrenocorticotropic hormone (ACTH); prolactin; growth hormone (GH); thyroid-stimulating hormone (TSH); and the gonadotropins—luteinizing hormone (LH) and follicle-stimulating hormone (FSH). Beta endorphins, the functions of which have not yet been fully determined, are probably also secreted by the pituitary as are hormones that control lipolysis.[1]

ACTH regulates the release of cortisol and androgens from the adrenal cortex. Prolactin is essential for lactation.

GH stimulates skeletal development, increases protein synthesis, and decreases the rate of carbohydrate metabolism. TSH regulates the synthesis and release of active thyroid gland hormones. LH induces ovulation and stimulates the testes to produce androgens. FSH stimulates the development of the ovaries or maturation of the testes.

Hormone secretion by the adenohypothysis is controlled by specialized cells in the hypothalamus, which produce hypophysiotropic hormones that reach the anterior pituitary via the hypophyseal-portal circulation and stimulate or inhibit the release of a given tropic hormone.[2] Control of hypophysiotropic secretion is complex and comes in part from neuronal and chemical input from higher brain centers. (See Figure 2.2.) The principal neurotransmitters involved in the control of hypophysiotropic neurons are dopamine, norepinephrine, and serotonin.[3]

The posterior lobe is actually a component of the hypothalamus and is thus connected through an axonal system to the nuclei of the median eminence. Upon stimulation, it releases oxytocin and vasopressin (antidiuretic hormone, ADH). Vasopressin acts on the distal tubule of the kidney by increasing permeability of the responsive epithelium to water. Thus, urine is more concentrated as water is reabsorbed. ADH is an integral part of the homeostatic mechanism that controls water balance and effective blood volume.[1]

Oxytocin is synthesized predominantly by the paraventricular nuclei. It stimulates contraction of the myoepithelial cells of the breasts and thus aids in the ejection of milk. Although oxytocin in pharmacologic doses causes contraction of uterine smooth muscles and is widely used in labor, it does not appear to play a physiologic role in the delivery process.[4]

Pituitary Disorders

Panhypopituitarism

Total pituitary deficiency in man is probably incompatible with survival unless replacement therapy is instituted rapidly. The clinical presentation of panhypopituitarism may be dominated by either hypothyroidism or cortisol deficiency. If the syndrome occurs prior to puberty, short stature will result.[5] Adrenal function fails within a week after loss of the pituitary. Hypotension, hypothermia, vomiting, collapse, and death may occur if the patient does not receive corticosteroid replacement. If the hypothalamus and stalk remain intact, recovery of ADH secretion takes place and diabetes insipidis may subside. Loss of pituitary gonadotropins leads to profound gonadal atrophy, with decreased potency and libido as sperm disappear from the semen.

Panhypopituitarism most commonly results from surgical hypophysectomy. Neoplasms of the pituitary, hypothalamic injury, the "empty sella syndrome," prolonged shock, radiation therapy, and trauma also produce hypopituitarism and deficiency states.[6]

Neoplastic Disorders

The growth of pituitary neoplasms may produce endocrine disturbances or subtle neurologic signs. The diagnosis is eventually provided by the history, physical examination, and anatomic and functional studies. Anatomic studies include skull films, sellar tomograms, visual field testing, and computerized tomography of the head. Occasionally, contrast studies such as angiography and pneumoencephalography may be needed for diagnosis. Assessment of pituitary function and evaluation of parathyroid and endocrine pancreatic functions are also essential.[7]

Cushing's Disease and Cushing's Syndrome

Patients with Cushing's disease develop bilateral adrenal hyperplasia secondary to secretion of ACTH by basophilic or chromophobic pituitary adenomas. These individuals must be differentiated from patients with

Cushing's syndrome, which results from tumors of the adrenal gland or the ectopic production of ACTH by nonpituitary tumors.[8] The pituitary gland was first suspected as a pathologic source of hormone secretion in the early description of the disease by Harvey Cushing in 1932.[9]

The salient features of Cushing's syndrome are truncal obesity, thin extremities, cutaneous striae, hirsutism, moon facies, amenorrhea, osteoporosis, hypertension, hypokalemia, and hyperglycemia. Diagnosis is confirmed by lack of diurnal variation in ACTH levels and lack of suppression of ACTH levels by high or low doses of dexamethasone. The metyrapone challenge test helps differentiate between cases caused by tumors of the adrenals and those caused by the pituitary.[10]

It is estimated that 50–80% of patients with Cushing's syndrome have a pituitary-dependent cause. Bilateral adrenalectomy has been abandoned as a first-line treatment because of its surgical mortality and subsequent adrenal insufficiency. Nelson's syndrome, the development of biologically aggressive ACTH-secreting tumors, occurs in about 10% of patients after adrenalectomy.[11]

Prolactin-Secreting Neoplasms

The most common symptom of prolactin-secreting tumors is amenorrhea, occurring in 75% of cases. Galactorrhea occurs in 50% of patients and the remainder seek medical attention because of headache. Some hyperprolactinemic women will have noted spontaneous galactorrhea and many will complain of weight gain, decreased libido, oily skin, hirsutism, and inability to conceive. Men usually complain of impotence and decreased libido.

The primary clinical impairment resulting from elevated serum prolactin levels is the suppression of the menstrual cycle and resulting infertility, which may be caused by the inhibitory effect of prolactin on gonadotropin-releasing hormones. Serum prolactin levels may also be elevated by phenothiazine therapy and hypothyroidism.[12] FSH- and LH-secreting tumors are rarely seen; thyrotropin-secreting tumors are also very rare.[3]

Acromegaly

Acromegaly is caused by excess secretion of GH, usually from a microadenoma of the anterior pituitary. This produces a general overgrowth of skeletal, connective, and soft tissues. Facial features become coarse and the hands and feet become markedly enlarged.

The most specific diagnostic test is measurement of GH before and after glucose administration. Normally, glucose will markedly suppress the GH level, but this does not occur in patients with active acromegaly. In those patients, GH levels show little or no suppression or occasional

TABLE 2.1. Clinical features of hypersecreting pituitary tumors.

Syndrome	Hormonal excess	Clinical features
Cushing's disease	Adrenocorticotropic hormone (ACTH)	Centripetal obesity ("moon" facies, supraclavicular fat pad) Striae, ecchymoses Hirsutism Hypertension, glucose intolerance Psychiatric disturbances
Prolactin-secreting tumors	Prolactin	Amenorrhea or oligomenorrhea Infertility Loss of libido Galactorrhea
Acromegaly	Growth hormone (GH)	Enlarged hands and feet Distortion of facial features Gigantism (prepubertal) Visceromegaly Osteoarthritis Glucose intolerance Peripheral neuropathy Skeletal muscle weakness

paradoxic increase. GH secretion is normally stimulated by α-adrenergic influences from norepinephrine or dopamine.[1]

Manifestations of acromegaly reflect parasellar extensions of the anterior pituitary adenoma (macroadenoma) and peripheral effects produced by the excess GH. Cardiomegaly occurs frequently, occasionally with symptoms of congestive failure.[13] Glucose intolerance may aggravate cardiovascular problems and decrease the lifespan of patients.

Treatment of acromegaly depends on the stage at which the disease is detected, as well as presence of visual impairment. Transsphenoidal hypophysectomy is a frequent option, along with radiation therapy or transcranial approach if necessary. (See Table 2.1.)

Nonfunctioning Tumors

Nonsecreting tumors of the pituitary gland are frequently larger than secreting tumors, presenting with headache, visual disturbances, and increased intracranial pressure. Hypopituitarism may occur as evidence of endocrine dysfunction.[14] The most common tumors of this category are craniopharyngiomas and chromophobe adenomas. Craniopharyngiomas may develop as a cystic or solid mass and may occur at any age but are often seen in children.[15]

Pituitary apoplexy is a life-threatening condition caused by sudden changes that occur in pituitary neoplasms.[10] Spontaneous hemorrhage or infarction of a tumor presents with sudden headache, loss of consciousness, cranial nerve deficits, and meningeal symptoms.[17] Prompt differentiation must be made from subarachnoid aneurysm rupture, as pituitary insufficiency and death may follow pituitary apoplexy. Therapy includes rapid steroid administration and surgery for decompression of the optic chiasm and nerves.[17]

Preanesthetic Assessment

Preoperatively, patients should have been evaluated for endocrinologic and anatomic aspects of hypothalamic-pituitary disease. If the endocrine studies indicate a need for replacement therapy, it should begin about two weeks before surgery. The surgical procedure usually involves removal or manipulation of the anterior pituitary. For this reason, patients must receive steroid replacement therapy to provide adequate glucocorticoid levels for the perioperative period. Normal blood levels of pituitary hormones are listed in Table 2.2.

Premedication should be appropriate to relieve anxiety without causing undue sedation. Diazepam (5–10 mg orally) the morning of surgery is often used without problems in patients who are not obtunded. It is more important to prepare the patient for the postoperative period, when he or she will awaken with nasal packing and be required to breathe through the mouth and follow commands.

Cushing's Disease: Anesthetic management of the patient with Cushing's disease requires awareness of the physiologic effects of excess cortisol secretion. Preoperative evaluation and control of blood pressure, electrolyte imbalance, and plasma glucose levels are indicated. Choice of anesthetics will not significantly alter the intraoperative release of cortisol due to stress.

Acromegaly: Management of anesthesia for the patient with acro-

TABLE 2.2. Normal blood levels of pituitary hormones.

Hormone	Blood level (nl)
Cortisol (morning level)	$4.9\mu g/dl$ $(7-18\mu g/dl)$
Tetraiodothyronine (T4)	$6.1ug/dl$ $(4-11\mu g/dl)$
Triiodothyronine (T3) uptake	25.2% (25-36%)
Follicle-stimulating hormone (FSH)	$7.4\mu U/ml$ $(1-15\mu U/ml)$
Thyroid-stimulating hormone (TSH)	$3.5\mu U/ml$ $(10\mu U/ml)$
Luteinizing hormone (LH)	$3.1\mu U/ml$ $(1-15\mu U/ml)$
Prolactin	12.7ng/ml (1-20ng/ml)
Estradiol	16pg/ml (0.8-24pg/ml)
Growth hormone (GH)	2-5ng/ml

Note: nl = normal range.

megaly involves careful attention to the symptoms induced by GH excess. Of primary importance are changes in the upper airway. Distortion of facial features usually results in a difficult mask fit. The tongue and epiglottis are enlarged, predisposing to airway obstruction and difficult visualization of the vocal cords. The glottic opening may be narrowed secondary to vocal cord enlargement and possible subglottic narrowing.[18]

Preoperative airway evaluation is crucial, especially if the patient presents with hoarseness or dyspnea on exertion. Indirect laryngoscopy and x-rays of the neck should be obtained for thorough assessment. Fiberoptic or awake intubation may be preferred if difficulties are anticipated; the nasotracheal route should be approached cautiously because of frequent turbinate enlargement.[19]

If the acromegaly patient has diabetes mellitus, intraoperative monitoring of glucose levels is essential. A vigorous osmotic diuresis could mimic signs of early diabetes insipidis.[21] Hypertension should be well controlled during transphenoidal hypophysectomy as the surgeons frequently must use cocaine and epinephrine-containing solutions during the procedure. Allen's test should be performed before placement of a radial artery catheter because there may be inadequate collateral circulation caused by hypertrophy of the carpal ligament.[21] Choice of anesthetic is not influenced by acromegaly; however, a technique that allows for smooth extubation and rapid neurologic assessment is preferred and recommended.

Anesthetic Plan

Anesthetic management of patients undergoing pituitary surgery is not fundamentally different from that for other craniotomies except that cerebral dehydration with diuretic agents is not necessary. Rather, if better visualization is necessary, cerebrospinal fluid may be drained from a lumbar subarachnoid catheter.

Whether the transsphenoidal or transcranial approach is used, basic neuroanesthetic principles apply in terms of preparation and induction of anesthesia. Transsphenoidal surgery using the operating microscope is usually preferred except when tumors are mainly outside the sella.[21] (See Figure 2.3.)

Monitoring should include that normally required during craniotomies or appropriate for the patient's medical condition. Placement of a central venous catheter and Doppler probe may be required if the patient is to be placed in an upright position or cavernous sinus exploration is anticipated.[21] A smooth induction with thiopental (3–4 mg/kg) or midazolam (0.1–0.15 mg/kg) should be followed by intravenous lidocaine (1.5 mg/kg) or intratracheal spray of 4% lidocaine. If no problems are anticipated, a nondepolarizing relaxant may be used to facilitate intubation.

Some clinicians prefer the use of an armored (anode) endotracheal tube. A well-placed flexible tube is usually sufficient as long as breath sounds are continuously monitored, especially during positioning (and repositioning) of the head. Anesthetic agents should provide for intra-operative hemodynamic stability and rapid postoperative neurologic evaluation.

Frequently a catheter is placed in the lumbar subarachnoid space through which air can be instilled. The surgeon can then under fluoro-scopic inspection monitor the removal of the tumor.

As pertains in all other cases in which air is placed in a closed space, the use of nitrous oxide is not justified.

Preparation of the nasal mucosa with cocaine and epinephrine may precipitate hypertension, tachycardia, and dysrhythmias. Drugs for treat-

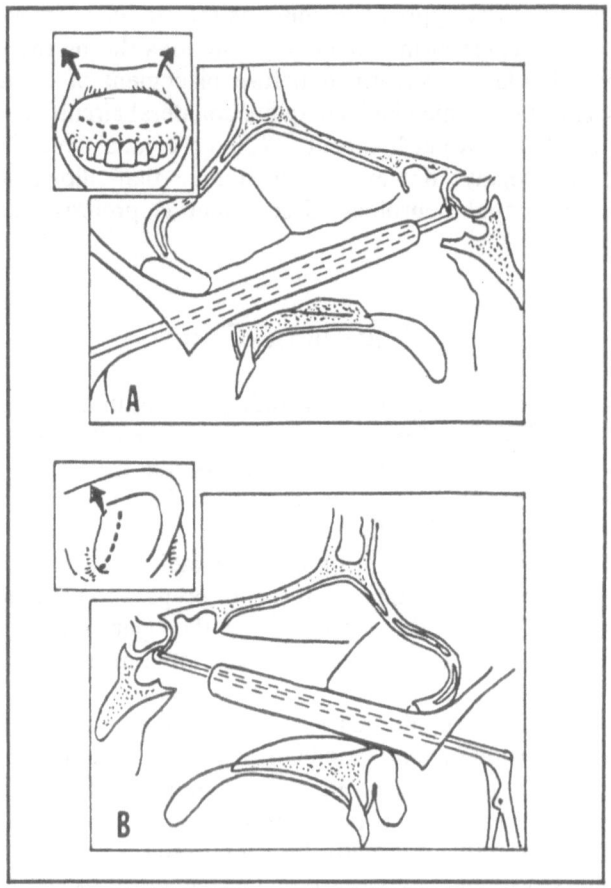

FIGURE 2.3. Different approaches to the sella. A. Sublabial, transseptal. B. Endonasal transseptal.

ment of those conditions should be readily available. The possibility of diabetes insipidus developing soon after the extirpation of the gland requires that vasopressin replacement therapy also is readily available.

References

1. Abhoud CF, Laws ER: Clinical endocrinological approach to hypothalamic-pituitary disease. J Neurosurg 1979;51:271–91.
2. Besser GM (ed): The hypothalamus and pituitary. London, WB Saunders, Clin Endocrinol Metab 1977;6:281.
3. Tindall GT: Surgery of the pituitary gland. Curr Probl Surg 1981;43:609–79.
4. Edwards CR: Vasopressin and oxytocin in health and disease. Clin Endocrinol Metab 1977;6:223–59.
5. Wright JC, Basel JA, Wilkins L: An evaluation of 75 patients with hypopituitarism beginning in childhood. Am J Med 1965;38:484–98.
6. Smith RR: *Essentials of Neurosurgery*. Philadelphia: J.B. Lippincott Co., 1980.
7. Hardy J: Transsphenoidal hypophysectomy. J Neurosurg 1971;34:582–94.
8. Kohler J: *Clinical Endocrinology*. New York: John Wiley and Sons, 1986.
9. Cushing H: The basophilic adenomas of the pituitary body and their clinical manifestations. Bull Johns Hopkins Hosp 1932;50:137–95.
10. Tyrell JB, Brooks RM, et al: Cushing's disease: selective transsphenoidal resection of pituitary microadenomas. N Engl J Med 1978;298:753–58.
11. Zervas NT, Martin JB: Management of hormone-secreting pituitary adenomas. N Engl J Med 1980;302:210–4.
12. Franks S, Jacobs HS: Hyperprolactinemia. Clin Endocrinol Metab 1983;12:641–63.
13. McGuffin WL, Sherman BM, et al: Acromegaly and cardiovascular disorders: a prospective study. Ann Intern Med 1974;81:11–8.
14. Majesko MJ: Anesthetic considerations in patients with neuroendocrine disease. In: *Anesthesia and Neurosurgery*, Cottrell J, Turndorf HT (eds). St. Louis: C.V. Mosby, 1986;224–45.
15. Shapiro K, Till K: Craniopharyngiomas in childhood: a rational approach to treatment. J Neurosurg 1979;50:617–23.
16. Wakai JC, Fukushima T: Pituitary apoplexy: Its incidence and clinical significance. J Neurosurg 1981;55:187–93.
17. Mitsumoto H, Coning JP: Spontaneous infarction in pituitary tumors: neurologic and therapeutic aspects. Neurology 1975;25:580–7.
18. Kitahata LM: Airway difficulties associated with anesthesia in acromegaly. Br J Anaesth 1971;43:1187–90.
19. Cucchiara RF, Messick JM: Airway management in patients with acromegaly. (letter) Anesthesiology 1982;56:157.
20. Laws ER, Abhoud CF: Perioperative management of patients with pituitary microadenomas. Neurosurgery 1980;7:566–70.
21. Messick JM, Laws ER: Anesthesia for transphenoidal surgery of the hypophyseal region. Anesth Analg 1978;57:206–15.

CHAPTER 3

The Patient with Sickle Cell Anemia*

Gary Hartstein

Case History. *A 31-year-old black man, an intravenous cocaine abuser with a history of sickle cell anemia (SCA), presented to the hospital with headache, stiff neck, and left hemiparesis of 5 days' duration.*

The patient was last admitted to the hospital 7 years earlier for painful sickle cell crisis, and was reportedly transfused at that time. He last used cocaine intravenously 2 weeks before this admission. He had no allergies, took no medication, and had only occasional sickle crises (2–3 per year, requiring only analgesics).

The patient was thin, drowsy but arousable, and in no acute distress. Vital signs were: temperature 100.3°F, pulse 48/min, blood pressure 130/80 mmHg, respiratory rate 18/min. Mild scleral icterus, nuchal rigidity, and positive Kernig's and Brudzinski's signs were noted, as was a right carotid bruit, a III/VI systolic murmur, and digital clubbing. A left hemiparesis with decreased appreciation of light touch and pinprick sensation on the left were also present.

Laboratory studies showed white blood cell count 24,000, hemoglobin 8.3 gm/dl, hematocrit 25.3%, and SMA-6 within normal limits. SMA-12 was significant for total:direct bilirubin 6.3:1.5, LDH 404. Lumbar puncture showed elevated opening pressure, xanthochromia, and many red cells. CT scan of the head showed multiple right parietooccipital infarcts. Carotid angiography revealed right carotid occlusion and a left posterior cerebral artery aneurysm. Hemoglobin electrophoresis was not performed.

The patient was scheduled for urgent clipping of a posterior cerebral artery aneurysm.

Introduction

Sickle cell anemia (SCA) is a genetic, molecular disease involving a mutation in one of the genes coding for hemoglobin (Hb). This mutation changes the behavior of the Hb molecule and affects all organ systems.

The disease is marked by a chronic hemolytic anemia and is punctuated

---

* Reviewed by Dr. Maria Santorineou, Professor of Medicine, Division of Hematology, Albert Einstein College of Medicine, and Director of Hematology at the Bronx Municipal Hospital Center.

by clinical crises. The significance of this entity for the anesthesiologist goes beyond the deranged physiology in the affected systems; clinical crisis in a patient can be triggered by several factors under the direct control of the anesthesiologist, namely oxygenation, pH, temperature, and patient position.

Genetics

Hb is a tetrameric protein, with each subunit (a globin peptide) containing one heme prosthetic group. Several forms of Hb exist in the course of normal development, from embryonic through adult life, differing in the nature of their subunits. The genes coding for the subunits are located on chromosomes 11 and 16, and are activated sequentially. After the embryonic hemoglobins (formed from two subunits coded by chromosome 16 and two coded by chromosome 11), fetal Hb is synthesized.

Fetal Hb (HbF) is formed from two alpha subunits, whose genes are located on chromosome 16, and two gamma subunits, coded on chromosome 11. Adult Hb (HbA) contains the same alpha subunits, with two beta globin chains (also coded on chromosome 11).[1]

SCA is caused by a point mutation in the beta gene. The codon for the sixth amino acid of the beta globulin peptide (glutamic acid) is GTG; a point mutation changes this codon to GAG, a triplet that codes for valine. Hb containing this altered beta chain is called HbS.

The homozygous individual has two HbS genes, which results in sickle cell disease or sickle cell anemia. The heterozygous individual inherits both a normal HbA and an abnormal HbS; thus, he carries the sickle cell trait (but does not have the disease) and has an essentially normal life. The SCA patient has 85–90% HbS; the remainder is HbF. Patients with sickle cell trait have 30–50% HbS, with the balance composed of HbA. Because sickle cell trait causes clinical problems only under very special circumstances (eg, exposure to high altitudes), we will concern ourselves here with the homozygous state—SCA.

Another condition of interest in this context is sickle-C disease. These patients have one beta gene coding for HbS, and the other gene coding for another mutant Hb, HbC. The clinical expression of sickle-C disease differs somewhat from that of SCA, but because both HbS and HbC cause sickling, both disorders will be included in our discussion. The anesthetic considerations are similar for both.

The gene for HbS apparently originated in West and Central Africa, areas where Falciparum malaria is endemic. Heterozygosity for HbS (the sickle cell trait) confers resistance to Falciparum malaria, probably by inhibiting intraerythrocytic multiplication of the parasite. This explains the persistence of this gene in the indigenous population. The slave trade is responsible for the appearance of the gene in the United States. The sickle cell trait is observed today in 8–9% of American blacks; SCA is estimated to affect 1 in 625 live births. Sickle-C disease, in the same population, is present in approximately 1 in 800 live births.[1]

Pathogenesis

Each subunit of normal adult hemoglobin is folded into a complex tertiary structure, with nonpolar, hydrophobic amino acids located toward the interior of the molecule, and hydrophilic polar residues outside. The heme group, with its iron atom, is located in the central hydrophobic pocket. This is important in maintaining the iron in its reduced (ferrous) state, the only state that binds oxygen. The polar surface of the globin chain interacts with the aqueous environment of the red blood cell (RBC).

The four subunits interact with each other to form the Hb molecule. Binding of an oxygen molecule causes the subunits to shift position with respect to each other, inducing a change in the molecule's affinity for oxygen, which is responsible for the S-shaped oxyhemoglobin saturation curve. Individual HbA molecules do not interact. The substitution of valine (a hydrophobic amino acid) for glutamic acid (a hydrophilic residue) at position 6 of the beta chain radically changes this series of reactions.

Position 6 is located on the outside of the Hb molecule; in the deoxygenated form, two small hydrophobic areas are normally exposed on any Hb molecule's surface. The beta-6 valines of one HbS molecule fit perfectly into the hydrophobic areas of two adjacent deoxy-HbS molecules, whose beta-6 valines in turn bind to two adjacent HbSs. This intermolecular bonding leads to rapid polymerization, with formation of long double-stranded fibers of HbS.[1] (See Figure 3.1.)

These fibers, called tactoids, lead to dramatic increases in the viscosity of the RBC contents and severely reduce the cell's deformability, which then prevents adequate passage of the RBC through the microcirculation. Further polymerization of HbS leads to sickling, where the RBC assumes a crescentic shape.

The red cell's deformability is decreased earlier in the polymerization process than the occurrence of morphologic sickling. Initially, the sickling phenomenon is reversible when the cell is oxygenated, but repeated cycles of polymerization and depolymerization damage the cell membrane, with increased loss of intracellular water and potassium. This leads to a very high mean corpuscular hemoglobin concentration (MCHC), and the cell becomes irreversibly sickled. [2] These sickled cells are cleared from the circulation by the reticuloendothelial system, leading to chronic hemolytic anemia.

A study of the kinetics of HbS polymerization (also called gelation) shows that the presence of nucleation sites is necessary for the process to proceed rapidly. These sites consist of chains of 15–30 molecules of polymerized HbS.[1] The time necessary for the formation of these nucleation sites accounts for the delay observed between the occurrence of conditions necessary for polymerization and its onset.

This delay is shortened, and the rate of gelation is increased by the following factors: (1) increasing concentration of HbS in the deoxy form; (2) increasingly acidic pH; (3) increasing temperature; and (4) increased levels of 2,3-diphosphoglycerate (2,3-DPG). The presence of other Hb species acts to inhibit gelation of interfering with formation of the cross-linked Hb lattice. HbF is particularly efficacious in inhibiting the polymerization process. Temperature, pH, and 2,3-DPG act by favoring the deoxy state of HbS.[1,2]

The clinical disturbances in SCA are brought about by altered rheologic

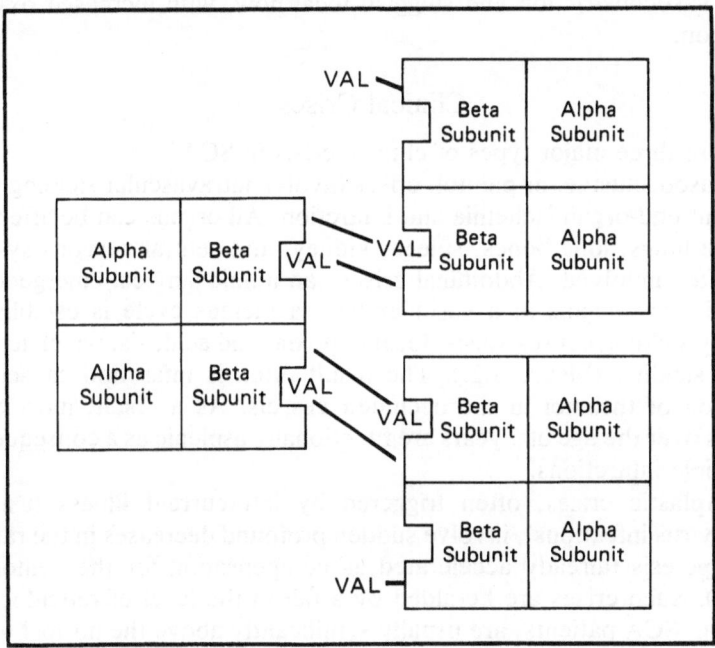

FIGURE 3.1. Schematic hemoglobin S polymer. The beta-6 valine is shown binding to the hydrophobic area present on all forms of deoxygenated hemoglobin.

properties that lead to diminished blood flow in the microcirculation, with ischemic damage to the involved structures. The rheologic problem is threefold. First, as mentioned above, the RBCs are less deformable because of increased membrane rigidity, increased cytosolic viscosity, and changes in the surface area–volume relationship of the RBC itself. Second, the RBCs show increased adhesiveness. These two phenomena operate primarily in the microcirculation. Third, plasma viscosity, which occurs mainly in large vessels,[2] can increase (especially with increases in acute-phase reactants during infections, which are known clinically to result in crises).

Clinical Aspects

General Effects

SCA is a chronic hemolytic anemia with superimposed crises. Since only the deoxygenated form of HbS polymerizes, localized or systemic hypoxia and Hb desaturation are necessary for sickling to occur. Patients with SCA show sickling at an O_2 saturation of 80%, corresponding to a PaO_2 of 50 torr. Thus, sickled RBCs are usually present in the mixed venous blood. Other conditions that favor sickling are acidosis, local capillary stasis, and increases or decreases in temperature. Elevations in temperature favor the deoxy form of HbS, while lowering of temperature causes vasoconstriction and sluggish local flow, with increased oxygen extraction.

Clinical Crises

There are three major types of clinical crisis in SCA.

(1) Vasoocclusive, or painful, crises involve intravascular sickling with attendant end-organ ischemia and infarction. All organs can be affected, with the lungs, long bones, spleen, kidney, and central nervous system most often involved. Abdominal crises can mimic surgical emergencies. Once sickling begins in a vascular bed, a vicious cycle is established whereby sickling causes stasis, local hypoxia, and acidosis, which lead to further sickling (Figure 3.2.). The result often is infarction caused by formation of thrombi in the occluded vessels. As a result, most SCA patients over the age of 5 years are functionally asplenic as a consequence of multiple infarctions.

(2) Aplastic crises, often triggered by intercurrent illness (usually papovavirus infections), involve sudden profound decreases in the rate of erythropoiesis (already accelerated as compensation for the hemolytic anemia). Such crises are heralded by a fall in the level of reticulocytes (which in SCA patients, are usually significantly above the normal value of 1-2%), followed by precipitous declines in Hb/Hct values.

(3) Sequestration, usually seen in children between the ages of 6 months

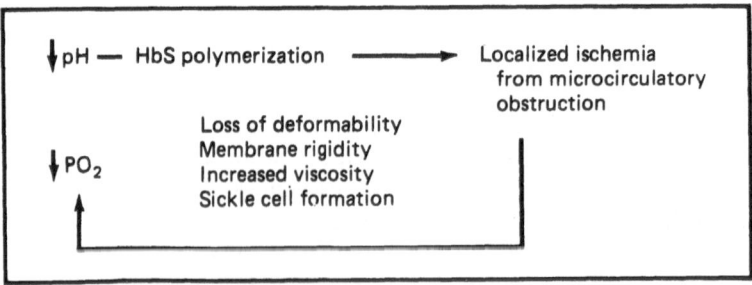

FIGURE 3.2. The Vicious Cycle of Vasoocclusion.

to 5 years (when not yet asplenic), involves sickling and obstruction of the venous drainage of the spleen, along with massive pooling of blood. In these circumstances, the spleen can become huge, reaching into the pelvis, and the clinical presentation can be that of hypovolemic shock.[3]

Laboratory values reflect the chronic hemolytic anemia, with Hb usually between 7 and 9 gm/dl, hematocrit around 25%, and signs of accelerated erythropoiesis, with elevated reticulocyte counts. Platelet and white cell counts are also often increased. Increased mean corpuscular volume (MCV) may reflect folate deficiency secondary to hyperactive erythropoiesis or may simply be a result of the presence of young red blood cells in the circulation. Haptoglobin is decreased, while bilirubin (both total and direct) is usually mildly elevated.

Pathophysiology

SCA has a pronounced effect on several organ systems.

Cardiorespiratory System

Cardiac output increases to compensate for the chronic anemia, ultimately resulting in dilated cardiomegaly and a variety of functional murmurs, usually systolic. Multiple ECG changes have been described (changes in PR interval, ST-segment and T-wave changes, etc). Cor pulmonale can result from SCA-induced pulmonary hypertension.[3]

In an autopsy study of 72 patients with sickle cell disease, necrosis of the pulmonary alveolar wall was noted in 17% of patients, but in only 6% of controls. In the SCA patients, the necrosis was associated with sickled cells in the adjacent pulmonary capillaries, and with local alveolar exudate or edema. This suggests that sickling with localized infarction occurs in areas of poor gas exchange. Focal areas of fibrotic scarring were found in 26% of patients and in 8% of controls—findings consistent with the idea that the persistent pulmonary infiltrates (despite adequate antibiotic therapy) often seen in SCA patients reflect localized areas of alveolar wall necrosis. Massive emboli consisting of necrotic bone marrow were seen only in SCA patients (13%), and were the cause of death in 7%. All were associated with long-bone infarction; marrow emboli were necrotic, and thus were not due to resuscitative efforts. Progressive amputation of pulmonary vascular reserve can lead to pulmonary hypertension; 7% of patients in this series had anatomic evidence of cor pulmonale.[4]

Renal System

SCA produces functional alterations of the kidneys with considerable clinical consequences. Both tubular and glomerular lesions have been described.[5,6]

A tubular defect—a loss of urinary concentrating ability called hyposthenuria—is the most commonly described renal lesion. Early in the course of SCA this defect can be reversed by exchange transfusion, suggesting that it is a result of sickling in the vasa recta, with a loss of the renal medullary concentration gradient. The loss of this gradient also explains why this lesion does not respond to antidiuretic hormone (ADH) administration. Later in the disease the vasa recta and the tubules are destroyed, and the renal defect becomes fixed. Hyposthenuria places the SCA patient at increased risk of dehydration, especially when exposed to situations associated with increased fluid losses (eg, fever, tachypnea, diarrhea, vomiting). Further, urine volume and specific gravity are no longer valid gauges of fluid status in these patients.

Another tubular defect is the inability to excrete an acid or potassium load. This is similar in some ways to a distal renal tubular acidosis; problems can arise in situations involving potassium loads (eg, blood transfusions, administration of potassium penicillin), or in situations where an acidic urine must be produced (eg, diarrhea with increased losses of bicarbonate). These functional tubular deficits correspond to the anatomic lesion of chronic tubulointerstitial nephritis, seen in many SCA patients in their 30s and 40s, even when blood urea nitrogen (BUN) and creatinine are normal.

The glomerulus is also involved. Occasionally, patients have the classic nephrotic syndrome (massive proteinuria, hypoproteinemic edema, and hyperlipidemia). Others show an immune-complex glomerulonephritis (usually the membranoproliferative form). The antigen in the immune complexes is hypothesized to be derived from ischemic tubular cells. nonimmune glomerulonephritis is also seen, and may be due to phagocytosis of sickled cells by the mesangium.

Papillary necrosis may occur in up to 40% of adult patients, and may be asymptomatic. Similarly, hematuria is common in SCA patients, with or without associated papillary necrosis.

Hepatobiliary System

Liver function tests in SCA patients generally show increased total and conjugated bilirubin, to which both increased hemolysis and liver dysfunction contribute.[7] Up to 50% of adult SCA patients have elevated alkaline phosphatase, but isoenzyme fractionation shows bone to be the origin of this enzyme. Abnormal liver function tests are common in older SCA patients, with some worsening during crises. This could imply progressive liver impairment in this disease.

10% of all hospital admissions for SCA are for hepatic crises. The symptoms of this type of vasoocclusive episode are fever, nausea and vomiting, jaundice, right upper quadrant pain, and elevations of liver function tests. Differential diagnosis includes hepatitis; in hepatic crisis, serology remains normal, and elevated SGOT and SGPT return to normal within 7–10 days.

As in any disease with increased hemolysis, gallstones are common in SCA.[7] The average incidence of cholelithiasis in three series of SCA outpatients was 14% for patients under 10 years of age, and 36% for those between 10 and 20. Fifteen percent of those patients with cholelithiasis develop common bile duct obstruction from stones. If sonography shows dilated intrahepatic bile ducts, or if clinical suspicion is high, diagnosis can be confirmed by percutaneous transhepatic cholangiography (PTC) or endoscopic retrograde cholangiopancreatography (ERCP). Endoscopic sphincterotomy can be performed for the patient who presents a prohibitive operative risk.

Cholecystitis must be differentiated from hepatic crisis since the symptoms are very similar. Cholescintigraphy ("HIDA" scanning) is probably the best technique for making the diagnosis. Cholecystectomy is indicated for acute cholecystitis.

With confirmed gallstones in an asymptomatic SCA patient, the decision to operate is difficult because of the increased surgical morbidity in SCA patients. The combined results of several reported series, most of which used preoperative transfusions, showed 14 of 97 patients with serious complications, including one death.[7] Complications were primarily pneumonia, atelectasis, and pulmonary infiltrates. The consensus seems to favor cholecystectomy for asymptomatic patients who have documented gallstones, recurrent abdominal pain, and who present a difficult problem in differentiating between recurrent hepatic crisis and pain due to cholelithiasis.

Diagnosis

Diagnosis is suggested by the patient's history, and confirmed by a "sickle cell prep"—the microscopic examination of blood after the addition of a reducing agent (usually sodium metabisulfite). Blood from patients with either SCA or sickle trait will sickle in this preparation; hemoglobin electrophoresis reveals the percentage of HbS present (the nonpolar valine residue alters the electrophoretic mobility of the Hb molecule).

Treatment

Several attempts at etiologic treatment of SCA have been proposed, but genetic manipulations remain highly controversial and are not yet possible.

As noted earlier, HbF inhibits sickling. It has been shown that certain chemotherapeutic agents that act at specific phases of the cell cycle (eg, cytarabine and hydroxyurea) increase the synthesis of HbF in SCA patients. These drugs cause a considerable decrease in cycling erythropoietic cells, with a secondary burst of increased erythropoiesis. This wave of increased RBC-formation includes a predominance of cells

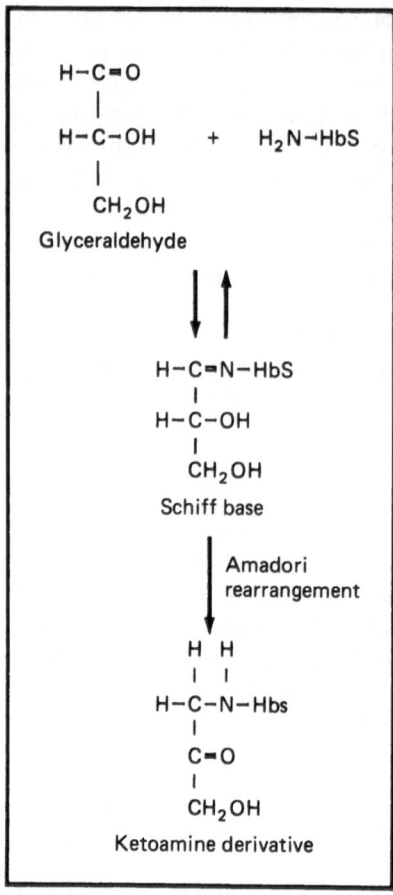

FIGURE 3.3. Glyceraldehyde Reaction with Hemoglobin S.

synthesizing HbF. The clinical utility of this approach, however, has not yet been demonstrated.[8]

Bepridil, a peripheral vasodilator with antianginal properties, has been shown to inhibit sickling in vitro. It appears to work by increasing membrane permeability to water and sodium, which causes cellular swelling and a decrease in MCHC.[9] Lowering the MCHC reduces the rate and extent of sickling (see above). Clinical trials have not yet been reported.

Cetiedil citrate, another agent with vasodilator properties and membrane activity, has been tested in SCA patients in vasoocclusive crisis. A dose of 0.4mg/kg I.V. every 8 hours for 4 days resulted in a significant decrease in the number of painful sites and in the length of crisis.[10]

The HbS molecule can also be modified chemically. Glyceraldehyde reacts with side-chain amine groups of HbS (Figure 3.3.) to form a ketoamine derivative. This modified HbS molecule shows decreased polymerization. Studies of RBCs treated ex-vivo with glyceraldehyde and then reinfused showed a significant increase in red cell survival. Untreated RBCs had a half life of 5.8 days; cells treated with 20 mmols of glyceraldehyde had a half life of 11.3 days. Potential problems with this agent include antigenicity of the chemically modified proteins, reactivity with molecules other than HbS, and decreased amino acid incorporation into other RBC proteins.[11]

Preanesthetic Management

Preoperative evaluation requires history taking (frequency of crises, last crisis, treatment), physical examination, routine laboratory studies, and if time permits, quantitative electrophoretic determination of HbS.[12] SCA patients undergoing elective surgery should receive transfusions sufficient to reduce HbS to 20–30% of total Hb, thus effectively eliminating the risk of sickling.[13]

Intercurrent infections must be treated, and preoperative teaching of deep breathing and the use of incentive spirometry are most useful. Pretreatment with bicarbonate was advocated in the past but easy availability of intraoperative blood gas analyses largely eliminates this need. Preoperative medication should be light enough to avoid respiratory depression with its attendant hypoxia and hypercarbia.

Anesthetic Management

Intraoperative management is keyed to avoidance of those factors that predispose to sickling, ie, hypoxia, hypotension, hypothermia, acidosis, and vascular stasis. No single anesthetic technique has been found to be preferable, as long as strict attention to the above factors is exercised.[14]

Struggling, breath-holding, and laryngospasm on induction are undesirable. In patients with no evidence of cardiorespiratory compromise, inspired oxygen concentrations of at least 30% should be adequate; with any evidence of compromise, at least 45% should be used.[14] Ventilation/perfusion mismatch should be minimized by maintaining appropriate alveolar ventilation and cardiac output. Fluid overload and electrolyte imbalance should also be avoided. Frequent intraoperative measurement is essential.

Positioning must be accomplished to minimize stasis. Use of tourniquets should be avoided if possible; if necessary, careful exsanguination of the limb should be carried out.[15] Low-molecular-weight dextran has been suggested in this setting to improve local rheology, but no studies demonstrating its effectiveness have been published.[14]

Deliberate hypotension in SCA patients has not been well addressed in the literature. Although one source counsels avoidance of such techniques, others point out that techniques which lower blood pressure while preserving local perfusion (via vasodilation) should, in theory, be safe.[14]

Intraoperative sickling, unless massive and accompanied by cardiovascular collapse, is difficult to diagnose. Arbitrary timed blood sampling for smear might disclose ongoing sickling, but this would not be reliable. Close attention to oxygenation, temperature control, and perfusion should decrease the chance of sickling and make sampling unnecessary. The possibility of intraoperative sickling should, however, be retained on the list of differential diagnoses if unexpected complications occur during anesthesia.

Monitoring

Monitoring should include ECG and placement of an intraarterial cannula to allow frequent determinations of blood gas values and serum electrolytes. Pulse oximetry is essential as a constant real-time display of arterial

O_2 saturation. Temperature must also be monitored. Bladder catheterization is useful; the possible presence of hyposthenuria must be remembered in evaluation of urine output.[13]

Postoperative Care

Postoperative care requires avoidance of hypoxia and prophylaxis of pulmonary infection, the two greatest risks facing SCA patients after anesthesia.[14] Most deaths in these patients occur postoperatively. Regional techniques (eg, intercostal blocks, epidural narcotics) are preferable to systemic narcotics for pain relief, and supplemental oxygen for 24–48 hours is necessary. Early ambulation is important.

References

1. Gibson JR: Anesthetic Implications of Sickle Cell Disease and Other Hemoglobinopathies, in Barash PG (ed): ASA Refresher Courses, Philadelphia, JB Lippincott, 1986, pp 139–57.
2. Embury SH: The clinical pathophysiology of sickle cell disease. Annu Rev Med 1986;37:361–76.
3. Scully RE, Mark EJ, McNeely BU: Clinicopathological conference. Case 52–1983. N Engl J Med 1983;309:1627–36.
4. Haupt HM, Moore GW, Bauer TW, et al: The lung in sickle cell disease. Chest 1982;81:332–37.
5. Pogue VA, Feinfeld DA: Renal and electrolyte problems in sickle cell anemia. Hosp Phys 1986(Dec);pp 69–75.
6. Strauss J, Zilleruelo G, Abitbol C: The kidney and hemoglobin S. Nephron 1986;43:241–45.
7. Schubert TT: Hepatobiliary system in sickle cell disease. Gastroenterology 1986;90:2013–21.
8. Veith R, Galanello R, Papayannopoulou T, et al: Stimulation of F cell production in patients with sickle cell anemia treated with cytarabine or hydroxyurea. N Engl J Med 1985;313:1571–75.
9. Reilly MP, Asakura T: Antisickling effect of bepridil. Lancet 1986;1(8485):848.
10. Benjamin LJ, Berkowitz LR, Orringer E, et al: A collaborative double-blind randomized study of cetiedil citrate in sickle cell crisis. Blood 1986;67:1442–47.
11. Benjamin LJ, Manning JM: Enhanced survival of sickle erythrocytes upon treatment with glyceraldehyde. Blood 1986;67:544–46.
12. Pearson HA: Hemoglobinopathies, in Conn HF, Conn RB (eds): Current Diagnosis, ed 5. Philadelphia, WB Saunders, 1977, pp 447–52.
13. McNiece WL: Anemia, in Stoelting RL, Dierdorf SF (eds): Anesthesia and Coexisting Disease. New York, Churchill Livingstone, 1983, pp 532–35.
14. Aldrete JA, Guerra F: Hematologic Diseases, in Katz J, Benumof J, Katz LB (eds): Anesthesia and Uncommon Diseases. Philadelphia, WB Saunders, 1981, pp. 325–31.
15. Gilbertson AA: Anaesthesia in West African patients with sickle cell anaemia, haemoglobin SC disease, and sickle cell trait. Br J Anaesth 1965;37:614–22.

CHAPTER 4

The Patient for Percutaneous Transluminal Coronary Angioplasty*

Alrick Brooks

Case History. *A 65-year-old man with a history of inferior wall myocardial infarction (M.I.) in 1979 and 1986 was admitted because of unstable angina. He had percutaneous transluminal coronary angioplasty (PTCA) in 1986 following the second MI.*

The patient had a 38-year history of insulin-dependent diabetes mellitus. His medical history was unremarkable for any other disease except congestive heart failure (CHF) in 1986 following the MI. No allergies were known. He did not smoke or drink.

The patient was taking diltiazem 60 mg q.i.d.; nifedipine 20 mg t.i.d.; furosemide 40 mg q.d.; nitropaste 5 cm² q.d.; insulin NPH 12U and regular insulin 6U in the morning and NPH 12U and regular 4U in the evening.

The electrocardiogram showed normal sinus rhythm, old inferior wall MI changes, and nonspecific STT-wave changes in the precordial leads. Chest X-ray was unremarkable.

The patient weighed 70 kg. Vital signs were: blood pressure 100/60 mmHg, pulse 72/min, respiratory rate 18/min, temperature 36.6°C. Physical examination was unremarkable. Serum chemistries and hematologic indices were within normal limits.

Cardiac catheterization showed: ejection fraction of 58%, left ventricular end-diastolic pressure (LVEDP) within normal limits, 70% occlusion of right coronary artery, 50% left anterior descending (LAD) occlusion, and 50% occlusion of the first diagonal artery. The patient was scheduled for PTCA and possible coronary artery bypass graft (CABG).

---

* Reviewed by Dr. Ingrid Hollinger, Associate Professor, Department of Anesthesiology, Albert Einstein College of Medicine.

Introduction

About 10 million people in the United States suffer from coronary artery disease (CAD). Annually, there are approximately 1,300,000 new myocardial infarctions, 150,000 coronary artery bypass grafting procedures (CABG), and 700,000 deaths related to CAD.[1] Percutaneous transluminal coronary angioplasty (PTCA) has become an alternative treatment modality for selected patients with CAD who would otherwise undergo CABG. Since its introduction by Andres Gruntzig in 1977, its safety and benefits have been verified by many studies worldwide.[2] (See Table 4.1.)

Cardiovascular Physiology

A basic understanding of cardiovascular physiology is important for proper assessment of the CAD patient for PTCA and possible CABG.[3,4]

The primary function of the heart is to pump blood at a rate sufficient to meet the metabolic requirements of peripheral tissues. Therefore cardiac output (CO) is considered the key test of myocardial function. Cardiac output is heart rate multiplied by stroke volume (CO = HR × SV).

Normal values of these indices are: CO, 5–6 L/min in a 70-kg person; SV, 60–90 ml/beat; HR, 80 beats/min. To compare the cardiac function of patients, CO is related to body surface area and expressed as the cardiac index (CI). Therefore CI = CO/BSA. Normal CI is 2.5–3.5 L/min/m^2.

Heart rate is determined primarily by the sinoatrial node rhythmicity caused by spontaneous phase 4 depolarization of its pacemaker. Phase 4 depolarization is regulated by the sympathetic and parasympathetic nervous systems. Stroke volume is affected mainly by four factors: preload, afterload, contractility, and wall motion abnormalities.

Central venous pressure (CVP) is a reasonably good reflection of right ventricular preload under normal conditions. Factors affecting preload include total blood volume, body position, intrathoracic pressure, intrapericardial pressure, venous tone, pumping action of skeletal muscles, and the atrial contribution to ventricular filling. There is often a 10–30%

TABLE 4.1. Pros and cons of performing PTCA versus CABG.

Benefits	Possible complications
Sustained relief of ischemia	Prolonged angina and myocardial infarction
Cost one third that of CABG	Coronary, dissection, occlusion, spasm, emboli
Shorter hospital stay	Coronary rupture and perforation (rare)
	Restenosis requiring repeat PTCA

decrease in blood pressure and CO with loss of atrial contraction. This condition is seen most often in patients with aortic stenosis or idiopathic hypertrophic subaortic stenosis who develop atrial fibrillation.

Afterload of the left ventricle is the wall stress affecting the myocardium during left ventricular (LV) ejection. Clinically this is assessed by calculating the systemic vascular resistance (SVR):

$$SVR = MAP - CVP/CO$$

(MAP = mean arterial pressure.)

If preload and afterload are held constant, stroke volume is a function of the contractile state of the myocardium. Several factors increase myocardial contractility including sympathetic stimulation, parasympathetic inhibition, and positive inotropic drugs. Contractility is decreased by hypoxia, acidosis, beta-adrenergic blockers, slow calcium channel blockers, inhalation anesthetics, myocardial ischemia, and infarction.

Left ventricle wall motion abnormalities (dyssynergy) occur when localized areas of the left ventricle are hypokinetic, akinetic, or dyskinetic. This phenomenon can significantly decrease stroke volume.

CO, the key test of myocardial function, is measured on the basis of the Fick principle, which states:

$$CO = VO_2/CaO_2 - CvO_2,$$

where VO_2 is oxygen consumption, CaO_2 is oxygen content of blood leaving the lung, and CvO_2 is oxygen content of blood entering the lung.

Alternative techniques for measuring CO are: (1) thermodilution, via pulmonary artery catheter, which measures only right side CO and is not useful in the presence of intracardiac shunts; (2) the dye dilution technique using indocyanine green, which does not require a pulmonary artery catheter and is useful in the presence of intracardiac shunts.

Coronary Circulation

Understanding the physiology of coronary circulation is important in assessing patients with CAD. Resting coronary blood flow averages 4–5% of total CO. Most of the coronary blood flow to the ventricle occurs in diastole. Autoregulation of coronary blood flow occurs in the range of 60–150 mmHg. The balance between myocardial oxygen demand and oxygen supply is the overall controlling factor in the coronary circulation. The heart extracts approximately 65% of the arterial blood oxygen, ie, almost maximal oxygen extraction. Therefore, if the heart requires more oxygen, coronary blood flow must be increased, which, in patients with coronary artery disease may not be possible due to atherosclerotic processes or coronary artery spasm.

Decreased myocardial oxygen supply is caused by: (1) decreased coronary blood flow secondary to tachycardia, diastolic hypotension, increased preload, hypocapnia, and coronary spasm; (2) decreased oxygen delivery as in anemia, hypoxia, and decreased 2,3-diphosphoglycerate (2,3-DPG).

Increased myocardial oxygen demand is caused by tachycardia, increased wall tension (eg, increased preload and afterload), and increased contractility.

Percutaneous Transluminal Coronary Angioplasty

PTCA is the actual enlargement of a stenotic vessel lumen. There are three components to the coronary angioplasty system: a guiding catheter, a nonelastomeric balloon dilation catheter filled with contrast medium, and a leading guidewire. Patients selected for PTCA must be suitable for cardiac surgery and willing to undergo CABG if necessary.[5] Preoperative preparation is similar for both procedures except for the use in CABG of antiplatelet therapy (dipyridamole) and intravenous heparinization (approximately 10,000 units).

PTCA can be performed via a femoral or brachial artery approach. Most procedures are performed under local anesthesia with oxygen

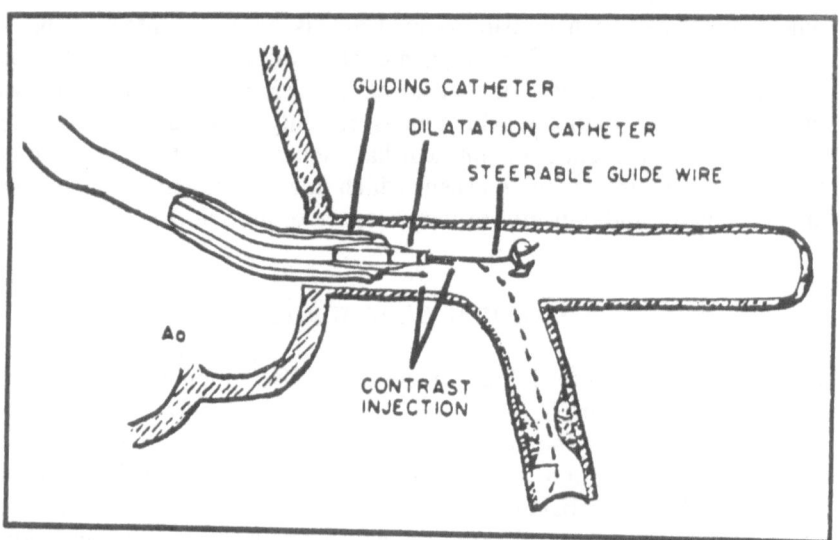

FIGURE 4.1. Schematic diagram of the three components of angioplasty: guiding catheter positioned in ostium of coronary artery; dilatation catheter positioned in the left main artery ready to be advanced over the guidewire, and soft-tip shapable guidewire which can be steered to enter the desired vessel and advanced gently across the target stenosis. Adapted from Ref. 6 (Baim and Faxon, 1986).

supplementation and intravenous sedation. Actual dilation of the vessel is preceded by coronary angiography and ventriculography. Nitroglycerin is injected to determine if spasm is a significant component of stenosis and to reduce the incidence of spasm of the coronary vessels. Intravenous verapamil or sublingual nifedipine can also be used.

Angioplasty is carried out according to Figures 4.1. and 4.2. The bulk of improvement in vessel lumen is effected by overstretching of the vessel by the PTCA balloon. Compression of the atheromatous plaque accounts for approximately 5% improvement, and extrusion of plaque contents even less in increasing the vessel lumen.[6]

Approximately 25% of the candidates for CABG are also candidates for PTCA.[5] Table 4.1 lists benefits versus complications of PTCA. If PTCA is unsuccessful because of coronary dissection, occlusion, rupture, perforation, or myocardial infarction, general anesthesia is required for revascularization. Acute myocardial infarction occurs after 5-10% of all PTCA and nearly all such patients are candidates for emergency revascularization.[7] There are two groups of patients, those who are urgent, ie, requiring surgery in less than 24 hours and those who are elective

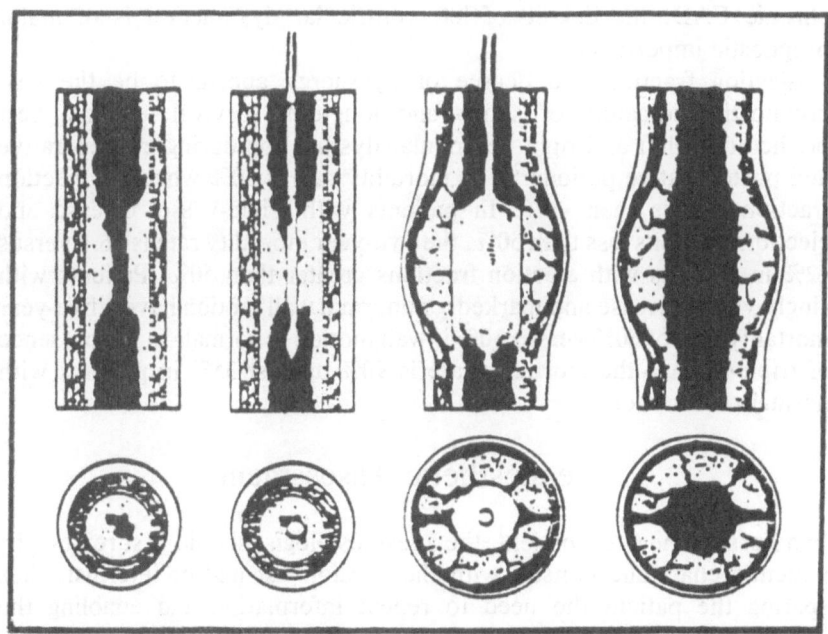

FIGURE 4.2. Proposed mechanism of angioplasty: Inflation of the balloon catheter within the stenotic segment produces cracking of the intimal plaque and stretching of the media, adventitia, and diameter of the vessel. Compression of the plaque material and extrusion of liquid plaque contents appear to contribute only slightly to the increase in luminal diameter. Adapted from Ref. 6 (Baim and Faxon, 1986).

candidates. In the urgent group there is a reported complication rate 54% versus 18.8% in the elective group.[8] The mortality rate was 4.4% for urgent patients and 3.2% for the elective group. All deaths were cardiac related.[8]

Recently there has been new interest in providing general anesthesia for PTCA in those patients experiencing acute MI.[9] Proper preoperative assessment is imperative because of significant morbidity and mortality associated with CAD. Mortality rate after CABG is between 0.3 and 6.2%. Prognosis in CAD is related to the development and severity of dysrhythmias, myocardial infarction, and venticular dysfunction. Studies have demonstrated that in patients with prior myocardial infarction, the risk of reinfarction is 36–100% with a mortality of 54–70%. Recent studies by Rao[10] have indicated a significantly reduced six-month reinfarction rate of 5% and mortality rate of 2% when aggressive preoperative monitoring and therapy are used.

Because the indications for PTCA have been extended from single-vessel disease and are being applied to patients with advanced ischemia, more patients will require emergency operations. In this group of patients, prompt use of the intraaortic balloon pump is used to control myocardial ischemia and diminish the risk of MI. In patients with acute or chronic CAD, the degree of left ventricular dysfunction is of major prognostic importance.

Ejection fraction and degree of dyssnergy appear to be the best prognostic indicators of short- and longterm survival and the best predictors of left and right ventricular dysfunction during intraoperative and postoperative periods.[7] The mortality rate is 30% when the ejection fraction is less than 40%. In patients with triple-vessel disease and ejection fractions less than 50%, the two-year mortality rate is 36% versus 12% in patients with ejection fractions greater than 50%. Patients with single-vessel disease and markedly abnormal wall motion have a five-year mortality rate of 60% versus 10% if wall motion is normal. In the presence of triple-disease the mortality rate is 90% against 35% in patients with normal wall motion.[1]

Preanesthetic Assessment

In assessing the CAD patient, the anesthesiologist should first review the patient's chart and consult with the cardiologist and/or internist, thus sparing the patient the need to repeat information and enabling the anesthesiologist to concentrate on discussing the anesthetic management and process with the patient and trying to allay some of his anxiety. A brief history and physical examination and inspection of pertinent laboratory data are imperative.

In addition to identifying and treating systemic and localized infections, coagulopathies, and anemia, the following major evaluations are essential.

Cardiac Assessment

Significant coronary disease usually presents with a history of chest pain. Angina is a symptom of myocardial ischemia and implies a relative imbalance between oxygen supply and demand. Typical angina involves pain, heaviness or pressure retrosternally, related to stress or exertion and relieved by rest or nitroglycerin. Other symptoms associated with ischemic episodes, referred to as "epiphenomena," include sweating, nausea, numbness, shortness of breath, palpitations, dizziness, and syncope. It is important to note that some patients may identify these symptoms more easily than classic chest pain.

Such a history may be incidentally obtained in patients undergoing regional anesthesia for procedures such as transurethral resection of the prostate or in patients with peripheral vascular disease undergoing amputation or debridement of extremities. Epiphenomena symptoms are also important in patients receiving local anesthesia with sedation, such as for cataract surgery, PTCA, or pacemaker insertion.

Description of these symptoms may be the only way to assess if these patients are experiencing myocardial ischemia. For instance, shortness of breath may indicate a significant degree of left ventricular failure. Dizziness or syncope may be related to decreased cardiac output secondary to dysrhythmias or the onset of left ventricular failure or a combination of both. The most serious dysrhythmias are ventricular fibrillation, ventricular tachycardia, and premature ventricular contractions. In patients with PVCs, the greatest risk of developing ventricular fibrillation occurs when the R and T waves coincide or a multifocal pattern develops. Ventricular dysrhythmias are predictive of multiple-vessel disease. Atrial dysrhythmias associated with CAD have significant risk in the presence of ischemia, left ventricular failure, and left ventricular outlet obstruction.[11]

The most common cause of left ventricular failure is hypertension. Evaluation includes complete history of the disease and determination of any end-organ changes. Exact information on drugs used should be obtained, because of increased morbidity and mortality in inadequately or untreated hypertensive patients during anesthesia. Acute withdrawal or omission of drugs such as propranolol may precipitate angina that may progress to myocardial infarction. Acute cessation of clonidine therapy can produce a hypertensive crisis because of loss of a central inhibitory effect on the sympathetic nervous system.

Cerebrovascular Disease

A history of stroke, syncope, lightheadedness, convulsions, diabetes, or hypertension is not uncommon and may indicate carotid and/or cerebrovascular disease. Anesthetic management of these patients is directed at maintaining cerebral autoregulation as close to a normal range as possible, ie, MAP close to preanesthetic pressures, relatively high oxygen tension, and normocarbia.

Endocrine Disease

Diabetes, another important disease often seen in CAD patients, can have significant morbidity. Management aims at maintaining blood glucose levels between 125 and 175 mg/dl and avoiding hypoglycemia regardless of the regimen used. It is very important to probe for ischemic epiphenomena in diabetics because the neuropathy that accompanies this disease can diminish and abolish the patient's sensation of angina.[7]

Respiratory Assessment

The presence of any existing pulmonary disease must be evaluated. If there is any indication of pulmonary dysfunction, testing should include arterial blood gas analyses, pulmonary function tests with and/or without bronchodilators. It is important to stress to patients with pulmonary disorders the importance of deep breathing and coughing, and discontinuation of smoking to decrease carbon monoxide levels. These measures help decrease the incidence of postoperative complications such as atelectasis, pneumonia, and hypoxia.

Hepatic/Renal Assessment

Detecting and determining the severity of significant hepatic and/or renal disease may help in reducing perioperative morbidity and mortality in the patient with CAD and also help in choosing appropriate fluid replacement and anesthetic agent or technique. Testing should include SMA-12, serum proteins, liver enzymes, BUN/creatinine levels, and creatinine clearance.

Physical Examination

An abbreviated physical examination limited to the foregoing disease states and systems should include assessment of vital signs such as blood pressure and heart rate to help determine the effects of antihypertensive and antiarrhythmic drugs. Temperature evaluations indicate the presence of infection. Airway examination is crucial. Should PTCA fail, emergency CABG is indicated and this requires prompt, flawless intubation. Chest examination should evaluate chronic obstructive pulmonary disease (COPD) and asthma.

Cardiac examination should include determination of heart size, the detection of a third and fourth heart sound and any murmurs. The presence of S_3 indicates increased left ventricular end-diastolic pressure and S_4 is associated with decreased left ventricular compliance secondary to myocardial ischemia or infarction. Finally, examination of the extremities should determine venous and arterial accessibility.

Laboratory Data

Chest x-ray detects the presence of pulmonary edema, cardiomegaly, COPD changes, and pneumonia (which, if improperly treated, can significantly affect surgical outcome). The finding of a normal ECG does not preclude coronary artery disease. In 25–50% of CAD patients no abnormalities are detected electrocardiographically.[1] The ECG is only reliable as an indicator of cardiac disease when Q waves are present and ST-segment changes occur during anginal attacks.

Hemoglobin levels above 10 mg/dl or hematocrit above 30% are required. Prothrombin and partial thromboplastin time and platelet counts should be within normal limits to ensure adequate coagulation. Serum chemistry evaluation will detect the presence of hypo/hypernatremia and hypo-/hyperkalemia. Potassium levels must be maintained between 3.3 and 5.5 mg/dl to minimize the risk of cardiac dysrhythmias.

Stress test and echocardiography data can be used to assess ventricular function and anatomy. The "gold standards" for evaluation of coronary anatomy and quantification of ventricular function are coronary angiography and ventriculography. Information about ventricular function include ejection fraction, dyssynergy, cardiac output, and end-diastolic pressures. CI less than $2.2 \text{ L/m}^2/\text{min}$ and LVEDP greater than 15 mmHg indicate poor left ventricular function.

Significant stenosis means greater than 70% narrowing of a major coronary artery or greater than 50% reduction in size of the left main coronary artery. Problems in interpreting coronary catheterization data can arise with hypovolemia or a transient increase of LVEDP due to volume loading or ventricular dysfunction caused by contrast dye. All catheterization data should be read to ensure proper perioperative management.

Drug Evaluation

It is extremely important to be aware of and maintain cardiac medications in the patient with cardiac ischemia. Continuation of beta-blocker medication up to the time of surgery may be beneficial in limiting intraoperative tachycardia, dysrhythmias, hypertension, and myocardial ischemia. Calcium channel blockers, which are widely prescribed in CAD patients for angina, dysrhythmias, and hypertension, also should be continued. Cardiac glycoside (digoxin) toxicity, which may be suspected by the presence of premature atrial contractions, second degree block, and frequent multifocal premature ventricular contractions, is a significant reason to postpone elective surgery. Therapeutic levels of digoxin and normokalemia should be ascertained. Digoxin and succinycholine may interact to produce ventricular dysrhythmias and may therefore require the avoidance of succinycholine in the patient on digoxin.[11]

Administration of diuretics prior to surgery is determined by the patient's cardiac status. Patients with significant CHF may require diuretic therapy prior to surgery while the hypertensive patient may benefit from withholding diuretics because of the chronic hypovolemic state associated with hypertension.

Anesthetic Plan

The choice of premedication should be individualized, based upon the patient's level of anxiety, extent of coronary disease, and general medical condition. Most patients may be given a minor tranquilizer or may not require premedication prior to PTCA. If PTCA is unsuccessful and emergency CABG is necessary, most such patients will arrive in the operating suite sedated from medications given during the PTCA.

Prior to and during revascularization the major objective is to optimize myocardial function by maintaining the balance between oxygen supply and demand. Pulse oximetry, electrocardiography, and blood pressure monitoring are standard during PTCA. Left ventricular ischemia is of greatest concern; therefore V_5 lead monitoring is preferable. Monitoring of lead II is useful for interpreting dysrhythmias and right ventricular ischemia.

If emergency CABG is required after failed PTCA or for PTCA following acute MI, a radial arterial line placed after documentation of a satisfactory Allen Test will provide continuous blood pressure monitoring, electrolyte sampling, and blood gas estimations. Measurement of pulmonary artery or direct left atrial pressure may be indicated if mitral regurgitation and/or significant left ventricular dysfunction is present. Esophageal stethoscope and temperature monitoring are standard for general anesthesia. Recent studies have shown reliable determination of left ventricular function by transesophageal echocardiography. This may become routine in the future.

In the patient for emergency CABG after failed PTCA, there is an increased need for the use of the intraaortic balloon pump and lidocaine, inotropic support, and the requirement for large amounts of blood products.[8] The increased use of blood products may be related to the prior antiplatelet therapy and heparinization plus the emergent nature of the surgery.

After failed PTCA during which the patient received thrombolytic therapy with streptokinase, urokinase, or tissue plasminogen activator, any of which may lead to bleeding, placement of a pulmonary artery catheter or central venous catheter should be limited to the brachial or external jugular routes. In addition to bleeding problems, allergic reactions and fever may also occur after thrombolytic therapy. Inhibition of the thrombolytic agents can be accomplished by alpha-epsilon aminocaproic acid.[12]

Two groups of patients undergoing CABG have been identified: (1) those with a history of angina and hypertension but without symptoms of CHF, ejection fractions greater than 55%, LVEDP less than 12 mmHg, no ventricular dyssynergy, and normal cardiac output; and (2) those patients with CAD and poor left ventricular function, ie, history of multiple MI, signs and symptoms of CHF, ejection fractions less than 40%, LVEDP greater than 18 mmHg, multiple areas of dyssynergy, and decreased cardiac output.

Narcotic techniques, especially with sufentanil and fentanyl, combined with muscle relaxants like vecuronium and atracurium that have minimal to no cardiovascular effects are generally suitable for the second group of patients. Nitrous oxide should be avoided because of its myocardial depressant effect. In the first group of patients an inhalation technique or a mixed narcotic inhalation technique with muscle relaxants may be more appropriate to attenuate tachycardia and hypertension that often occur following surgical stimulation, especially sternotomy.

As stated earlier, there is increasing interest in using general anesthesia for PTCA in patients with acute MI. In a recent study by Kates and associates,[9] it was shown that general anesthesia may offer an advantage (over the usual local anesthesia with sedation) by providing complete pain relief, including that from cardioversion, thus lowering rate pressure product and improving arterial oxygenation, which may favorably balance myocardial oxygen supply and demand. The high O_2 tension provided by general anesthesia may be beneficial in ischemic myocardial border zones.[13] This may be extremely important since most of the cardiac complications of urgent operations are ischemia and infarction. Finally, endotracheal intubation may also prevent aspiration of gastric contents in acute MI patients undergoing emergency PTCA.

Despite lack of widespread use of general anesthesia for PTCA, there are clinical situations such as emergency PTCA or after failed PTCA, in which good preanesthetic assessment can be crucial to satisfactory myocardial revascularization.

References

1. Mangano D: Assessment of the patient with myocardial ischemia. American Society of Anesthesiologists Annual Refresher Course Lectures, No. 140, 1983.
2. Gruntzig AR, Senning A, Stiegenthaler WE: Nonoperative dilation of coronary angioplasty. N Engl J Med 1979;301:61–8.
3. Kaplan J. Cardiovascular Physiology. In: Anesthesia, 2nd ed, Miller RD (ed). New York: Churchill Livingstone, 1986, pp 1165–97.
4. Tinker J: Preoperative Assessment of the Adult with Cardiac Disease. In: Manual of Cardiac Anesthesia, Thomas SJ (ed). New York: Churchill Livingstone, 1984, pp 153–71.

5. Warren SC, Warren SG: Coronary angioplasty: Current concepts. Am Fam Physician 1985;32(2):145–49.
6. Baim DS, Faxon DP: Coronary Angioplasty—Cardiac Catherization and Angiography, 3rd ed, Grosman W (ed). Philadelphia: Lea & Febriger, 1986, pp 473–80.
7. Caplan R. Preoperative evaluation of the patient with ischemic heart disease. ASA Annual Refresher Course Lectures, No. 141, 1985.
8. Brahos GJ, Baker NH, Ewy HG: Aortocoronary bypass following unsuccessful PTCA: Experience in 100 consecutive patients. Ann Thorac Surg 1985;40(1):7–10.
9. Kates RA, Stack RS, Hill RF: General anesthesia for patients undergoing percutaneous transluminal coronary angioplasty during acute myocardial infarction. Anesth Analg 1986;65:815–18.
10. Rao TLK, El-Etr AA: Myocardial reinfarction following anesthesia in patients with recent infarctions. Proc 55th Cong Int Anesthesiol Res Soc, Atlanta, 1981, pp 131–32.
11. Rogers MC: Diagnosis and Treatment of Cardiac Dysrhythmias. In: Anesthesia, 2nd ed, Miller RD (ed). New York: Churchill Livingston, 1986, pp 510–12.
12. Lake CL: Anesthesia for emergency surgery in the cardiac patient. ASA Annual Refresher Course Lectures, No 116, 1986.
13. Maroko PR, Radvany P, Braunwald E, et al: Reduction of infarct size by oxygen inhalation following acute coronary occlusion. Circulation 1975;52:360–69.

CHAPTER 5

The Infant with Meningomyelocele*

Randall D. Wilhoit

Case History. *The patient, a 24-hour-old infant girl weighing 3.2 kg at birth, was delivered by cesarean section at 39 weeks' estimated gestational age. The lecithin/sphingomyelin ratio obtained before delivery was 3:1. The mother had a routine pregnancy, except for a fetal ultrasound obtained at 20 weeks that showed a mass in the lumbar area. The patient has two brothers, one of whom had a lumbar meningomyelocele. There is no family history of muscular dystrophy or anesthetic difficulties.*

The patient has had no respiratory or feeding difficulties since delivery. Physical examination shows normal vital signs and skin turgor. A large membranous sac filled with fluid is located in the lumbar area. She has gross motor paralysis below the L3 level, and no evidence of sensation below the L3 level. The anus is patulous on physical examination.

The lower extremities and pelvis appear grossly normal. There is no sign of kyphosis or scoliosis on physical examination. The lungs are clear to auscultation, and the heart has a normal rate and rhythm with no audible murmurs or clicks. The airway appears normal on external examination.

The head circumference measures 39 centimeters, which is greater than the 95th percentile, and has remained stable since delivery.

Hematocrit is 49%, hemoglobin 16.8 gm/dl, electrolytes are all within normal limits. Chest x-ray shows a normal cardiac silhouette with clear lung fields. Urinalysis is normal with a specific gravity of 1.015.

Introduction

Meningomyelocele is a congenital deformity that arises during closure of the neural tube in the embryo, resulting in a defect in the spinal column from which a sac of meninges protrudes containing spinal cord elements.

---

* Reviewed by Dr. Robert McKay, Associate Professor, Department of Anesthesiology, University of Alabama at Birmingham.

The anesthesiologist encounters such patients frequently, when they present for closure of the primary defect and for shunting procedures to correct hydrocephalus, as well as for later orthopedic and urologic procedures.

Patients with meningomyelocele present management problems, as they often have other congenital defects and may require surgery at a very young age, frequently when they are only 1–2 days old. They require precise care intraoperatively to maintain temperature homeostasis and an adequate blood volume. An additional consideration in their care is the prone position in which they must be placed for surgery.

Incidence

The incidence of meningomyelocele is reported at 0.2–4 per 1000 live births, with a slight preference for females and Caucasians. It is highest in the Irish and Welsh populations.[1] In the United States it is estimated at 0.5 per 1000 births.[2] The incidence rises with increasing parity, and is also higher in lower socioeconomic classes. Families in which there is a child with meningomyelocele have an increased risk of recurrence in subsequent pregnancies—the odds are 1 in 20 if there is one previously affected child and 1 in 10 when there are two previously affected children.[3] The incidence is also increased in the offspring of consanguineous marriages.

Etiology

The etiology of meningomyelocele is unknown but is believed to be multifactorial. Although the increased familial occurrence indicates a possible genetic defect, identical twins do not always share the abnormality. Other evidence for an environmental etiology includes geographic differences in the occurrence rate as well as a seasonal variation. However, since no specific teratogen has been proved to cause meningomyelocele,[3] both genetic and environmental factors probably play a role in the etiology.

The basic defect in meningomyelocele is a failure of the posterior neuropore to close in the embryo. The neural groove forms at about 20 days of gestational age and fuses into a tube by about 23 days. Failure of the anterior portion to close causes either anencephaly or an encephalocele; failure of the posterior portion to close causes meningomyelocele.[4]

Spina bifida is a commonly used term that encompasses meningomyelocele, and refers to failure of the vertebral arches to fuse. It can present as *spina bifida occulta,* in which skin and soft tissues cover the defect, or in two other forms that involve protrusion of the meninges out of the defect with no skin or soft tissue covering. *Meningoceles* have no nervous tissue within the sac, and are very rare. *Meningomyeloceles* have all three possible components of spina bifida: a bony defect, a meningeal sac, and nervous tissue within the sac.

Clinical Aspects

Often there is no nerve function below the level of the lesion.[5] The most common position of the defect is in the lumbosacral area, less frequently in the thoracic area, and more rarely in the cervical area. (Figure 5.1.) Major paralysis in one study was defined as paralysis above the third

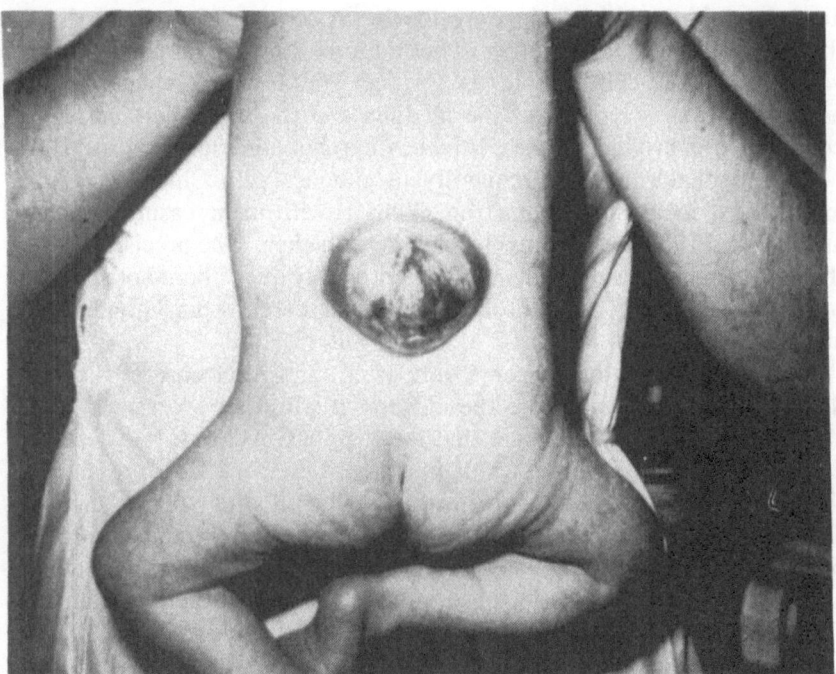

FIGURE 5.1. Infant with a lumbar meningomyelocele.

lumbar segment with, at most, only active hip flexion remaining.[6] The nerve damage often results in a neurogenic bladder and an incontinent anal sphincter, as well as paralysis of the lower extremities. Only about 20% of infants with menigomyeloceles have no paralysis evident at birth. Some children do have minimal reflex activity in the lower extremities at birth, but this often disappears within a few days and has not been shown to improve the longterm prognosis of the nerve lesion.[5] The sensory lesion is easily documented by pinprick testing.

Orthopedic malformations are commonly associated with meningomyelocele. The worst of these, kyphosis and scoliosis, can be severe; congenital hip dislocation and talipes equinovarus have also been described.[4] Other congenital abnormalities include cardiac defects, diaphragmatic hernia, omphalocele, gastroschisis, and Down's syndrome (mongolism).[6]

Neurologic Abnormalities

The most common neurologic abnormality associated with meningomyelocele is the Chiari II or Arnold-Chiari malformation. In one review of 33 infants with meningomyelocele, none had a normal computed tomography (CT) scan. McLone et al state that this defect is the major cause of death in children with meningomyelocele.[7] It consists of an elongation of the cerebellar vermis, resulting in herniation of the caudal portion of the vermis and the choroid plexus through the foramen magnum. The herniation causes kinking of the medulla and the upper cervical spinal cord and a disturbance of the cortical cytoarchitecture (polymicrogyria).[1]

Hydrocephalus occurs frequently in patients with Chiari II malformations, the incidence ranging from 62–85%, with an increasing incidence as the level of the meningomyelocele moves higher.[8] The precise cause of the hydrocephalus is unknown, but it is probably due either to obstruction of the aqueduct of Sylvius or to failure of cerebrospinal fluid (CSF) absorption.

Hydrocephalus often presents only after surgical closure of the back defect. If it is present before the closure, it will often worsen after the surgery. Linder et al postulate that the meningomyelocele sac acts as a distensible space that provides dampening of elevated CSF pressure; in their study, CSF pulse pressures rose significantly after surgical closure. This indicates that a change in the elasticity of the intracranial contents occurs with closure of the defect, which may in turn precipitate or accelerate hydrocephalus in these infants.[8] A second theory postulates that the Chiari II malformation causes a partial obstruction of CSF circulation, which worsens after closure of the back lesion.[5]

The deleterious effects of hydrocephalus may be secondary to both the degree of increased intracranial pressure (ICP) and the rapidity with which it develops.[3] The newborn has a very pliable skull with open fontanelles and unfused sutures, and thus is less likely to have a rapid increase in ICP. It has also been shown that ICP measurements in these patients are not constant, and therefore are not reliable indicators for the decision to place a shunt. The surgeon generally bases such a decision on serial head circumference measurements, serial CT scans, or ultrasound scans.[3]

The Chiari II malformation directly causes brainstem dysfunction in some patients. The most severe symptoms are apnea, stridor, and gastroesophageal reflux. McLone et al found these symptoms in 32% of the patients they studied; in 13% the symptoms were life threatening. Problems directly stemming from the Chiari II malformation caused 11 of the 14 deaths in the series.[7]

The natural history of this dysfunction leads to improvement over time in those patients who survive the initial problems. Posterior fossa decompression has been tried as therapy for the symptomatic Chiari II malformation, but it does not appear to change the natural course of the disease or to increase survival.[7] The problems of stridor, apneic spells, and gastroesophageal reflux are of particular concern to the anesthesiologist; the preanesthetic evaluation should carefully review these areas.

Intellectual Development

Patients with meningomyelocele have a high incidence of decreased intelligence, which in the past was attributed to both the Chiari II malformation and to the hydrocephalus. Recently Mapstone compared two groups of children with meningomyelocele, one with shunts and one without shunts. He found the inteligence quotient (IQ) to be in the low-normal to normal range in both groups. He then compared children having shunt complications, usually infection, with those having no shunt complications. In the group having shunts with complications, he found a significantly decreased IQ.[9] This finding has since been substantiated by others.[5]

Thus, it is currently assumed that a patient with a Chiari II malformation and hydrocephalus, if adequately treated, will not necessarily have a decrease in intellect. These studies also point to the necessity of meticulous care of patients requiring shunts, as complications may markedly decrease the patient's future quality of life.[9] Many patients with meningomyelocele have good intelligence and may lead productive lives.

Surgical Candidates

One of the important controversies in the management of meningomyelocele deals with selection of children for surgery. In the 1960s Sherrard et al, operating on "all comers," reported excellent results in regard to the longterm social functions of their patients.[10] On later review, these results were found to be far too optimistic. When these children reached school age, a large number of them showed a decreased intelligence with minimal social skills.[5]

In response, in 1971, Lorber devised four adverse criteria (Table 5.1.), which he used to exclude selected infants from active treatment (ie, surgery). Infants were excluded from aggressive surgical management if they had one or more of the adverse criteria. Of his first 37 patients, the 25 receiving no active treatment died within 9 months. Of the remaining 12 patients receiving active treatment, 11 survived.[11]

TABLE 5.1. Parameters for selection of meningomyelocele infants for treatment.

Degree of paralysis—The most severe infants are those with no voluntary muscle activity in the lower limbs or at most hip flexion only.

Head circumference—Hydrocephalus is considered severe if the head circumference at birth is ≥90th percentile.

Kyphosis—Kyphosis is considered severe if the defect is so gross as to require corrective osteotomy at the time of closure of the meningomyelocele.

Associated gross congenital anomalies or major birth injuries—Examples are heart defects or severe birth hypoxia.

Adapted from Ref. 11: (Lorber, 1972).

In the late 1970s several studies incorporated new concepts.[6,7,12] Shunt therapy had improved markedly over this time, and improved the prognosis for meningomyelocele patients. McLone in 1985 published a study in which all patients had early surgery, within 48 hours of birth.[7] The longterm functional results in these patients were as good as those in the patients reported by Lorber in 1981.[13] However, in Lorber's study, patients with one or more adverse criteria had been excluded from surgical therapy. Also, only 14% of McLone's patients died.[7]

Charney et al in 1985 published a series in which they used modified selection criteria to decide on early surgical intervention. They required that two or more serious problems be present before surgery was denied. Their overall mortality rate was 18.2%.[6] In that study, 84 of the infants were operated on within 7 days of birth. In 12 infants late closure was performed after 7 days of age, when the parents reversed their earlier decision to withhold surgery. Fourteen infants had no surgery and all died within 7 months. Thus, similar mortality rates have been achieved in modern studies of selected versus nonselected patients, and this debate continues today.[5]

Another point of contention among surgeons is whether immediate surgery—within 48 hours of birth—is essential, or whether closure of the defect can safely be delayed for 2–7 days. Delaying closure in the past was thought to be associated with an increased risk of ventriculitis and sepsis.[7] Early closure was thought to improve neurologic functions.[10]

Charney et al, in 1985, did not find an increased incidence of ventriculitis associated with delaying closure up to 7 days. They found that prophylactic perioperative antibiotics were useful in infants having closure between 2 and 7 days, but that they were not needed in infants having closure before 2 days of age. Charney and associates also substantiated earlier reports that neurologic function was not worsened by delaying surgery, nor improved by early intervention.[6]

Many moral, social, and legal issues have arisen regarding management of infants with meningomyelocele. In most states, surgery is not mandated in children with overwhelming life-threatening anomalies. The team involved in medical care, including also risk management and ethics groups, should be assembled to discuss with the parents the benefits and anticipated outcome. Delaying surgery even for several days while such consults and decisions are established has not been shown to worsen outcome or increase morbidity.[6]

Preoperative Evaluation

History

The preoperative evaluation should include a thorough history, including information on the family medical history, the course of the pregnancy, and the type of delivery of the child. Chervenak et al[2] recommend cesarean section, as there are reports of cerebral injury in approximately 14% of neonates with meningomyelocele born vaginally. These cerebral birth injuries may be reversible, and some of the improvments seen in the neurologic status of neonates in the first few days of life may be due to recovery from these birth injuries.[2] Also, a history of apnea, stridor, or gastroesophageal reflux consistent with a symptomatic Chiari II malformation should be sought.[7]

Physical Examination

The physical examination should include a thorough check for other congenital lesions, especially congenital heart defects.[6] The vital signs, especially temperature, should be checked, as many infants have had inadequate thermal protection and are hypothermic.[14] The patient should be examined for orthopedic defects, especially scoliosis and kyphosis. Orthopedic defects of the lower extremities should also be noted.[6]

A complete neurologic examination covering sensory and motor levels, as well as the level of the meningomyelocele lesion, is important. It is also important to note the baby's head circumference, checking for changes since birth. Head circumference should also be compared with the normal values for gestational age and birth weight.[11] Infants with high lumbar, thoracolumbar, and cervical meningomyeloceles may have paralysis of the intercostal and abdominal musculature, yielding a limited respiratory reserve.[15]

Laboratory Tests

Preoperative laboratory studies should include a hemoglobin and hematocrit to establish a preoperative baseline, and a urinalysis to help evaluate the fluid and volume status of the infant. The newborn is an obligate sodium excreter, and thus will not be able to concentrate urine.[16]

Electrolytes should be checked as these babies may lose a significant amount of fluid from the meningomyelocele defect and therefore may be dehydrated preoperatively.[14] A chest x-ray may be helpful if there is a question of aspiration or of a cardiac abnormality. A CT scan and a cranial ultrasound obtained preoperatively will provide a baseline for follow-up studies.[5]

Medication

Preoperative medication regimens are a controversial subject in pediatrics. In the neonate, however, most authorities would use only an anticholinergic agent. This class of drugs reduces vagal tone, lessens oral secretions, and may reduce the tendency for laryngospasm.[17] Another advantage of these drugs is that they reduce gastric fluid volume and the acidity of gastric secretions. Most authorities would avoid narcotics or sedatives for neonates. Atropine in a dose of 0.02 mg/kg given intramuscularly on call to the operating room (OR) is the anticholinergic most often recommended.[17]

Anesthetic Plan

OR Temperature

The OR should be warmed prior to the patient's arrival. Warmed cleansing solutions should be available, as well as a blood/fluid warmer that will heat the intravenous fluids administered. A heating mattress should be in place, and heating lamps available in the OR. The infant's head should be covered after induction to prevent heat loss. Once the induction is completed, the anesthetic gases should be warmed and humidified.[16] The baby should also be transferred to and from the OR in a warmed environment such as an incubator.

These precautions are important for all neonates, but especially for babies with a meningomyelocele.[14] All infants have a high surface area to volume ratio and only a thin layer of subcutaneous fat for insulation, and thus lose heat more rapidly than adults do. Also, infants do not shiver and can only generate heat by brown-fat utilization, which is mediated by the sympathetic nervous system.[16]

Neonates with meningomyelocele often have paralysis of their lower extremities, which leads to a lower metabolic rate and thus to a decreased ability to maintain body temperature. Meningomyelocele may also be accompanied by a decrease in the temperature-regulating ability secondary to hypothalamic dysfunction that may occur with the Chiari II malformation.[14] This abnormality, when added to the disruption of temperature control at the central level caused by anesthetics, can cause the neonate to become extremely hypothermic in the OR. Hypothermia is a complication that is easier to avoid than to treat.[16]

Monitoring

The deployment of appropriate monitors is an important consideration in these patients. Monitors may assist the anesthesiologist in detecting any previously unrecognized anomalies, such as cardiac or respiratory defects. Essential monitoring includes a stethoscope, a continuous ECG, core body temperature, and noninvasive blood pressure measurement. Usually temperature monitors and stethoscopes are placed in the esophagus.

Pulse oximetry warns of decreasing arterial oxygen saturation before clinical signs such as bradycardia can occur. Transcutaneous oxygen monitoring, which is influenced by arterial oxygenation and the adequacy of tissue perfusion, can be of assistance by providing an indirect monitor of the intravascular volume status of the patient.[16] End-tidal CO_2 monitoring may help detect esophageal intubation or unintended extubation. An intravenous (I.V.) catheter adequate for blood transfusion must be placed preoperatively in all infants undergoing surgery for meningomyelocele. However, for most infants, an indwelling arterial catheter and central venous cathether have not been found essential.[14,15]

Intubation and Induction

Most authors recommend awake intubation of the neonate with meningomyelocele prior to the induction of anesthesia.[1,14,15] Intubation with the patient lying left side down is recommended. An awake intubation is necessary because endotracheal tube placement in the lateral position can be difficult, especially in infants. Intubation in the supine position is possible if pads are used to prevent pressure on the meningomyelocele; however, most authors consider the lateral position safer.

In older patients, an I.V. induction with thiopental and a shortacting relaxant such as atracurium can be employed. Nondepolarizing muscle relaxants are preferred as the use of succinylcholine in the presence of neurologic deficits may lead to hyperkalemia.

As an alternative in the patient without I.V. access, an inhalation induction may be performed with nitrous oxide and a potent volatile agent. An I.V. catheter may then be placed and a muscle relaxant given to facilitate endotracheal intubation. Induction with intramuscular methohexital may also be used. If the patient has a history of gastroesophageal reflux or aspiration, the intubation should be performed using cricoid pressure.[17]

The anesthetic may then be continued using any agents desired, but most anesthesiologists prefer a low dose of volatile agents. Intravenous agents such as benzodiazepenes, narcotics, or barbiturates can be used; however, these longacting agents may cause respiratory depression postoperatively.[14] A longacting muscle relaxant may be used only if the surgeon is not going to use nerve stimulation during the case.

In the absence of nitrous oxide, air should be mixed with the anesthetic gases delivered, to decrease the inspired oxygen concentration. Prolonged delivery of a high concentration of oxygen can predispose the infant to the development of retrolental fibroplasia. Current guidelines suggest that an infant is at risk for developing retrolental fibroplasia until older than 44 weeks' estimated gestational age.[16]

The anesthesiologist must consider the effect of the anesthetic on ICP. Milligan studied a group of critically ill preterm infants and found them to have a failure of autoregulation of cerebral blood flow. In these infants, cerebral blood flow followed changes in mean arterial blood pressure directly and proportionately.[18] Rogers et al, in a review of neonatal control of cerebral blood flow, found marked sensitivity to changes in the arterial partial pressure of oxygen. This sensitivity appears to be much greater than that seen in adults. Conversely, they noted that infants appear to have a reduced responsiveness of cerebral blood flow to changes in arterial partial pressures of carbon dioxide.

In healthy preterm infants, they found that autoregulation of cerebral blood flow occurs at a lower mean arterial blood pressure range than in adults. Finally, in adults the sympathetic nervous system, especially in the pons and mesencephalon, plays a large role in regulating cerebral vasomotor responses; this system is not fully developed in infants.[19] The Chiari II malformation, with its resultant brainstem dysfunction, may also compromise the sympathetic nervous system.

Thus, the infant has less reserve to respond to stress and maintain homeostasis of cerebral blood flow in control of ICP. The usual anesthetic precautions to control ICP should apply: avoid hypoxia, avoid positive end-expiratory pressure, and maintain normotension. The partial pressure of carbon dioxide should not be allowed to rise markedly, and should be maintained at or slightly below normal by assisted or controlled ventilation. If these precausions are taken, the cerebral vasodilatory actions of the volatile anesthetics appear to be well tolerated by the neonate.

In the past local anesthesia had been used on these infants, supplemented by a whiskey nipple or pentobarbital gavage. These types of anesthetics, used in the 1940s and early 1950s, were associated with a period of high perioperative infant mortality rates.[14] A direct spinal technique has been described to anesthetize these infants, producing potentially hazardous hypotension in several cases. Although no instances of respiratory compromise were reported, this would be a significant risk to consider.[20] In patients with uncertain spinal fluid dynamics, a brainstem abnormality, and possible hydrocephalus, spinal anesthesia seems unwise. It would also appear to increase the risk of ventriculitis, although no such cases have been reported. These methods are now only of historical interest.

Prone Position

The challenge of administering anesthesia in the prone position can be minimized by careful attention to detail. The endotracheal tube must be well secured to prevent slippage. The breath sounds must be carefully checked following each change in position. Placement of transverse bolsters, under the shoulders and under the pelvis, is recommended.[14,21] No pressure should be placed on the abdomen or chest. The chest must be free to expand with inspiration.

The lack of pressure on the abdomen is especially important for two reasons. First, abdominal compression can limit diaphragmatic excursion, decreasing both tidal volume and functional residual capacity. Secondly, increased abdominal pressure may limit venous return from the lower extremities through the inferior vena cava; this would divert increased amounts of blood from the vena cava to the lumbar and paravertebral venous plexuses.[21] In this way abdominal compression may markedly increase intraoperative blood loss.[14]

Significant blood loss can occur during this procedure as the tissues around the defect are undermined to develop the flap. Schroeder and Williams found that 52% of patients had a loss of greater than 10% of the total blood volume, and that eight patients had greater than a 20% loss.[14] Because of the small blood volume of the neonate, accurate assessment of blood loss is critical. It is often hard to know how much blood has seeped into the drapes; thus, careful monitoring of blood pressure and heart rate is essential. As previously mentioned, transcutaneous oxygen monitoring can also be of assistance.[14,16]

Calculations should be done to estimate erythrocyte mass and acceptable red cell loss in order to maintain the hematocrit at greater than 40%. Maintaining the hematocrit at such levels compensates for the infant's decreased cardiovascular reserve, and for the left shift of the fetal hemoglobin dissociation curve.[16] An alternative approach is to replace with blood any blood loss in excess of 10% of the total blood volume.[14] Blood loss up to 10% should be replaced with isotonic crystalloid solutions in a ratio of 3 cc of crystalloid to each 1 cc of blood loss. Maintenance I.V. fluids and correction of any deficit should be administered in the routine fashion of the individual anesthesiologist.[17]

Postoperative Management

Postoperatively, most of these infants can be extubated after discontinuation of the anesthetic. Precautions should be taken to maintain the patient's core temperature in the recovery room and nursery. The patient will be nursed in the prone position postoperatively, and care should be taken to ensure that no pressure is placed on the chest or abdomen. The use of the prone position postoperatively dictates that the infant should be wide awake before extubation.[14] Those patients with high defects involving the thorax or those with brainstem dysfunction may require respiratory support after surgery.

Oozing of blood may continue, necessitating close monitoring of the hematocrit. These patients should have a respiratory monitor (apnea monitor) applied postoperatively. Because these infants are often premature, anesthesia may expose them to an increased risk of apnea for up to 24 hours after the anesthetic.[22] This occurs in addition to the previously mentioned stridor and apnea associated with the Chiari II malformation.[7]

References

1. Katz J, Steward DJ: *Anesthesia and Uncommon Pediatric Diseases*. Philadelphia: W.B. Saunders Company, pp 52–5, 1987.
2. Chervenak FA, Duncan C, Ment LR, et al: Perinatal management of meningomyelocele. Obstet. Gynecol 1984;63:367–80.
3. Katzen M: The total care of spina bifida cystica. Surg Annu 1981;13:325–39.
4. Nelson WE, Vaughan VC, McKay, RJ, et al: *Textbook of Pediatrics*. Philadelphia, W.B. Saunders Company, 1979, pp 1747–50.
5. Guthkelch AN: Aspects of the surgical management of meningomyelocele: A review. Dev Med Child Neurol 1986;28:525–32.
6. Charney EB, Weller SC, Sutton LN, et al: Management of the newborn with meningomyelocele: Time for a decision-making process. Pediatrics 1985;75:58–64.
7. McLone DG, Dias L, Kaplan WE, et al: Concepts in the management of spina bifida. Concepts Pediatr Neurosurg 1985;5:97–106.
8. Linder M, Nichols J, Sklar FH: Effect of meningomyelocele closure on the intracranial pulse pressure. Childs Brain 1984;11:176–82.
9. Mapstone TB, Rekate HL, Nulsen FE, et al: Relationship of CSF shunting and IQ in children with meningomyelocele: A retrospective analysis. Childs Brain 1984;11:112–18.
10. Sharrard WJW, Zachary RB, Lorber J, et al: A controlled trial of immediate and delayed closure of spina bifida cystica. Arch Dis Child 1963;38:18–22.
11. Lorber J: Spina bifida cystica: Results of treatment of 270 consecutive cases with criteria for selection for the future. Arch Dis Child 1972;47:854–73.
12. Kaiser G, Rudeberg A: Comments on the management of newborns with spina bifida cystica—active treatment or no treatment. Z Kinderchir 1986;41:141–43.
13. Lorber J, Salfield S: Results of selective treatment of spina bifida cystica. Arch Dis Child 1981;56:822–30.
14. Schroeder HG, Williams NE: Anesthesia for meningomyelocele surgery: Some problems associated with immediate surgical closure in the neonate. Anesthesia 1966;21:57–65.
15. Singh CV: Anesthetic management of meningocele and meningomyelocele. J Indian Med Assoc 1980;75:130–32.
16. Dierdorf SF, Krishna G: Anesthetic management of neonatal surgical emergencies. Anesth Analg 1981;60:204–15.

17. Salem MR, Bennett EJ: Anesthetic care of pediatric surgical patients. Crit Care Med 1980;8:541–47.
18. Milligan DWA: Failure of autoregulation and intraventricular hemorrhage in preterm infants. Lancet 1980;i:896–98.
19. Rogers MC, Nugent SK, Traystman RI: Control of cerebral circulation in the neonate and infant. Crit Care Med 1980;8(10):570–74.
20. Calvert DG: Direct spinal anesthesia for repair of meningomyelocele. Br Med J 1966;2:86–7.
21. Meridy HW, Creighton RE, Humphreys RP: Complications during neurosurgery in the prone position in children. Can Anaesth Soc J 1974;21:445–53.
22. Steward DJ: Pre-term infants are more prone to complications following minor surgery than are term infants. Anesthesiology 1982;56:304–6.

CHAPTER 6

The Infant with Tracheoesophageal Fistula and Esophageal Atresia*

Sylvia McMullan

Case History. *A baby girl was delivered by normal spontaneous vaginal delivery after 35 weeks of uncomplicated gestation. Apgar scores were 9 at 1 minute and 10 at 5 minutes. Birth weight was 2250 gm. Shortly after delivery, the baby had several episodes of cyanosis and bradycardia and a "barking" type of cough. Large amounts of secretion were noted about the mouth and nose.*

An attempt to pass a nasogastric tube was unsuccessful; obstruction was met at approximately 10 cm from the nares. A chest x-ray revealed the tube coiled in the upper esophagus. Right upper lobe atelectasis and air in the stomach were seen.

Physical examination revealed some respiratory distress and a deformity of the right arm. Sinus tachycardia was 192/min and tachypnea 55 breaths/min; ECG was otherwise normal. Initial laboratory values were as follows: hematocrit 62%; WBC 7000/mm³; glucose 85 mg/dl; PaO_2 55 mmHg (FiO₂ .35); $PaCO_2$ 37 mmHg. Other values were within normal limits.

The patient was scheduled for surgical repair of the tracheoesophageal fistula and esophageal atresia.

Introduction

The first case of tracheoesophageal fistula and esophageal atresia (TEF and EA) was described in 1967 by Thomas Gibson, but it was not until 1939 that a patient survived a multiple-staged surgical repair. Two years later Haight reported the first successful single-stage repair.[1]

Survival has improved dramatically over the past the past few years because of anesthetic, surgical and medical advances, and improved postoperative care. Patients with TEF and EA have been categorized as:

---

* Reviewed by Dr. Elizabeth Brodman, Associate Professor of Anesthesiology, Montefiore Medical Center, Bronx, New York.

Group A: full-term infants over 2500 gm, without pulmonary complications or other associated anomaly

Group B: infants weighing 1800-2500 gm, with moderate pneumonia and/or associated anomalies

Group C: infants weighing less than 1800 gm, with severe pneumonia or severe associated anomaly

Prematurity, pulmonary complications, and associated anomalies comprise the most important factors that affect survival.[2] Three risk groups have been described.[3]

Survival of group A patients approaches 100%, whereas survival in group C is only 50%.[4] The overall survival for all patients is 65–75%.[4-9]

Pathophysiology

TEF and EA have been reported in 1/3000 to 1/4000 live births.[5] The abnormality begins to develop embryologically shortly after conception. At about 3 weeks of gestational age, the lungs start forming as an outpouching of the ventral wall of the foregut. Initially, this outpouching is attached to the foregut but eventually is separated by the development of the esophagotracheal septum. The trachea and lung buds migrate caudad and the larynx cephalad.

In normal development, the only communication between the gut and the respiratory tract is the laryngeal aditus. Normally by the 26th day, the trachea and esophagus have separated as two parallel tubes up to the level of the larynx. If the separation between the trachea and the esophagus is interrupted, the more rapidly growing trachea divides the proximal from the distal esophagus, forming a fistula. Esophageal atresia results when the lateral esophageal grooves continue distally in the process of separating the dorsal esophagus from the ventral trachea.

Anomalous vessels may also cause discontinuity of the esophagus by mechanical obstruction of the developing esophagus.[5,6] Several types of TEF and EA are described. It is important to know the patient's abnormal anatomy prior to surgery because the anesthetic management and surgical repair vary with the different types. In the presence of a communication between the gastrointestinal tract and the respiratory system there is increased risk of aspiration, which can be avoided by appropriate active precautions. In less than 10% of cases, EA exists without a fistula and aspiration is less likely to occur.

The most commonly used classification of EA and TEF is that described by Gross[7]: (Figure 1)

Type A: EA without fistula

Type B: EA—with the upper segment of the esophagus communicating with the trachea

Type C: EA—with the upper segment blind and the lower segment communicating with the back of the trachea

Type D: EA—with both upper and lower segments communicating with the trachea

Type E: TEF without EA (also called type H)

Type F: Esophageal stenosis

Type C is by far the most common and accounts for 80–90% of all cases. Fewer than 10% of cases described are type A. The other types occur even less commonly.[8]

Clinical Presentation and Diagnosis

Polyhydramnios is usually present in the mother and raises suspicion before delivery that some form of intestinal obstruction exists in the fetus. Premature delivery occurs in about one third of cases.[2] Associated anomalies occur in 50% of cases and are the most significant cause of morbidity and mortality.[8]

At birth these infants have large amounts of foamy oral secretions. If the diagnosis is missed at this time, it should be realized during the first feeding. Crying, gagging, choking, coughing and/or cyanosis and apnea will accompany any attempts to swallow. The aspiration of food is soon followed by pneumonia. The pulmonary problem is magnified by gastric juice refluxing through the fistula (gastric acidity develops within 24 hours after delivery), and by regurgitation and aspiration of secretions from the

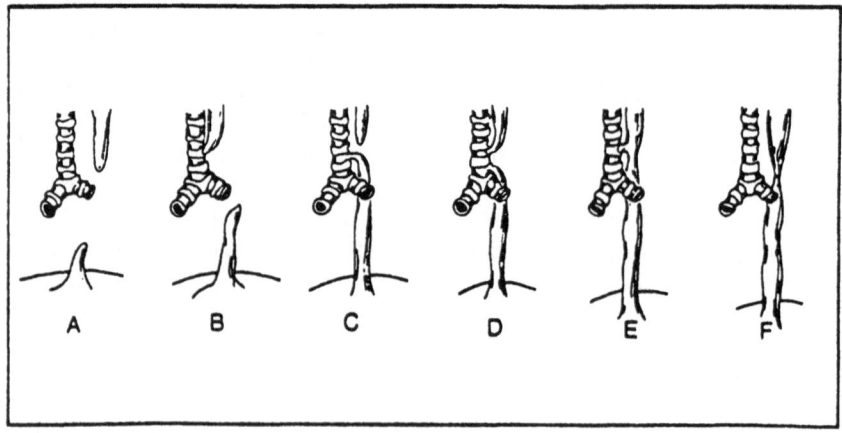

FIGURE 6.1. Gross' classification of esophageal atresia and tracheoesophageal fistula: A = esophageal atresia without fistula; B = esophageal atresia with proximal fistula; C = esophageal atresia with distal fistula; D = esophageal atresia with proximal and distal fistula; E = tracheoesophageal fistula without atresia; and F = esophageal stenosis.

upper esophageal pouch. The infant then becomes tachypneic and develops abdominal distention (in types C, D, and E), which further interferes with ventilation.

Rapid measures including intubation and head-up position should be taken to protect the airway and prevent progression of respiratory and metabolic acidosis and possible cardiorespiratory arrest. In EA, the distended upper pouch compresses the cartilage of the tracheal wall, weakening the structure and causing tracheomalacia. Airway obstruction results and gives rise to a characteristic "barking" cough.[9]

The diagnosis is strongly suggested if a catheter cannot be passed into the stomach. The catheter will stop at 10–12 cm from the gum line. A chest x-ray confirms the diagnosis and shows a curled catheter in the upper pouch of the esophagus. Injection of contrast media is not recommended because of the possibility of aspiration and subsequent increased morbidity and mortality.[5]

The chest x-ray also demonstrates the presence of pneumonia, which is more common in the right upper lobe as the result of aspiration of feedings and secretions. In addition, if the chest x-ray shows an air bubble in the stomach, this is evidence of a TEF. The absence of air in the stomach is pathognomonic of EA (types A and B). The chest x-ray may also aid in the diagnosis of associated congenital anomalies, especially if cardiac or bony anomalies are present. In rare instances, symptoms may be subtle. Bronchoscopy may be necessary to identify a fistula in the posterior wall of the trachea.

TEF and EA are part of the well-recognized association of anomalies called VATER: Vetebral anomalies, Anal atresia, Tracheoesophageal fistula, Esophageal atresia, and Radial limb anomalies. Gastrointestinal defects (eg, pyloric stenosis) and genitourinary anomalies (particularly renal) may also be associated with TEF and EA.

Treatment

Affected infants should not be fed and should be placed in 30° upright position. Contents of the upper esophageal pouch are put on continuous suction by means of a sump catheter. Antibiotic therapy is started if pneumonia is present.

Gastrostomy is sometimes indicated emergently in the management of these infants and can be performed prior to definitive repair of the esophagus. The procedure may be life-saving if severe distention of the stomach elevates the diaphragm and acutely compromises ventilation. Ventilatory mechanics are improved, the stomach decompressed, and the possibility of reflux of gastric contents decreased. Also, gastrostomy is usually performed in critically ill, low-birth-weight premature babies with or without pulmonary complications or associated anomalies.

Gastrostomy may be performed under local anesthesia. The procedure may be accompanied by insertion of a transpyloric or jejunostomy tube for feeding[10] or a central cannula for hyperalimentation.

Division of the TEF and esophagoesophagostomy are performed at a later date when the infant has gained weight or has recovered from his pneumonia and all associated anomalies have been appropriately evaluated. Other pediatric surgeons believe that the respiratory status will not improve until the fistula is ligated and, therefore, perform a staged approach with gastrostomy and fistular division followed by esophageal anastomosis weeks or months later.[10]

If the infant weighs more than 1800 gm, has no other congenital anomalies, and has not developed pneumonia, then primary repair can be undertaken. The surgical approach is through a right thoracotomy with the infant in a left lateral decubitus position. The fistula is ligated and esophageal anastomosis performed.

Preanesthetic Assessment

General preoperative evaluation of the neonate should include assessment of the factors listed in Table 6.1.

Electrolyte status should be assessed and corrected and a blood type and crossmatch performed to ensure availability of packed red blood cells.

Respiratory Status

Since these infants have increased risk of aspiration and pneumonia, it is important to evaluate respiratory function preoperatively, including physical examination, chest x-ray, and blood analyses. If pulmonary disease is present, placement of an indwelling arterial catheter and frequent analyses of blood gases are helpful in following pulmonary function. Administration of supplemental O_2 with or without intubation is often needed. Hyperoxia in premature infants should be avoided because of the potential for retinopathy and retrolental fibroplasia. Use of pulse oximetry to monitor oxygen saturation provides a continuous assessment of safe levels of oxygen.

Prematurity

Prematurity adversely affects survival. Infants who weigh less than 1800 gm or have severe lung disease or associated anomalies may not tolerate a definitive procedure. In such cases, it is safer to perform a gastrostomy under local anesthesia, and stabilize and nourish the infant before the corrective surgery is performed.

TABLE 6.1. Preanesthetic evaluation
of the TEF/EA infant: factors to be
assessed.

- weight
- gestational age—premature or term
  infant
- weight vs gestational age—small for
  gestational age (SGA), appropriate for
  gestational age (AGA), large for
  gestational age (LGA)
- heart rate, respiratory rate, pattern, and
  blood pressure
- hematocrit, WBC
- BUN, Na^+, K^+, Cl^-, HCO_3^-
- physical anomalies
- glucose
- urine output
- pH, PO_2
- calcium
- ECG
- chest x-ray
- presence of cyanosis

Other problems of prematurity to be evaluated include hypoglycemia, hypocalcemia, respiratory distress syndrome (RDS), and hyperbilirubinemia. Abnormalities should be corrected prior to surgery. All attempts must be made to keep the infant as close to normothermic as possible.

Cardiac Status

Fourteen percent of TEF patients have associated cardiac anomalies,[11] the most common of which is ventricular septal defect, followed in decreasing order of frequency by patent ductus arteriosus, atrial septal defect, coarctation of the aorta, dextrocardia, tetralogy of Fallot (more frequent in patients with associated gastrointestinal abnormalities), truncus arteriosus, transposition of the great vessels, atresia, and pulmonary stenosis. A pediatric cardiac consultation should be sought. Rarely correction of the cardiac anomaly may take precedence over repair of the TEF. Intubation and tracheostomy and gastrostomy are palliative emergency measures.

Associated Anomalies

The presence of other congenital anomalies is common, especially anal atresia, renal deformities, and radial limb dysplasia (which may limit arterial and venous access). Any vertebral abnormalities should be assessed, particularly if they may hamper endotracheal intubation.

Anesthetic Plan

Routine monitors include ECG, blood pressure, pulse oximetry, capnography, and temperature. A precordial stethoscope is placed in the left axilla to monitor breath sounds. Every effort should be made to maintain normothermia by warming the operating room with heating lamps, warming blankets, and humidified warmed gases. Warmed, intravenous fluids with dextrose are given at 4 ml/kg/h. An additional 6.8 ml/kg/h is given for intraoperative evaporation and "third-space" loss. Replacement of blood loss should be on an ml-for-ml basis. Atropine (0.02 mg/kg) is all the premedication that is needed and it can be given intravenously in the operating room prior to induction.

The upper esophageal pouch is suctioned prior to intubation. Awake tracheal intubation is performed with the patient breathing spontaneously in a semiupright position. The bevel of the endotracheal tube should be facing anteriorly to help avoid intubating the fistula[5] (most fistulas are located posteriorly, just proximal to the carina). Some advocate intubating the right main stem bronchus and then pulling back slowly until breath sounds are bilaterally equal and the stomach is not inflated.[11] The ideal position for the tube is above the carina and distal to the TEF.

After intubation, anesthesia is induced and maintained with O_2, air, or N_2O, and halothane. All inhalation agents depress blood pressure in neonates both because of the intrinsic properties of the agents and the susceptibility of the infant's heart, which has a less compliant ventricle, a decreased contractile mass, and decreased extent and velocity of shortening. The MAC of halothane in the newborn is 0.87% compared to 1.2% in babies aged 1–6 months.[12] Positive pressure ventilation must be cautiously attempted before administering a muscle relaxant.[10]

If gastric distention through the fistula occurs, the N_2O is discontinued and the patient is allowed to breathe spontaneously with gentle manual assistance until the chest is opened and the fistula closed. If spontaneous breathing with or without assisted ventilation does not provide adequate ventilation, then decompression of the stomach by percutaneous needle or gastrostomy may be necessary before the thoracotomy is performed.

Complete relaxation, required for the esophageal anastomosis, can be achieved with a nondepolarizing muscle relaxant and positive pressure ventilation. Although not currently recommended by the manufacturer for use in children below the age of 2, atracurium may be the muscle relaxant of choice, especially for babies with a renal anomaly. Adequate arterial blood gas values confirm the adequacy of ventilation. In premature infants it is important to maintain the PaO_2 level between 60–80 mmHg; 30–70% O_2 concentration is usually adequate for this purpose. Oxygen can be diluted with air if N_2O is contraindicated, eg if air has been demonstrated in the stomach preoperatively.

Postoperatively, vigorous healthy neonates without associated anomalies should be awake and extubated at the end of the procedure.

Complications

Acute airway obstruction may occur at any time, secondary to secretions, clots, or surgical manipulation. Periodic expansion of the right lung may be necessary, with frequent tracheal suctioning.

If there are pulmonary complications pre- or postoperatively, controlled ventilation and antibiotics should be continued. The most frequent complications in the immediate postoperative period are the development of atelectasis and pneumonitis from retained secretions in the tracheobronchial tree.[13] The pharynx should be suctioned gently with a soft catheter that has been measured and clearly marked to prevent crossing and possibly damaging the anastomotic site.

Several complications may occur secondary to the surgery such as anastomotic leaks and strictures. Esophageal strictures are treated with repeated dilatations. Recurrent laryngeal nerve injury and tracheomalacia have been described. When tracheomalacia occurs, a soft segment of the trachea collapses causing airway obstruction that often requires tracheostomy.

Although most babies have complete recovery, esophageal motility abnormalities may occur and can lead to aspiration pneumonia, asthma, bronchitis, and fibrosis. Mucociliary clearance of the tracheobronchial tree is impaired and can increase the incidence of upper and lower respiratory infections.

References

1. Gregory GA: Pediatric Anesthesia, vol 2, New York: Churchill Livingstone, 1983, p 655.
2. Calverley RK, Johnson AE: The anaesthetic management of tracheoesophageal fistula: a review of 10 years experience. Can Anaesth Soc J 1972;19:270–82.
3. Waterston DJ, Bonham Carter RE, Aberdeen E: Oesophageal atresia: tracheoesophageal fistula: a study of survival in 218 infants. Lancet 1962;1:819–22.
4. Koop CE, Schnaufer L, Broennle AM: Esophageal atresia and tracheoesophageal fistula. Supportive measures that affect survival. Pediatrics 1974;54:558–64.

5. Haight C: Congenital esophageal atresia and tracheoesophageal fistula. Pediatric Surgery, 2nd ed, ed by WT Mustard. Chicago: Year Book Medical Publishers, 1969.
6. Cumming WA: Esophageal atresia and tracheoesophageal fistula. Radiol Clin North Am 1975;13:277–95.
7. Gross RE: The Surgery of Infancy and Childhood. Philadelphia: WB Saunders, 1953, p 76.
8. Katz J, Steward DJ: Anesthesia and Uncommon Pediatric Diseases, Philadelphia: WB Saunders, 1987, p 72.
9. Davies MR, Cywes S: The flaccid trachea and tracheoesophageal congenital anomalies. J Pediatr Surg 1978;13:363–67.
10. Ito T, Sugito T, Nagaya M: Delayed primary anastomosis in poor-risk patients with esophageal atresia associated with tracheoesophageal fistula. J Pediatr Surg 1984;19:243–47.
11. Greenwood RD, Rosenthal A: Cardiovascular malformations associated with TEF and EA. Pediatrics 1976;57:87–91.
12. Lerman J, Robinson S, Willis MM, et al: Anesthetic requirements for halothane in young children 0–1 month and 1–6 months of age. Anesthesiology 1983;59:421–24.
13. Milligan DW, Levison H: Lung function in children following repair of TEF. J Pediatr 1979;95:24–7.

CHAPTER 7

The Burned Patient

Gerald Scheinman*

Case History. *A 58-year-old man was brought to the emergency room with 30% second- and third-degree burns involving his chest, arms, neck, and face. He had fallen asleep while smoking in bed. Approximately 40 minutes had elapsed between the time of the fire alarm and the patient's arrival at the hospital. He had a history of alcohol abuse. No other medical history was available.*

Physical examination showed an obese man in moderate respiratory distress, with a harsh, dry cough. Eyebrows and eyelashes were singed and black soot particles were noted in the nose. The patient was able to respond to his name but was not oriented to time or place. His arms and neck had been covered with first-aid dressings.

Vital signs were: blood pressure 180/110 mmHg; pulse 115/min; respiratory rate 28/min. Laboratory data included: hemaglobin 18 gm; hematocrit 47%; SMA-6 within normal limits. Arterial blood gas analyses on room air were: pH 7.3; PaO₂ 56; PaCO₂ 38. Urine specific gravity was 1.030.

Fiberoptic endoscopy revealed some laryngeal edema and the decision was made to intubate. Venous access was achieved through both saphenous veins and fluid resuscitation was begun. The posterior tibial artery was cannulated. Sedation with morphine sulfate was adequate.

Over the next 2 hours, circulation to both hands seemed to be compromised and the patient was taken to the operating room for fasciotomy and debridement and dressing of the chest and neck wounds.

Introduction

The anesthesiologist's involvement in the management of the burn patient begins in the emergency room. Over 2 million people in the United States seek medical care each year because of burns, and 100,000 are hospital-

---

* Reviewed by Dr. Jasu Mehta, Associate Professor of Anesthesiology, Albert Einstein College of Medicine, Bronx, New York.

ized. Despite improvements in both acute and chronic care of these patients, there are over 10,000 deaths per year.[1-4] It is estimated that there is a 1 in 70 chance that a resident of the United States will be hospitalized for a burn.[3]

The care of a burned patient involves acute and chronic phases. Initial care is concerned with the pulmonary and cardiovascular systems and loss of fluid and electrolytes. Subsequent attention focuses on immune system abnormalities, metabolism, temperature regulation, and cosmetic and functional abnormalities, in addition to continued support of cardio-respiratory function.

A severe burn imposes tremendous physiologic stress on the victim, because the skin is the largest organ in the body. The two layers of the skin, the epidermis and dermis, have different functions. Although the outermost part of the epidermis is dead, it provides an essential mechanical barrier against the environment, protecting against bacterial invasion and regulating the loss of heat and fluid. Within the dermis are the nerves and blood vessels to the skin. Thus, a partial-thickness burn that leaves parts of the dermis intact is painful, but a full-thickness burn is completely anesthetic.[5]

Classification of Burns

Both patient age and severity of the burn have major roles in determining outcome. Mortality is higher at either end of the age spectrum. The severity of burn relates both to the depth of skin and the extent of body surface area involved.

First-degree burns cause minimal damage to the epidermis and are characterized by pain and erythema. Treatment is symptomatic and is directed toward relief of discomfort and fever. The wounds usually heal within 5–10 days.[5]

Second-degree burns involve the entire epidermis and extend partially into the dermis. Because of the exposure of the nerve endings, this type of wound is very painful. If the damage to the dermis is superficial, the wound will heal rapidly because of the presence of epidermal elements in the surviving sweat glands and hair follicles, and scarring is usually minimal. With a deep burn, the majority of the epidermal cells are damaged, scarring is common, and functional and cosmetic problems are frequent.[5]

Third-degree burns result in total destruction of the dermis and epidermis. As a result they are avascular and anesthetic, and the wound, which does not heal spontaneously, requires skin grafting. There tends to be a zone of ischemia present beneath these burns, composed of injured but viable tissue. With further hypoxia, ischemia, or the development of infection, this underlying tissue may become nonviable and increase the extent of third-degree burn. Aggressive management from the start is, therefore, warranted to salvage this viable tissue.[5]

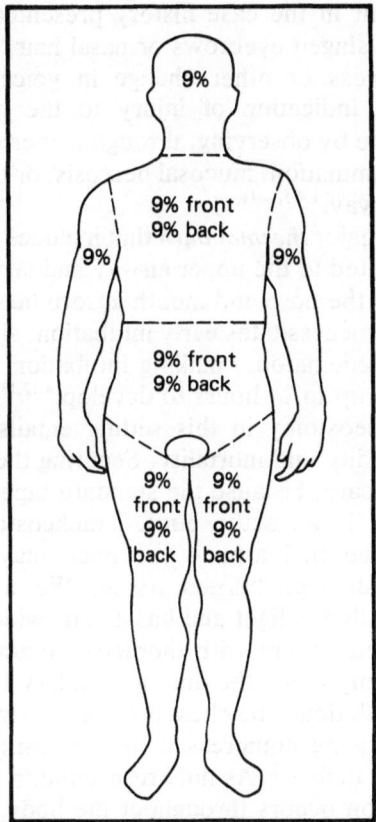

9%

9% front
9% back

9%

9%

9% front
9% back

9%
front
9%
back

9%
front
9%
back

FIGURE 7.1. "Rule of Nines" for estimating extent of burns, showing relative percentage of body surface area (BSA) in adults.

The percentage of the total body surface area (BSA) damaged by the burn can be calculated by a number of methods. The "rule of the nines," which breaks the body down into areas of 9% or multiples of 9%, is probably the simplest[6,7] (see Figure 7.1.). The total BSA involved and the severity of the burns are important in calculating the fluid requirements necessary for resuscitation.[6-8]

Airway Management

Airway Injury

The major cause of mortality in the fire victim is *inhalational injury*, which accounts for more than 50% of deaths.[8,9] Management of those survivors presenting to the emergency room is based on both history and clinical examination. A history of involvement in a closed-space fire or impaired sensorium should increase the suspicion of an inhalational injury, as was evident in the case history presented. The presence of facial or neck burns, singed eyebrows or nasal hair, carbon deposits on the mucosa, hoarseness or other change in voice, or carbonaceous sputum is a further indication of injury to the respiratory system. Diagnosis can be made by observing, through a fiberoptic bronchoscope, airway edema or inflammation, mucosal necrosis, or the presence of soot or charring in the airway.[1,4,5,9–11]

The patient with a major *thermal burn* that includes injury to the airway often has damage limited to the upper airway and larynx, because of the efficiency with which the nose and mouth absorb heat. Any suspicion of an upper airway burn necessitates early intubation, since the airway may become increasingly edematous, making intubation more difficult. Airway edema may take up to 24 hours to develop.[4,12,13]

Performing a tracheostomy in this setting entails a significantly increased risk of morbidity and mortality. Securing the endotracheal tube should be done with care, because the standard tape may not adhere to the skin when there is an acute burn. Tracheostomy "cord"[12,13] or venous extension tube tied around the neck may be a satisfactory substitute but may damage burned tissue. We use a commercially available tube holder that is light and has a soft, wide elastic band.

The severely burned patient with thoracoabdominal burns may need emergency escharotomy along the anterior axillary lines of the chest to allow for normal ventilation. The chest may be constricted by the burned tissue as if it were being compressed by a tourniquet, resulting in a restrictive ventilatory defect.[13] As fluid resuscitation progresses, marked tissue edema formation occurs throughout the body, further decreasing chest wall compliance and increasing the work of breathing.

Burns that involve the respiratory tract of young children are more dangerous than similar lesions in adults: The child's airway is smaller in diameter and more prone to become obstructed by edema; children have less respiratory reserve and become fatigued more rapidly with the increased work of breathing in respiratory burns; and children have increased baseline metabolic demands and O_2 consumption that are compounded by any surface burn.

Carbon Monoxide

The partial combustion of fuels by fire results in the generation of carbon monoxide, a toxic colorless and odorless gas, the adverse effects of which are due to an increased affinity of hemoglobin for carbon monoxide, resulting in a decrease in the amount of oxygen transported by hemoglobin; impairment of the use of oxygen by cells; and a shift in the hemoglobin-oxygen dissociation curve to the left. There is less available oxygen at the site of a fire because of consumption of oxygen by the fire itself, and this aggravates the hypoxemia of the fire victim.[11]

Carbon monoxide has a 200-fold greater affinity for hemoglobin than does oxygen. Normally, 0–5% of hemoglobin is bound tightly to carbon monoxide, and even at low concentrations this tight binding between carbon monoxide and hemoglobin decreases the amount of hemoglobin available to bind with oxygen, significantly reducing the oxygen-carrying capacity and oxygen content of the blood even though the arterial PO_2 and oxygen saturation remain normal. Since the carotid bodies are sensitive to PaO_2 and not oxygen content, tachypnea is frequently absent. Owing to the shift of the hemoglobin-oxygen dissociation curve to the left, a lower level of oxygen tension must be reached at the tissue level before oxygen is released from the hemoglobin molecule.[2,11,14,15]

The half-life of carboxyhemoglobin in a person breathing room air is approximately 4 hours, but this period can be reduced to 40 minutes when 100% oxygen is administered. Thus, supplemental O_2 should be given in emergency situations to all victims of major fires.

The symptoms of carbon monoxide exposure may be subtle: for example, headache, dizziness, nausea, and confusion with even moderately severe intoxication (carboxyhemoglobin levels of 20–40%). Levels of 60% are frequently fatal. A high index of suspicion from the history is essential. The only reliable means of diagnosis is by direct measurement of the carboxyhemoglobin level in the blood. Pulse oximetry or cooximetry will reveal an inaccurate oxygen saturation.

Other Combustion Products

The presence of carboxyhemoglobin in the blood may indicate the possibility of exposure to other toxic products of combustion that may be present at the scene of a fire and can cause a chemical burn of the airway.

Water-soluble gases such as chlorine, ammonia, hydrogen chloride, and sulfur dioxide can damage the upper airways by reacting with the aqueous part of the mucous membrane to form strong acids and alkalis that can cause ulceration and edema. The lipid-soluble gases tend to travel farther down the respiratory tract and cause deep burns. Soot and carbon particles may absorb these gases and help carry them down to the lower respiratory tract.

All of these agents tend to impair the function of the respiratory cilia, which normally act to clear mucus and debris, resulting in small-airway obstruction and exacerbation of respiratory dysfunction and favoring the proliferation of bacteria in a host who is already immunocompromised. Both direct chemical stimulation of the airways by the toxic gases and stimulation of neural reflexes can cause bronchospasm. The surfactant activity of the lung tends to be reduced, resulting in further congestion and atelectasis. Steroids increase the risk of infection and are contraindicated in patients with inhalational burns.[11,15]

Fluid Resuscitation

Since the survival of the patient with a major burn depends on appropriate fluid resuscitation, this should begin in the emergency room. The leading cause of death prior to our current management protocols were hypovolemic shock or subsequent renal failure. The loss of plasma in patients with burns that involve more than 30% of the BSA may exceed 4 ml/kg/hr.[6] Insufficient fluid replacement can also increase the extent of third-degree burns by allowing the transition of a viable ischemic deep burn to a nonviable full-thickness burn.

The resulting hypovolemia is due to several factors:

● increased microvascular permeability at the burn site;
● a generalized cell membrane defect that shifts large volumes of extracellular fluid into the cell, with further exacerbation of the intravascular volume depletion;
● increased vascular permeability and the evaporation of fluid due to loss of the protective skin layers, leading to an increase in interstitial oncotic pressure relative to intravascular pressure; and
● release of vasoactive mediators from the burned tissue.[5]

Edema

Fluid replacement may cause generalized burn edema that can also increase morbidity. Tissue edema in burned areas can result in a decreased O_2 tension because of an increased diffusion distance, leading to further insult to cells already ischemic.[5] Edema also increases tissue pressure and may increase ischemia by compromising blood flow to affected areas. This is especially important in the extremities, where circumferential burns may increase tissue pressure under the deep fascia and totally occlude the vascular supply to the limb. Immediate fasciotomy may be necessary to reestablish blood flow.[13,14]

Thermal injury to tissues causes an initial decrease in blood flow. Edema begins with the resolution of this transient decrease in blood flow through the heat-damaged vessels. The rate at which the edema develops and its severity depend on the adequacy of flow through the microcirculation and, therefore, the adequacy of fluid resuscitation. Systemic hypovolemia that results after a large injury may delay the rate of edema formation, which may not peak until 18–24 hours after the injury. In smaller burns, the edema is usually maximal 8–12 hours postinjury.

Large gaps between endothelial cells occur in vessels in burned areas. These histologic changes present minutes after the injury and may persist for several days to weeks in those vessels that remain patent. The microvasculature becomes permeable to macromolecules the size of fibrinogen and larger. Vasoactive agents that are released from the burned tissue, leukotrienes, O_2 radicals, and prostaglandins are also thought to be responsible for the vascular changes that occur. Fluid resuscitation has to be done carefully, because increases in the hydrostatic pressure can markedly increase the fluid losses to the interstitial compartment that result from these vascular changes.[5,6]

Tissues that are distant from the immediate burn site also become edematous during fluid resuscitation. The severe hypoproteinemia that results from both the burn and fluid resuscitation alters the Starling forces, favoring an outward shift of the intravascular fluid. There also appears to be a loosening of the interstitial matrix that facilitates the movement of intravascular fluid into the interstitial space.[5,6]

Burns involving more than 30% of the BSA (combined deep partial thickness and full thickness) cause a generalized decrease in the cellular transmembrane potential that is especially prominent in muscle. This allows a shift of extracellular sodium and water into the intracellular space and causes generalized cellular swelling, thus increasing the volume needed for adequate resuscitation. If the fluid replacement is adequate, the membrane changes resolve after 24–36 hours; otherwise cell death may follow.[5,6]

Clinical Management

Adequate resuscitation of the burned patient with the large volumes of fluid that are frequently necessary requires appropriate monitoring. The vascular instability after a burn is short-lived (approximately 24–48 hours), and it is important to support the patient during this period with the least morbidity possible. The volume of fluid needed for resuscitation depends on the age of the patient, BSA, and the size and depth of the burn. The various formulas used to calculate fluid replacement are guidelines to be used while monitoring hemodynamic status and urine output.

The use of hypertonic saline minimizes postburn edema; however, close monitoring of serum electrolytes is mandatory. The presence of inhalational injury markedly increase the fluid requirements, since the injured lung acts as an additional fluid reservoir. After the first 18–24 hours, the rate of fluid loss decreases markedly if perfusion is maintained.

Blood pressure is not a reliable parameter with which to follow the adequacy of fluid replacement, because of a marked increase in catecholamine release. The maintenance of a heart rate less than 110/min usually indicates adequate fluid resuscitation, except in the older patient, in whom the heart may not respond appropriately to hypovolemic stress.

In those patients urine output is a more valuable guide to the degree of fluid replacement, because it reflects the maintenance of renal blood flow. Indirectly, urine output may also be used to guage the degree of perfusion of other organs.

The adult burn patient tends to be glucose intolerant because of the high levels of circulating catecholamines. The fluid used for resuscitation should be glucose-poor to avoid an osmotic diuresis, which would eliminate one of the ways to assess the appropriateness of fluid replacement. Children lack equivalent glycogen stores or the ability to convert fats or protein to glucose; therefore, resuscitation fluid in the pediatric patient should contain glucose, the concentration of which should be decreased if glycosuria occurs.

The urine output in adults should be 0.5–1.0 ml/kg/hr and in children 1.0 ml/kg/hr.[7,14,16] Children also have a greater fluid requirement than adults for the same degree of burn, and they tend to require formal fluid resuscitation with burns involving smaller percentages of BSA than do adults.

The use of central cannulae or pulmonary artery catheters in burned patients entails a higher risk of complications than in other patients. Adequate perfusion may be accomplished with low filling pressures; the risks of empirically increasing the pressures must be weighed against those of overhydration.

Along with the severe hypovolemia that occurs secondary to the fluid shifts, cardiac output is also decreased by a myocardial depressant factor present in plasma. This is most apparent in patients with severe burns involving BSA of more than 40%. The cardiovascular system subsequently becomes hyperdynamic, with a 2- to 3-fold increase in cardiac output. This may continue for several months after injury and is caused by an increase in catecholamine and renin activity.[13]

The use of arterial blood gas analyses to measure acid-base balance provides valuable information about the adequacy of perfusion. The persistence of a base deficit indicates inadequate perfusion. However, in circumstances in which there has been inhalation of either carbon monoxide or cyanide, there may be inhibition of mitochondrial enzymes leading to anaerobic glycolysis and a persistent base deficit.

Some of the commonly used resuscitation formulas in the first 24 hours following a burn injury are listed in Table 7.1.

Infection

In patients hospitalized with burns, the major cause of death remains infection, most commonly of the burn wound itself and the pulmonary system. Burn patients have significant alterations in both the humoral and cellular components of the immune system as well as loss of the physical barrier provided by intact skin.

Other potential sites for the development of infections include points of intravenous access. The detection of suppurative thrombophlebitis may

TABLE 7.1. Several protocols used in the fluid resuscitation of burned patients.

Name	Solution
Brooke	Ringer's lactated solution 1.5ml/kg/% burn + colloid 0.5ml/kg/% burn + 5% dextrose in water, 2000ml
Modified Brooke	Ringer's lactated solution 2.0ml/kg/% burn
Parkland	Ringer's lactated solution 4.0ml/kg/% burn
Evans	Normal saline 0.1ml/kg/% burn + colloid 1.0ml/kg/% burn + 5% dextrose in water, 2000ml
Hypertonic sodium chloride	Volume of fluid containing 250mEq/L sodium to promote a urinary output of 30ml/hr

be difficult, and extreme care has to be taken with all intravenous cannulae in burn patients. Cartilage, because of its poor blood supply, may become infected if it underlies a full-thickness burn. The prolonged use of urinary catheters may cause urinary tract infections. The insertion of invasive cardiac monitors may cause bacterial endocarditis. Finally, prolonged nasotracheal intubation or the use of nasogastric tubes may cause sinusitis or middle ear infections.[16]

Systemic antibiotic prophylaxis in the immediate postburn period has been shown to cause the rapid emergence of resistant organisms and has therefore been discontinued. Tetanus prophylaxis is necessary, because the wound is an anaerobic environment. Hyperimmune globulin may be required initially, since tetanus antibodies require time to be produced by the vaccine.

Currently, topical antibiotics are used to slow bacterial growth. Since the burn wound contains dead cellular material, it is an excellent culture medium for all microorganisms. Any organism may be a pathogen in the burn patient, and it is usually one that is already present. Potential sources are the gastrointestinal tract, nonburned skin, or the vaginal flora. Early closure of a large burn wound decreases the chance of infectious wound complications.

Examination of serial biopsies of the burn wound for the presence of organisms beyond the original wound margin, as well as routine culturing, will enable selection of appropriate antibiotics to decrease or eliminate pathogens. Concentrations of organisms greater than 10^5/gm tissue from a full-thickness-wound biopsy are associated with an increased likelihood of hematogenous dissemination and "burn-wound sepsis."

The burn patient requires careful monitoring of antibiotic levels because of the several aspects of his altered physiology: changes in cardiac output, levels of binding proteins, plasma volume, metabolic rate, and renal function; and loss of the protective skin layer.[15-19]

Topical agents are important because the blood supply to burned areas may range from poor in partial-thickness burns to nonexistent in full-thickness burns. Systemic antibiotics may not reliably reach the sites of infection. Topical application places the drugs at the sites where the risk of bacterial contamination is highest, limits the diversity of wound flora, and prevents the conversion by bacterial action of superficial burns to deeper ones. However, with burns there is the significant potential for systemic toxicity because of the large absorptive surfaces that may be present. Some of the more common agents are discussed below.

Silver sulfadiazine is the most commonly used topical agent and can be applied to the wound once or twice daily. It is easy to apply, causes minimal discomfort on application, and does not stain unburned areas or linen. Its penetration into the wound is intermediate between that of mafenide and of silver nitrate. Significant toxicity is rare because of its poor absorption. A transient leukopenia that resolves even with continued use can occur, and has not been found to be clinically significant. Silver sulfadiazine is a reasonably effective agent, especially against gram-negative organisms.[17]

Silver nitrate does not cause significant pain upon application but stains everything with which it comes in contact. The hypotonic solution that is used causes a significant leaching of sodium, potassium, and other solutes from plasma. Replacement is based on careful monitoring of the electrolyte concentrations. A potential but rare complication is methemoglobinemia due to the reduction of nitrate to nitrite by the bacteria present.[17]

Mafenide is used twice a day as a cream, and in spite of causing significant pain on application this drug has been used widely as a prophylactic agent. It is active against most gram-positive and a broad spectrum of common gram-negative bacteria. Penetration of the burn wound is both rapid and of high degree. Mafenide is a potent inhibitor of carbonic anhydrase, leading to renal bicarbonate wasting; a metabolic acidosis results, compounded by the presence of an acidic metabolite. There is a compensatory increase in alveolar minute ventilation that may limit its use. These side effects, as well as the appearance of superinfection with resistant organisms, have decreased the routine use of mafenide.[17]

Metabolic Changes and Nutritional Needs

The burn patient experiences a greater increase in metabolic rate than any other stressed patient—as much as a 100% increase with burns affecting more than 50% of the BSA. Burn patients cannot increase their metabolic rate further, and additional stresses, such as hypothermia or sepsis, may increase mortality. The mediators of this response (ie, the increased metabolic rate) are in part the stress hormones that are increased in burn patients.

Inadequate replacement of nutritional requirements, especially protein, can place a significant burden on the patient and may result in a rapid depletion of both skeletal and visceral protein as well as delayed wound healing and hindered immune response. Early wound closure has been shown to decrease the metabolic rate and protein catabolism.[5,20]

Patients suffering from burns that involve more than 20% of the BSA frequently suffer from decreased gastric emptying during the first 48 hours, caused by the increased levels of catecholamines as well as the edema of the bowel that occurs with fluid resuscitation. The ileus is usually self-limited. Burn patients are also are at risk for developing Carling's (stress) ulcer. Antacids have been found to be effective therapy. The H_2 antagonist cimetidine may also be helpful but may have additional side effects in the burned patient.[14,16,20]

Nutritional replacement may be attempted with a soft enteral feeding tube, which should be placed distal to the pylorus, because small-bowel function may be present despite the decrease in gastric motility. If this approach is not tolerated, as indicated by high gastric residual volumes or diarrhea, or if there is inadequate alimentation, parenteral nutrition may be necessary.

Anesthetic Plan

Preanesthetic Evaluation

Preanesthetic assessment includes documentation of medical history prior to the accident and, if possible, a list of current medications.

In patients requiring ventilatory support, note should be made of: 1) ventilator settings, especially if positive end-expiratory pressure (PEEP) is required; 2) the size of the endotracheal tube; 3) the length of the tube at the lips or nose; 4) means to secure the tube; 5) the cuff pressure; 6) the inspiratory pressure; and 7) the most recent arterial blood gas analyses.

If invasive monitoring is used, the trend of pressures, including cardiac output, should be noted.

The following laboratory values should be obtained prior to the operation: urinalysis, hematocrit, platelet count, coagulation profile, electrolytes, renal function tests, glucose, ionized calcium, and albumin and total protein.[2,13,21] Factor deficiencies in the clotting mechanisms should be corrected wherever possible. Hematologic consultation is usually wise.

The patient with a serious burn undergoes a number of debridement and reconstructive procedures in the weeks and months that immediately follow the accident. Recent experience has shown that survival is improved in those patients who undergo rapid closure of their wounds. This tends to require many debridement procedures in the first few weeks following the initial injury. Patients may experience considerable discomfort in the transfer from the burn unit to the operating room, which may thus be a very unpleasant experience. Premedication with a narcotic analgesic and a benzodiazepine may help to attenuate this problem.[2,13,21]

The Anesthetic Period

Monitoring: Significant alteration in physiologic status requires monitoring during the anesthetic period. The placement of the ECG patches may be difficult because commonly used areas may be devoid of skin or will be needed as skin-graft donor sites. It may be necessary, therefore, to place the patches at locations distant from the normal sites. Another option involves the use of needle electrodes but this is associated with increased electrical hazard to the patient. Use of an esophageal ECG may be advantageous.[2,13,21]

Recording the blood pressure may be a problem if there are extensive burns to all extremities. It may be necessary at times to place the cuff over burned areas. Placement of an intraarterial catheter is essential if major debridement is anticipated.[2,13,21] Recently, a device to monitor blood pressure from the finger (Finapres®, Ohmeda, Englewood, N.J.) has been introduced and is undergoing clinical trials.

Access to intravenous sites may traverse burned areas, but surgical placement should be avoided if possible because of the high risk of infection. Two large-bore intravenous cannulae are necessary, especially in major debridement where a significant blood loss may occur. Central pressure measurement is also important intraoperatively as a guide to fluid replacement.

The burned patient should have a urinary catheter in place if the operation is to occur during the period immediately following the acute event.[2,13,21]

The burned patient has a greater intraoperative problem with temperature control than a normal individual, for several reasons:

- Large areas of the body are exposed during the operative procedure.
- Hypermetabolism exists.
- There are increased evaporative and convective losses, owing to the destruction of the protective skin layer.
- Large volumes of cold or room-temperature blood and crystalloid are frequently administered during a major debridement.
- Procedures in cold operating suites are prolonged.
- The patient's thermoregulatory control mechanisms are disrupted during anesthesia.

The response of the body to hypothermia is to shiver, which places an additional stress on the burn patient with this further increase in oxygen consumption. It is important, therefore, to take appropriate measures to prevent unnecessary loss of heat by

- warming the operating suite to at least 25°C;
- warming all cleansing and intravenous solutions;
- covering as much of the exposed area as possible;
- humidifying and warming all inspired gases;
- using a radiant heater near the patient;
- applying aluminum foil to exposed areas.

Humidification is important in preventing the loss of heat caused by evaporation from the lung and in helping to protect the lung with decreased defense mechanisms from thermal injury.[2,13,21]

Induction: Induction can be especially challenging in the patient who has suffered burns to the face, neck, or upper chest, since such injuries may cause flexion contractures that limit neck and jaw mobility and make airway control difficult. Review of the patient's chart may provide valuable insight into prior successful management of the airway. Consideration should be given to intubating the patient awake, either orally or nasally. If the anesthesiologist is skilled, intubation over a fiberoptic bronchoscope should be the technique of choice.

The use of muscle relaxants should be carefully considered. Not only could intubation prove very difficult, especially if edema is severe, but administration of succinylcholine could result in a sudden fatal hyperkalemic response. The magnitude of the hyperkalemic response depends on the size of the burn, the dose of succinylcholine, and the time of administration relative to that of the injury. An abnormal response may occur as early as the first day after injury and last as long as 2 years. The risk tends to be greatest 5–90 days after the initial injury.

A third-degree burn involving as little as 10% of the BSA may be sufficient to induce this abnormal response. If succinylcholine is given and a cardiac arrest does indeed occur, CPR should be initiated and the patient treated appropriately for acute hyperkalemia. Therapy includes sodium bicarbonate, a glucose/insulin mixture, and hyperventilation, since these measures cause a rapid intracellular shift of the potassium ion. Calcium should be given to antagonize the cardiovascular effects.[22]

Since there is no method that has been shown to be effective in preventing or decreasing the hyperkalemic response in all patients, it is best to avoid using succinylcholine in burn patients.[23] The response appears to be due to a widespread distribution of the acetylcholine receptor on the muscle membrane that can respond to acetylcholine and release potassium extracellularly, as opposed to release only at discrete sites of the motor end-plate. A similar situation exists in patients who have suffered denervation injuries.[23]

In contrast with the response to succinylcholine, there tends to be a decreased sensitivity to the nondepolarizing muscle relaxants (NDMR). Doses of these muscle relaxants may need to be increased as much as 2.5–5 times.[23] Patients suffering burns of less than 10% of the BSA do not demonstrate this decreased sensitivity to NDMR. The peak decrease in sensitivity occurs 2 weeks after the burn but may last for up to a year after the burn has entirely healed. It is important to monitor the adequacy of neuromuscular blockade intraoperatively and to titrate the dose of relaxant appropriately. In spite of the need for increased doses of the NDMR, the doses of reversal drugs are unaltered.[23]

Once the trachea has been intubated, the cuff should be inflated just enough to prevent a leak. This is especially important when N_2O is being used as part of the anesthetic technique. The severely burned patient may undergo multiple intubations during the course of his hospitalization, and the tracheal cartilage is especially prone to damage after thermal injury.[2,13,21,24]

In the selection of induction agents the adequacy of volume replacement must be considered. If the patient has been appropriately volume-resuscitated, the use of a barbiturate is acceptable. Ketamine and etomidate are viable alternatives if hypovolemia exists.

Narcotics are required intraoperatively to prevent excessive pain at the end of the procedure. The use of narcotics also helps to reduce the need for higher concentrations of volatile anesthetic agents during graft harvesting and thereby avoids potential problems with control of blood pressure and cardiac output. Burn patients tend to have alterations in their ability to metabolize drugs, especially barbiturates.[23]

Following a burn, ventilation/perfusion mismatch abnormalities are common, especially if the airway has been traumatized. Anesthetic agents tend to increase this mismatch, and the typical anesthetic ventilator may be inadequate, especially if high inspiratory or positive end-expiratory pressures are required.

More sophisticated machines capable of providing high pressure and volume may be required, and this further underscores the need for intravenous agents. Venous admixture, which is common when there is inhalation injury, may become worse during anesthesia. Therefore, routine use of 50% N_2O is not advisable without the use of pulse oximetry and capnography or frequent blood gas analyses.

Blood Transfusions

Many burn patients are anemic because of increased destruction of the red blood cells by the reticuloendothelial system secondary to membrane damage. Multiple transfusions may be required during debridements, and therefore an adequate number of cross-matched units of blood should be available before the operation. It is often necessary to start the administration of blood before surgery begins. A major debridement may require a large number of transfused units, and there may also be a need to treat associated complications, such as deficiencies of clotting factors, thrombocytopenia, or citrate intoxication.[25-27] A general rule is that for each 1% BSA debridement planned, one unit of blood should be available for transfusion.

References

1. Haponik EF, Summer WR: Respiratory complications in burned patients: pathogenesis and spectrum of inhalation injury. J Crit Care 1987;2(1):49–74.
2. Lamb JD: Anesthetic considerations for the major thermal injury. Can Anaesth Soc J 1985;32(1):84–92.
3. Demling RH: Burns. N Engl J Med 1985;313:1389–98.
4. Formosa PJ, Waxman K: Inhalation injuries in burn patients. Hosp Phys July 1986;pp 69–82.
5. Demling RH: Pathophysiology of Burn Injury. In: Trauma: Clinical Care and Pathophysiology, JD Richardson, HC Polk Jr, LM Flint, eds, Chicago: Year Book Medical Publishers, 1987, pp 121–66.
6. Demling RH: Fluid replacement in burned patients. Surg Clin North Am 1987;67(1):15–30.
7. Merrell WE, Saffle JR: Fluid resuscitation in thermally injured children. Am J Surg 1986;152:664–69.
8. Lung CC, Browder NC: The estimation of areas of burns. Surg Gynecol Obstet 1944;79:352–58.
9. Wachtel TL, Long WB, Frank HA: Thermal Injuries of the Upper Respiratory Tract. In: Burns of the Head and Neck, TL Wachtel, DH Frank, eds, Philadelphia: WB Saunders, 1984, pp. 7–14.
10. Herndon DN, Langner F, Thompson P, et al: Pulmonary injury in burned patients. Surg Clin North Am 1987;67(1):31–46.
11. Cahalane M, Demling RH: Early respiratory abnormalities from smoke inhalation. JAMA 1984;251(6):771–73.
12. Heimbach D: Inhalation Injury. In: Burns of the Head and Neck, TL Wachtel, DH Frank, eds, Philadelphia: WB Saunders, 1984, pp. 15–23.
13. Cote CJ: Burn Debridement. In: Common Problems in Pediatric Anesthesia, LC Stehling, ed, Chicago: Year Book Medical Publishers, 1982, pp 131–43.
14. Solomon JR: Pediatric Burns. In: Burns, Critical Care Clinics., TL Wachtel, ed, Philadelphia: WB Saunders, 1985;1(1):159–73.
15. Luterman A, Sasco CC, Curreri PW: Infections in burn patients. Am J Med 1986;81(1A):45–52.
16. Hammond JS, Ward CG: Complications of the Burn Injury. In: Burns, Critical Care Clinics, TL Wachtel, ed, Philadelphia: WB Saunders, 1985;1(1):175–87.
17. Monafo WW, Freedman B: Topical therapy for burns. Surg Clin North Am 1987;67(1):133–45.
18. Moran K, Munster AM: Alterations of the host defense mechanism in burned patients. Surg Clin North Am 1987;67(1):47–56.
19. Dasco CC, Luterman A, Curreri PW: Systemic antibiotic treatment in burned patients. Surg Clin North Am 1987;67(1):57–68.

20. Pasulka PS, Wachtel TL: Nutritional considerations for the burned patient. Surg Clin North Am 1987;67(1):109–32.
21. Ward CF: Anesthesia for Head and Neck Burn Surgery. In: Burns of the Head and Neck, TL Wachtel, DH Frank, eds. Philadelphia: WB Saunders, 1984, pp 34–55.
22. Andreoli TE: Disorders of Fluid Volume, Electrolyte, and Acid-Base Balance. In: Textbook of Medicine, 16th ed, JB Wyngaarden, LH Smith Jr, eds, Philadelphia: WB Saunders, 1982, pp. 468–94.
23. Martyn J, Goldhill DR, Goudsouzian NG: Clinical pharmacology of muscle relaxants in patients with burns. J Clin Pharmacol 1986;26:680–85.
24. Stanley TH: Nitrous oxide and pressure and volume of high-low pressure endotracheal tube cuffs in intubated patients. Anesthesiology 1975;42:637.
25. Cullen B: Anesthesia for the patient with major burns. In: American Society of Anesthesiologists Annual Refesher Course Lectures #266, 1985
26. Szyfelbein SK, Drop LJ, Martyn JAJ: Persistent ionized hypocalcemia in patients during resuscitation and recovery phases of body burns. Crit Care Med 1981;9:454–58.
27. Tompkins RG, Burke JF: Burn therapy 1985: acute management. Intensive Care Med 1986;12:289–95.

CHAPTER 8

The Patient with Sepsis*

Gary Hartstein

Case History. *A 72-year-old man was admitted to the intensive care unit with hypotension, fever, and presumed sepsis. He had been in reasonably good health until one week prior to admission, when he noted decreased appetite and continuous hiccoughs. On the morning of admission his wife found him incoherent.*

Past medical history was significant for hypertension, treated with a diuretic, and a distant history of head and neck cancer treated with radiation therapy.

On admission to the ICU, the patient's blood pressure was 70 by Doppler measurement, pulse 115/min, and temperature 38.4°C rectally. Examination of the chest showed normal heart sounds and bilateral râles and rhonchi. The abdomen was diffusely rigid with marked right upper quadrant tenderness. Chest x-ray revealed a small right pleural effusion. Arterial blood gases on a 50% Ventimask showed pH 7.23, PCO_2 45, PO_2 65, O_2 saturation 47%. SMA-6 results were significant only for a serum bicarbonate level of 11.3 mEq/L. A scintigraphic scan with paraisopropylacetanilido-iminodiacetic acid (PIPIDA) failed to visualize the gallbladder after 4 hours.

The trachea was intubated and respiration was supported mechanically at an initial FiO_2 of 1.0. While preparations were being made to place arterial and pulmonary artery catheters, 500 ml of 5% albumin was infused over 15 minutes and was repeated once. After the fluid challenge, the blood pressure was 70/40 mmHg. A right heart catheterization was performed with the following results: right atrial pressure 0 mmHg, right ventricular pressure 24/2 mmHg, pulmonary artery pressure 26/14 mmHg, pulmonary artery wedge 14 mmHg. Cardiac output was 6.59L/min. Systemic vascular resistance was calculated as 607 dyne : sec : cm.

---

* Reviewed by Dr. Joanne Floyd, Assistant Professor, Department of Anesthesiology, Albert Einstein College of Medicine, Bronx, New York.

*The patient was scheduled for urgent exploratory laparotomy with a
presumptive diagnosis of sepsis from a gangrenous gallbladder.*

Introduction

Dorland's Medical Dictionary defines sepsis as "the presence in the blood
or other tissues of pathogenic microorganisms or their toxins; the
condition associated with such presence."[1] For our purpose, sepsis will
be defined as a characteristic systemic manifestation of infection, whether
or not bacteria are present in the blood (bacteremia). The syndrome
usually, but not always, consists of hypotension, with a normal or
elevated cardiac output and a low systemic vascular resistance. Septic
shock implies organ hypoperfusion, ie, central nervous system dysfunction, pulmonary failure, adult respiratory distress syndrome (ARDS),
renal insufficiency, and most significantly, progressive lactic acidosis.

The sepsis syndrome is occurring more frequently because of several
recent trends in medical practice, including more frequent use of invasive
monitors and catheters, aggressive cytotoxic and immunosuppressive
therapies, frequent use of corticosteroids, and the emergence of multiply
resistant strains of microorganisms. Furthermore, the patient population
is aging, and increased survival of patients with diseases such as diabetes
and cancer has dramatically increased the size of the population at risk.

Gram-negative bacteremia is one of the most common events leading to
the sepsis syndrome.[2] Approximately 70,000–300,000 cases of gram-
negative bacteremia occur each year.[3] Of these, 40–50% develop shock,
which is fatal in 40–90% of the cases in which it occurs. If sepsis caused
by gram-positive organisms, viruses, and fungi is included, up to 100,000
deaths from the sepsis syndrome occur annually in the United States.
From 1965 through 1974, 7–12 gram-negative bacteremic events per 1000
hospital admissions were estimated to have occurred.[4] This represents an
approximately 25-fold increase in incidence over two decades.[2]

Certain risk factors increase bacteremia, sepsis, and resultant death.
Patient characteristics associated with high risk of bacteremia include
advanced age, the presence of severe debilitating illnesses, and burns.
Latrogenic factors include: instrumentation of the genitourinary, respiratory, or gastrointestional tracts; intraarterial or intravenous cannulation;
mechanical ventilation; surgical or gastrointestinal endoscopic procedures; septic abortion or premature rupture of membranes; use of steroids
and or cytotoxic and antimetabolite drugs; and failure to drain purulent
collections.

Mortality from bacteremia is increased in the presence of cirrhosis, a
hematologic cancer, or surgery associated with steroid use, cancer, or
diabetes. Lack of a febrile response to bacteremia is also associated with
high mortality, as is hypotension.[5]

Gram-negative bacteremia carries a mortality of 7–10% if shock is not present, increasing to 47% if the patient is in shock. With gram-positive bacteremia, mortality with and without shock is 8% and 33%, respectively. In normotensive patients, polymicrobial bacteremia is associated with a higher mortality than is bacteremia where only one organism is isolated. If shock is present, the mortality is similar whether the infection is polymicrobial or monomicrobial, suggesting that once the full-blown syndrome of septic shock develops the shock state itself is the major determinant of outcome, rather than the bacterial insult.[6]

Diagnosis

Because of the high morbidity and mortality of the sepsis syndrome, the clinical index of suspicion must remain high, especially in patients at increased risk. Clinical findings may be those caused by infection itself and those related to the sepsis syndrome (ie, the systemic response to the infection).

Patients usually present with fever, often with rigors if bacteremia is present, and may have signs or symptoms relating to the source of the infection (eg, purulent sputum with râles, abdominal signs, urinary symptoms, etc). The following signs can all be associated with the sepsis syndrome, either as isolated findings or in groups.

The earliest sign of sepsis is often tachypnea with respiratory alkalosis. Altered mental status may occur, especially in the elderly in whom agitation or sudden onset or worsening of dementia may be seen. Seizures may also herald the sepsis syndrome; oliguria, thrombocytopenia, hypothermia, and leukocytosis or leukopenia may be noted. Hypotension is often a late sign, and may be associated with acidosis and shock. The need for a high clinical index of suspicion is apparent because of the subtlety of the above signs, especially if only one is present.

Of primary importance in treating sepsis are the rapid determination of the source of the infection and the prompt institution of appropriate definitive therapy for eradicating the infection (as contrasted with supportive therapy).[8] Studies have docuented that the prompt institution of appropriate antibiotic therapy significantly reduces mortality from gram-negative bacteremia, whether or not shock is present.[5]

When the diagnosis of sepsis is made or suspected, all invasive catheters should be changed, appropriate cultures should be obtained, and all suspected fluids should be stained and examined microscopically. Since certain groups of bacteria are often found in association with particular sites of infection, a knowledge of these relations is useful in initiating empiric antibiotic therapy (see Table 8.1.). Once cultures have been obtained, empiric antibiotic therapy should be instituted, taking into consideration the patient's status, the likely organisms, and the local

TABLE 8.1. Organisms frequently
associated with infection in various
organ systems.

Origin	Organisms
Respiratory tract	Pseudomonas
	E. coli
	Klebsiella
	Enterobacter
	Acinetobacter
	Serratia
Vascular system	Pseudomonas
	Serratia
	Enterobacter
Urinary tract	E. coli
	Klebsiella
	Enterobacter
	Proteus
	Serratia
Gastrointestinal tract	E. coli
	Klebsiella
	Enterobacter
	Serratia
	Bacteroides
	Salmonella
Biliary system	E. coli
	Klebsiella
	Enterobacter
	Serratia

epidemiology, including antibiotic sensitivities of endemic hospital species.

Intraabdominal sources present a special problem; they should be suspected in all surgical or trauma patients who have sustained even minimal violation of intestinal integrity. Diagnosis can be difcult. Ultrasound followed by PIPIDA scintigraphy will usually provide a correct diagnosis for acute acalculous cholecystitis, a not-infrequent cause of sepsis in the critically ill patient.[9] CT scan of the abdomen will demonstrate 80–90% of intraabdominal abscesses.[9] Laparotomy should be considered in high-risk patients (eg, those with trauma or previous surgery) if multiple organ failure develops without an apparent etiology. Percutaneous CT or ultrasound-guided catheter drainage of single abdominal abscesses is useful, if the access tract does not cross bowel.[10]

Another potential source of infection of particular interest to the anesthesiologist is paranasal sinusitis in the patient intubated by the nasotracheal route. Diagnosis is confirmed by CT scan of the head, sinus x-rays, or gallium scan. Treatment is with antibiotics and reintubation, either orally or with tracheostomy, to allow the sinus to drain.[11]

Pathophysiology

Not all bacteremic events lead to sepsis, and conversely, not all sepsis is associated with bacteremia. The crucial event leading to sepsis is the elaboration by the infecting organism of mediators, which in turn produce the clinical, biochemical, and pathophysiologic manifestations of sepsis. The nature and identity of these mediators is the subject of intensive and ongoing research, controversy, and interest, as is mediator involvement in sepsis, on which the literature is also extensive and often confusing.

The lipopolysaccharide component of the gram-negative bacterial cell wall (endotoxin), when injected into animals, reproduces several of the manifestations of sepsis. It is likely that endotoxin (in gram-negative infections) or some other structural bacterial component (in other bacterial infections) is involved in the release or activation of mediators in the patient.[3] Such mediators include the protein cascades (the complement, kinin, and coagulation systems), wherein inactive precursors are proteolytically activated.

Activation of complement, possibly via the alternate pathway, appears to occur early in septic shock,[12] although this has been questioned.[13] In a murine model of sepsis, a strain deficient in a complement (C5) survived longer and had reduced alveolar-arterial O_2 gradients and higher arterial O_2 tensions than C5-sufficient twins.[14] Activated C3 and C5 (C3a and C5a) are potent chemotactic substances for white blood cells, act to aggregate granulocytes, and dramatically increase vascular permeability, causing diffuse capillary leak. C3a and C5a are called anaphylotoxins because of the similarity of their effects to some of those of histamine. Complement-induced granulocyte activation and aggregation probably underlie several clinical consequences of sepsis, for example ARDS.[15]

Products of arachidonic acid metabolism (the prostanoids) include prostaglandins, prostacyclin, and thromboxane, and are probably also involved in the pathogeneis of sepsis.[16]

The cardiovascular response to sepsis seems to include a reversible decrease in myocardial performance, as indicated by a marked fall in ejection fraction. The serum from septic patients with low ejection fractions contains a peptide that produces myocardial depression in an in vitro preparation.[17]

Clinical Aspects

The hemodynamic, pulmonary, and metabolic effects of sepsis are complicated and varied.

The classic description of human septic shock defines two phases: "warm" shock with peripheral vasodilation, high cardiac output, and hypotension, followed by the preterminal phase of "cold" shock, characterized by cold, clammy skin, low cardiac output, and hypotension. This classic description, however, does not describe the clinical picture seen in most cases of human septic shock. It is based on a frequently used model of sepsis, the canine endotoxin model, in which dogs are injected with a lethal bolus of endotoxin, resulting in a low cardiac state with massive bloody diarrhea (which is rarely, if ever, seen in human sepsis).

Most human deaths from septic shock are from either refractory hypotension, with normal to high cardiac output maintained until death, or from multiple organ failure. Few humans die with a low cardiac output state.[3,18] Cardiac output is a rather poor indicator of global myocardial performance, since the intact organism is capable of altering rate, contractility, and loading conditions to maintain output in the face of compromised pump function.

Results of nuclear ejection fraction (EF) studies on patients in septic shock indicated that one half of the patients studied had EFs below 0.4, suggesting relatively severe depression of ventricular function. However, 76% of the survivors, but none of the nonsurvivors, had depressed EFs. Importantly, in those with depressed EFs, stroke volume was maintained by increase in both end-diastolic and end-systolic volumes. Survivors with depressed EFs gradually returned to normal by 10 days after the onset of shock.[19]

These findings were confirmed in a canine model that simulates accurately the hemodynamic findings in human sepsis.[20] This study showed reversible systolic dysfunction, with ventricular dilation and maintenance of stroke volume in response to volume infusion. Inadequate myocardial perfusion and global ischemia were ruled out as causes of the reversible ventricular dysfunction.[21] Septic shock can also give rise to segmental ventricular dysfunction, with ECG and echocardiographic findings similar to those of myocardial infarction.[22]

The sepsis syndrome is one of the major causes of ARDS. The mediators mentioned above are all capable of inducing damage to the alveolar-capillary membrane, the likely site of the initial injury of ARDS.

Septic patients are in a hypermetabolic, hypercatabolic state. Large amounts of endogenous protein are broken down, a process that is not inhibited by glucose administration. Relative insulin resistance is seen, as well as elevated rates of lipolysis. This metabolic situation can be reproduced by infusion of epinephrine, norepinephrine, cortisol, and glucagon in amounts similar to those present in septic patients.[23]

Supportive Treatment

The intial treatment consists of establishing the diagnosis of sepsis, obtaining appropriate culture materials, treating the infection (with antibiotics and drainage if necessary), and removal of any necrotic tissue.

At our institution, a hypotensive, septic patient receives a fluid challenge with 500–1000 ml of crystalloid. If this does not restore blood pressure to normal (at least 90 mmHg systolic), invasive hemodynamic monitoring is initiated, with placement of arterial and pulmonary artery catheters. Fluid resuscitation is carried out until a pulmonary artery wedge pressure of 12–18 mmHg is reached.

The rationale for this is threefold: 1) These patients are often dehydrated, as fever and tachypnea have usually increased insensible fluid losses, while decreased oral intake is often associated with the initial illness. 2) The diffuse capillary leak seen in sepsis necessitates large volumes of fluid to establish normal intravascular volume. 3) In sepsis, total body oxygen consumption becomes dependent on oxygen delivery over the wide range.[24–26] Thus, as long as calculated O_2 delivery (equal to the product of cardiac output $\times$ the arterial O_2 content) to the periphery increases, oxygen uptake rises, presumably reflecting improvement in the metabolic status of the tissues.

If restoration of adequate intravascular volume does not restore blood pressure to at least 90 mmHg systolic, vasopressor therapy is indicated. No controlled studies exist to determine the pressor of choice in sepsis. At our institution, if cardiac output is deemed to be "adequate" (admittedly a difficult assessment in sepsis!), a norepinephrine infusion is titrated to maintain a systolic blood pressure of 90 mmHg. Concomitantly, a low-dose dopamine infusion (1.5–2.5 μg/kg/min) is initiated to preserve renal perfusion. If cardiac output is low (ie, a mixed cardiogenic/septic picture), an acceptable blood pressure is established as above, at which point dobutamine is started, titrating until there is an effect on cardiac output.

All patients in shock in our ICU are mechanically ventilated to decrease the work of breathing. Standard goals are achievement of an arterial oxygen saturation of 90% or higher at an FiO_2 of no higher than 0.5; positive end-expiratory pressure (PEEP) is used as necessary to achieve this value, with careful attention to PEEP effect on cardiac output and O_2 delivery.

Nutritional support is initiated as soon as feasible after the septic insult, to minimize the adverse effects of excessive endogenous protein catabolism. The enteral route, while desirable, is often not possible in this group of critically ill patients. Nutritional goals, roughly speakiing, are to provide 35–40 nonprotein kcal/kg/day, and 1.5–2 gm protein/kg/day. The calories are divided between carbohydrate and fat with two constraints: 1) No more than 60% of total calories are given as lipid. 2) The rate of administration of carbohydrate should not exeeed 5–6 mg/kg/min.

Despite several anecdotal reports of favorable blood pressure responses to naloxone administration, and extensive literature reports on its use in various animal models of sepsis, we do not use this drug in septic patients. No controlled studies exist to document improved hemodynamics or, more important, improved outcome after naloxone administration.

Although the literature is replete with articles studying the effects of high-dose corticosteroids given before, during, and after sepsis, an article in 1984 reports the outcome of a randomized prospective trial of methyl-prednisolone vs dexamethasone vs placebo. The groups treated with steroids had higher percentages of patients with reversal of shock within 24 hours; overall mortality, however, was not different among the groups. The authors speculated that early in septic shock (within the first 4 hours), in certain subgroups of patients (as yet undefined), corticosteroids may be useful.[2] Two subsequent prospective, randomized, placebo-controlled, double-blind studies demonstrated a lack of effect of high doses of methylprednisolone when given early after the onset of the sepsis syndrome.[28] No effect of steroids on the evolution of ARDS was shown in a study reported in 1987.[30] These agents are thus not used routinely in our ICU for the sepsis syndrome.

Anesthetic Management

The goal of anesthetic management for septic patients consists of maintaining hemodynamic stability, assuring oxygen delivery to the tissues, and providing analgesia and amnesia as tolerated by the patient's condition. These goals can be met by continuing the plan of hemodynamic management outlined above and should be undertaken in consultation with the critical care specialist responsible for the patient. Septic patients usually require mechanical ventilation prior to arrival in the operating suite. Hemodynamic monitoring, including arterial and pulmonary artery catheters or noninvasive cardiac output monitoring, is essential.

No specific anesthetic plan has been shown to be superior for patients with sepsis. Although there is a resurgence of interest in epidural and spinal anesthetic techniques for reducing perioperative morbidity and mortality in high-risk patients,[27] major conduction blocks probably are not desirable for several reasons. The vasodilation produced by sympathetic blockade may not be tolerated by a patient already in a relatively hypovolemic, vasodilated state. Septic patients are often thrombocytopenic, with low-grade disseminated intravascular coagulation (DIC), a situation that contraindicates invasion of the neuraxis.

Nerve trunk block, eg, for upper extremity surgery, may be quite useful if no other contraindications are present. Limiting the sympathetic blockade would contribute to hemodynamic stability.

For general anesthesia, experience has shown ketamine to be a reasonable choice.[31] It is unlikely that volatile agents would be tolerated by these patients; the effect of high cardiac output on the uptake and distribution of inhaled agents should also be remembered. High-dose narcotics would probably be associated with hemodynamic stability, especially if careful attention is paid to filling pressure, and if the new potent narcotic agonists are used.

The need for postoperative ventilatory assistance is not a problem, inasmuch as mechanical ventilation should be used until the septic state resolves. Low doses of a benzodiazepine or low concentrations of a volatile agent should be added, if tolerated, to ensure amnesia, keeping in mind the cardiac-depressant effects of the benzodiazepine-narcotic combination.[32]

The use of intrathecal or epidural narcotics for postoperative pain relief and for blunting the hormonal stress response seems theoretically appealing but has not been studied in patients with sepsis.

References

1. Dorland's Illustrated Medical Dictionary; 26th ed. Philadelphia: WB Saunders, 1981, p 1189.
2. Greenman RL: Gram-negative Bacteremia, in LB Gardner (ed): Acute Internal Medicine. New York: Medical Examination Publishing, 1986, pp 393–99.
3. Parker MM, Parrillo JE: Septic shock: hemodynamics and pathogenesis. JAMA 1983;250:3324–27.
4. McCabe WR: Gram-negative bacteremia. Adv Intern Med 1974;19:135–58.
5. Kreger BE, Craven DE, McCabe WR: Gram-negative bacteremia. IV. Reevaluation of clinical features and treatment in 612 patients. Am J Med 1980;68:344–55.
6. Jacoby I: Septic Shock, in JM Rippe, RS Irwin, JS Alpert, et al (eds): Intensive Care Medicine, Boston: Little Brown and Co., 1985, pp 666–75.
7. MacLean LD: Shock: Causes and Management of Circulatory Collapse, in DC Sabiston (ed): Davis-Christopher Textbook of Surgery, 2nd ed. Philadelphia: WB Saunders, 1977, pp 82–92.
8. Altemeier WA, Todd CA, Wellford WE: Gram-negative septicemia: a growing threat. Ann Surg 1967;166:530–42.
9. Fox MS, Wilk PJ, Weissmann HS, et al: Acute acalculous cholecystitis. Surg Gynecol Obstet 1984;159:13–16.
10. Wilson RF: Special problems in the diagnosis and treatment of surgical sepsis. Surg Clin North Am 1985;65:965–89.
11. Deutschman CS, Wilton P, Sinow J, et al: Paranasal sinusitis associated with nasotracheal intubation: a frequently unrecognized and treatable source of sepsis. Crit Care Med 1986;14:111–14.
12. Sprung, CL, Schultz DR, Marcial E, et al: Complement activation in septic shock patients. Crit Care Med 1986;14:525–28.
13. Shatney CH, Benner C: Sequential serum complement (C3) and immunoglobulin levels in shock/trauma patients developing acute fulminant systemic sepsis. Circ Shock 1985;16:9–17.
14. Olson LM, Moss GS, Baukus D, et al: The role of C5 in septic lung injury. Ann Surg 1985;202:771–76.
15. Jacob HS, Craddock PR, Hammerschmidt DE, et al: Complement-induced granulocyte aggregation: an unsuspected mechanism of disease. N Engl J Med 1980;302:788–803.
16. Slotman GJ, Burchard KW, William JJ, et al: Interaction of prostaglandins,

activated complement, and granulocytes in clinical sepsis and hypotension. Surgery 1986;99:744–51.

17. Parrillo JE, Burch C, Shelhamer JH: A circulating myocardial depressant substance in humans with septic shock. J Clin Invest 1985;76:1539–53.

18. Groenwald AJ, Bronsveld W, Thijs G: Hemodynamic determinants of mortality in human septic shock. Surgery 1986;99:140–52.

19. Parker MM, Shelhamer JH, Bacharach SL, et al: Profound but reversible myocardial depression in patients with septic shock. Ann Intern Med 1984;100:183–90.

20. Natanson C, Fink MP, Ballantyne HK, et al: Gram-negative bacteremia produces both severe systolic and diastolic cardiac dysfunction in a canine model that simulates human septic shock. J Clin Invest 1986;78:259–70.

21. Cunnion RE, Schaer GL, Parker MM, et al: The coronary circulation in human septic shock. Circulation 1986;73:637–44.

22. Thomas F, Smith JL, Orm JF, et al: Reversible segmental myocardial dysfunction in septic shock. Crit Care Med 1986;14:587–88.

23. Shamoon H: Personal communication.

24. Haupt MT, Gilbert EM, Carlson RW: Fluid loading increases oxygen consumption in septic patients with lactic acidosis. Am Rev Resp Dis 1985;131:912–16.

25. Kaufman BS, Rackow EC, Falt JL: The relationship between oxygen delivery and consumption during fluid resuscitation of hypovolemic and septic shock. Chest 1984;85:336–40.

26. Bihari D, Smithies M, Gimson A: The effects of vasodilation with prostacyclin on oxygen delivery and uptake in critically ill patients. N Engl J Med 1987;317:397–403.

27. Sprung CL, Canalis PV, Marcial EH, et al: The effects of high-dose corticosteroids in patients with septic shock: a prospective controlled study. N Engl J Med 1984;311:1137–43.

28. Bone RC, Fisher CJ, Clemmer TP, et al: A controlled clinical trial of high dose methyl prednisolone in the treatment of severe sepsis and septic shock. N Engl J Med 1987;317:653–58.

29. Hinshaw L, Pedvzzi P, Young E, et al: Effect of high-dose glucocorticoid therapy on mortality in patients with clinical signs of systemic sepsis. N Engl J Med 1987;317:659–65.

30. Bernard GR, Luce JM, Sprung CL, et al: High dose corticosteroids in patients with the adult respiratory distress syndrome. N Engl J Med 1987;317:1565–70.

31. Yeager MP, Glass DD, Neff RK, et al: Epidural anesthesia and analgesia in high-risk surgical patients. Anesthesiology 1987;66:729–36.

32. Septic shock, in Rk Stoelting, SF Dierdorf, RL McCammon (eds): Anesthesia and co-existing disease. 2nd edition. New York: Churchill Livingstone, 1988, pp 664–66.

CHAPTER 9

The Patient for Pulmonary Lobectomy*

Jonathan S. Daitch

Case History. *A 63-year-old man with a history of chronic obstructive pulmonary disease (COPD) and angina was hospitalized for exacerbation of the COPD. His medications on admission included theophylline 300 mg b.i.d., metaproterenol inhaler q4h, diltiazem 30 mg q.i.d., and a 5 cm nitroglycerin patch. Chest x-ray revealed a right upper lobe (RUL) infiltrate that was treated with intravenous antibiotics. A subsequent x-ray showed an RUL mass. CAT scan revealed a 3 cm lesion and hilar adenopathy.*

Arterial blood gas analyses on room air showed: pH 7.35, PaCO$_2$ 42 mmHg, PaO$_2$ 56 mmHg. Hemoglobin was 16 gm/dl, hematocrit 48%; other chemical analyses were normal. ECG showed normal sinus rhythm with a vertical axis and incomplete right bundle branch block. Pulmonary function tests revealed moderate to severe obstructive lung disease, with a maximal breathing capacity (MBC) that was 55% of predicted, and a forced expiratory volume in 1 second (FEV$_1$) of 1.5L. A presumptive diagnosis of bronchogenic carcinoma was made, and the patient was scheduled for a right upper lobectomy. Isolation of the affected lung was requested.

Introduction

The use of positive pressure ventilators, double-lumen endobronchial tubes, and pulse oximetry has dramatically changed thoracic anesthesia over the past four decades. Before ventilators were introduced, a spontaneously breathing patient would exhibit mediastinal shift when the thorax was opened. Thus, the surgeon had to contend with a constantly moving surgical field, with the operative lung becoming small on inspiration and large on expiration. Prior to the availability of double-lumen

---

* Reviewed by Dr. Paul Goldiner, Professor and Chairman, Department of Anesthesiology, Albert Einstein College of Medicine, Bronx, New York.

tubes, single-lumen endotracheal tubes were placed endobronchially or Fogarty catheters were used for bronchial blockade. Double-lumen tubes now allow differential ventilation to each lung. Pulse oximetry has certainly made thoracic anesthesia safer by providing continuous assessment of arterial oxygenation. These new techniques allow safer anesthesia and better operating conditions.

Lung Tumors

About 90% of solitary pulmonary nodules are malignant. The remaining 10% of tumors that are benign are mainly hamartomas (80%), as well as angiomas, lipomas, leiomyomas, fibromas, and chondromas. The most common type of lung cancer is squamous cell carcinoma (60%). It is generally slow-growing and slow to metastasize. Large- and small-cell carcinomas each account for 15% of malignant tumors, and tend to grow rapidly and metastasize early. Adenocarcinomas, the majority of the remaining tumors, are usually small peripheral lesions with moderate growth rates.

Only small-cell tumors are considered unresectable: they spread rapidly via both blood and lymphatics, and metastisize early to brain, bone, and liver. The approach to patients with lung cancer consists first of staging, and then determination of physiologic operability. Finally, if appropriate, lung resection is performed, as this provides the only potential cure for lung carcinoma.

TABLE 9.1. Workup for lung carcinoma.

Symptoms and/or chest x-ray suspicious for lung cancer
History and physical examination
CBC, SMA-18, ECG, CXR, UA
PPD and anergy panel
Sputum for C&S and cytology
Hilar oblique tomograms
Thoracic CAT scan
Pulmonary function tests

Evidence of metastases:	No evidence of metastases:
1. Scans of liver, bone, brain	Achieve tissue diagnosis via
2. Consider biopsy of above	1. Bronchoscopy
3. If search for another primary is indicated: IVP, BE, UGI	2. Mediastinoscopy
4. Invasive diagnostic studies as indicated	3. Needle biopsy
	4. Mediastinotomy
	5. Scalene node biopsy

CXR = chest x-ray, UA = urinalysis, PPD = purfied protein derivative tuberculin test, C&S = culture and sensitivity, IVP = intravenous pyelogram, BE = barium enema, UGI = upper gastrointestinal series
Adapted from Ref. 6, (Miller, 1983).

Preoperative Staging

A standard evaluation of the patient with suspected lung cancer is outlined in Table 9.1. If metastatic disease is suspected, appropriate scans of liver, brain, and bone are performed. If there is any indication that the primary site is other than the lungs, additional studies must be undertaken.

Invasive procedures, such as mediastinoscopy, bronchoscopy, and needle biopsy, are performed to obtain a tissue diagnosis. Current staging utilizes the T (tumor), N (nodes), and M (metastasis) classification, as adopted by the American Joint Committee for Cancer Staging (Table 9.2). Patients with non-small-cell carcinomas with stage I or stage II disease are considered candidates for surgical resection. Thus, even cancers with

TABLE 9.2. TNM staging of lung cancer.

Primary tumor
T_x Malignant cells in cytology; site undetermined
T_0 No evidence of primary tumor
T_1 Tumor <3cm in size
T_2 Tumor >3cm in size
T_3 Tumor of any size with extension to chest wall, parietal pleura, diaphragm, or mediastinum, or within 2cm of carina

Nodal involvement
N_0 No lymph node metastases
N_1 Metastasis to peribronchial or ipsilateral hilum only
N_2 Mediastinal lymph node metastases

Distant metastasis
M_0 No distant metastasis
M_1 Distant metastasis present

Stage groupings
Stage I $T_1N_0M_0$
             $T_1N_1M_0$
             $T_2N_0M_0$

Stage II $T_2N_1M_0$

Stage III T_3 with any N or M
             N_2 with any T or M
             M_1 with any T or N

T = tumor, N = nodes, M = metastasis
From American Joint Committee for Cancer Staging and End-Result Reporting: System for staging of lung cancer. Chicago, 1979.

peribronchial and ipsilateral hilar adenopathy, as well as large tumors that have not extended beyond the pleura, are considered resectable provided there is no evidence of metastases. With appropriate staging, the incidence of unnecessary thoracotomy can be reduced to less than 20%.[1]

Contraindications to surgical resection include malignant pleural effusion, metastatic disease outside the thorax, superior vena cava syndrome, and recurrent laryngeal nerve palsy. Relative contraindications are poor general medical condition, phrenic nerve paralysis, oat cell carcinomas, and mediastinal involvement.

Types of Surgery

Segmental or wedge resection is indicated for small, peripheral lesions less than 3 cm in diameter, provided there is no hilar or metastatic involvement, or for patients with more extensive disease who have poor cardiovascular or pulmonary function.

Lobectomy is the operation of choice for lung cancer. It is appropriate in cases where there is peribronchial or hilar nodal involvement. The right upper lobe is most commonly resected, followed next by removal of the left upper lobe.

Pneumonectomy is indicated for more extensive disease, such as tumors involving the left or right main bronchus or tumors that have become fixed to the hilum. Mortality rates for segmental resection, lobectomy, and pneumonectomy are 0.5%, 1.3%, and 5%, respectively.[2]

Preoperative Evaluation

The preoperative evaluation for a lung resection is especially important because it assesses the ability of the patient to survive the planned procedure. In addition to the need for understanding the extent of pulmonary disease, it is also important to evaluate the cardiac status, since coronary artery disease (CAD), congestive heart failure (CHF), and chronic obstructive pulmonary disease (COPD) contribute significantly to postoperative morbidity and mortality. Most patients with poor outcomes succumb to respiratory insufficiency or cor pulmonale.

Pulmonary Assessment

A thorough history should specifically address the presence of dyspnea, smoking, cough, and wheezing. Dyspnea, a subjective sensation caused by a ventilatory effort out of proportion to physical activity, may result from either pulmonary or cardiac disease. If pulmonary in origin, severe dyspnea implies a markedly diminished respiratory reserve, with a forced expiratory volume in 1 second (FEV_1) of 1500 ml or less. A smoking history, quantified in terms of pack-years, is a risk factor for COPD and malignancy, with greater numbers of pack-years increasing the risk for both.

A productive cough lasting at least 3 months per year for at least 2 years is diagnostic of chronic bronchitis, which predisposes the patient to cor pulmonale. A history of asthma or wheezing raises the possibility that reversible airway obstruction is present.

Physical examination should include observation of the respiratory rate and pattern of breathing. A prolonged expiratory time, use of accessory muscles of respiration, diminished breath sounds, and poor diaphragmatic excursion imply emphysema and airway obstruction. Wheezing and plethoric habitus suggest chronic bronchitis. Consolidation from pneumonia can show dullness to percussion, egophony, bronchial breath sounds, and râles. Pulmonary fibrosis may also cause râles.

Any thoracic surgery patient should have pulmonary function testing both before and after inhalation of bronchodilators, as well as an arterial blood gas analysis. See Table 9.3. for normal values for pulmonary function tests.

The criteria for performing a pneumonectomy with minimum morbidity and mortality are well known (see Figure 9.1.). However, the criteria to ensure optimal results with a lobectomy are less well known.[2] Since less of the lung is resected, less preoperative pulmonary reserve is permissible than for a pneumonectomy. The minimum criteria for lobectomy include:
1) MBC (maximal breathing capacity) >40% of predicted
2) FEV, >1L
3) $FEV_{0.25-0.75}$ >0.6L

Patients who do not reach these minimum criteria may still be surgical candidates, depending on the results of split-lung function testing. Split-lung ventilation and perfusion studies help in determining the patient's

TABLE 9.3. Normal pulmonary function test values

(50-year-old man, 70kg, 180cm, sitting position)	
FVC (forced vital capacity)	4.74L
FEV_1 (forced expiratory volume in 1 sec)	3.87L
FEV_1/FVC	83%
PEFR (peak expiratory flow rate)	8.97L/sec
MMF (mid maximal flow rate: also called FEV $_{0.25-0.75}$)	3.08L/sec
D_{CO} (diffusion capacity for cardiac output)	32.1
ERV (expiratory reserve volume)	0.96L
RV (residual volume)	1.77L
TLC (total lung capacity)	6.51L
RV/TLC	27%
FRC (functional residual capacity)	2.73L
IC (inspiratory capacity)	3.78L

Adapted from Ref. 6, (Miller, 1983).

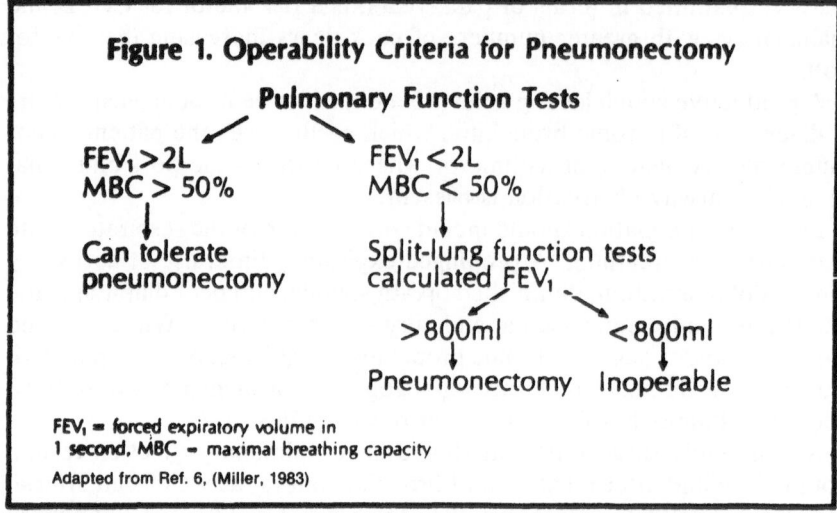

FIGURE 9.1.

calculated postoperative pulmonary reserve. Olsen et al have shown that
a calculated residual FEV_1 greater than 800 ml is compatible with a
reasonable ventilatory reserve, such that a patient can function normally.[3] Also, hypercarbia develops when FEV_1 is less than 800 ml.

This calculated lower limit of 800 ml for postoperative FEV_1 is
advocated because almost all patients who underwent lung resection with
a $PaCO_2$ greater than 45 mmHg died postoperatively of respiratory
failure.[4,5] Thus, patients scheduled for pneumonectomy with an FEV_1 of
2L or for lobectomy with an FEV_1 of 1L are evaluated with split-lung
function tests to ensure a postresection FEV_1 greater than 800 ml.

When such criteria are utilized to determine operability, mortality is
significantly reduced, yet less than 2% of patients are denied surgery.[6]
Nevertheless, even when these minimum criteria are not reached, thoracic procedures may still be performed for emergent or life-threatening
conditions, and mortality rates may be less than 35%.[7]

Cardiovascular Assessment

The history and physical examination should specifically seek evidence of
CAD and CHF. The patient should be questioned regarding anginal
patterns, dysrhythmias, hypertension, prior myocardial infarction (MI),
and symptoms of CHF (dyspnea on exertion, orthopnea, and paroxysmal
nocturnal dyspnea).

Physical examination may reveal distant heart sounds due to hyperinflation. A widened fixed split, a loud second pulmonic sound, or a gallop
rhythm heard best at the left sternal border that accentuates with

TABLE 9.4. Lung resection and cardiopulmonary risk.

Very low risk	Moderate risk	Very high risk
Cardiac	Cardiac	Cardiac
Normal cardiac size and function	CAD with angina, MI, or ECG changes	Intractable CHF or ventricular dysrhythmias
Normal blood pressure	Cardiac dysrhythmias	Uncontrolled MI
Normal ECG	Systemic hypertension	
	Valvular heart disease	
Pulmonary	Pulmonary	Pulmonary
Normal arterial blood gases	Hypoxia with a normal $PaCO_2$	Poor mechanical lung function ($FEV_1 < 35\%$)
Satisfactory mechanical lung function ($FEV_1 > 70\%$)	Reduced pulmonary function (FEV_1 of 35%-70%)	Irreversible CO_2 retention ($PaCO_2 > 45mmHg$)

Adapted from Ref. 10, (Ali and Ewer, 1980).

inspiration suggests pulmonary hypertension. A tender liver, jugular venous distention, and peripheral edema indicate decompensated cor pulmonale. In addition, an apical left ventricular gallop implies added cardiac risk.

Patients with a history of angina, previous MI, or suspected CAD should undergo an exercise stress test or thallium exercise scan preoperatively. Patients with a negative stress test can safely undergo pulmonary resection. Positive stress tests should be followed by coronary angiography to determine if the coronary arteries are amenable to bypass surgery. A successful coronary artery bypass graft (CABG) can be safely followed by lung surgery after 6 weeks.[6]

Ideally, thoracic surgery should be postponed until 6 months after an acute MI; cancer surgery, however, can be performed sooner, as clinical conditions dictate.

If the patient has a history of severe long-standing pulmonary disease or right- or left-sided CHF, then balloon occlusion of the pulmonary artery in the lung to be resected should be performed. Patients whose pulmonary artery pressure exceeds 35 mmHg with exercise will have greater than 50% mortality secondary to intractable cor pulmonale.[3,8] In addition, patients with a diffusion capacity less than 50% of predicted values have poorer outcome, since this reduced capacity implies significant reduction in the size of the pulmonary vascular bed.[9]

Overall cardiopulmonary risk for lung resection is summarized in Table 9.4.[10]

Laboratory Examination

The ECG may show evidence of pulmonary hypertension with right axis deviation, P-pulmonale, right ventricular hypertrophy, or complete (or incomplete) right bundle branch block. Indirect evidence of hyperinflation is indicated by low voltage, a vertical axis, or poor R-wave progression. Ischemic changes, evidence of prior MI, and dysrhythmias should also be noted on the ECG.

The chest x-ray should be reviewed looking specifically for hyperinflation, consolidation, pneumothorax, tracheal shift, location of the pathology, and vascular changes. Vascular markings are diminished in emphysema, and more prominent in patients who have chronic bronchitis with cor pulmonale. Also, the size of the heart and any evidence of pulmonary congestion should be noted.

An elevated hematocrit suggests hypoxemia or increased carboxyhemoglobin levels. Elevated bicarbonate levels probably indicate metabolic compensation for chronic respiratory acidosis. Arterial blood gas results should be evaluated specifically for hypoxemia and carbon dioxide retention.

Preoperative Preparation

Treatment of Existing Conditions

Patients with increased sputum production, change in sputum color, or any evidence of pneumonitis should receive antibiotic therapy as indicated. A regimen of bronchodilators should be used to treat wheezing, with therapeutic levels of theophylline being 10–20 $\mu g/ml$. Humidification, steroids, mucolytics, and expectorants may be helpful. Abstinence from smoking will decrease carboxyhemoglobin levels acutely; beneficial effects shown by pulmonary function tests require at least a month of abstinence. Dehydration and malnutrition must also be corrected preoperatively by enteral or parenteral means.

Medical therapy may also benefit patients with pulmonary hypertension and cor pulmonale. Right ventricular workload can be diminished by lowering pulmonary vascular resistance via normalization of PaO_2, $PaCO_2$, and pH. This, however, will be effective only if the pulmonary vasoconstriction is reversible, as is the situation with exacerbation of COPD. Therapy consists of supplemental oxygen, antibiotics, bronchodilators, digitalis, diuretics, or pulmonary vasodilators (eg, dobutamine, nitroglycerin, and nitroprusside).

Patients with dysrhythmias and hypertension should receive their medications on the morning of surgery. Preoperative digitalization for patients with CAD is advocated by some authorities.[6] Patients with angina or a history of MI should receive nitroglycerin preoperatively, with intravenous nitroglycerin available for intraoperative use.

Lastly, preoperative education of patients by respiratory therapists is helpful and should cover incentive spirometry, chest physiotherapy, and inhalation of bronchodilators.

Monitoring

Patients undergoing intrathoracic operations need monitoring that is specific for the procedure planned and appropriate for their underlying diseases. Standard monitoring should include ECG, blood pressure, oxygen saturation, heart and lung sounds, temperature, airway pressure, and neuromuscular transmission. A spirometer to measure tidal volume and calculate lung compliance is useful. Arterial blood gas analyses are essential at appropriate times.

Patients with advanced cardiopulmonary disease, patients requiring extensive procedures, or those cases in which a double-lumen endobronchial tube (DLET) is utilized require arterial cannulation for continuous blood pressure monitoring and frequent blood gas analyses. Capnography and mass spectrometry are also valuable. Monitoring of pulmonary capillary wedge pressures (PCWP), cardiac output (CO), and vascular resistance calculations may be helpful. Although not routinely available, transesophageal CO monitoring may prove valuable.

Normally, central venous pressure (CVP) is a good indication of intravascular blood volume. However, patients with advanced lung disease may have pulmonary hypertension and cor pulmonale such that CVP readings may not accurately reflect left-sided pressures. In those cases, only the PCWP accurately measures left ventricular filling pressures. Also, the pulmonary artery diastolic pressure may be significantly elevated above the wedge pressure, which indicates extensive pulmonary vascular disease.

Anesthetic Plan

To provide the best surgical exposure, the patient is usually placed in the lateral decubitus position (LDP), with the operative side nondependent. The incision is usually performed at the fifth or sixth intercostal space. The LDP may improve the ratio of ventilation to perfusion, since the diseased lung will be nondependent, and therefore less perfused.

If a patient has markedly reduced pulmonary reserve and might not tolerate the LDP very well, an anterior thoracotomy may be performed. The patient is placed supine and the incision is made through the third interspace. This approach, though technically more difficult for the surgeon, may be safer for specific patients.

A DLET may be used during an upper lobectomy to provide improved surgical exposure. Upper lobectomies are technically the most difficult to perform, and the surgeon will benefit greatly from one-lung anesthesia (OLA).

After appropriate monitors have been placed, the patient should be preoxygenated. Most patients tolerate a barbiturate-muscle relaxant induction, followed by inhalation of a volatile anesthetic agent until adequate relaxation has been achieved. Alternatively, ketamine, narcotics, or etomidate may be useful induction agents for patients who are more seriously ill. Intermediate-acting muscle relaxants are preferred because they lack cardiovascular effects and provide relaxation during further positioning of the patient.

For several reasons, a volatile agent is the cornerstone of anesthetic maintenance during intrathoracic surgery: It bronchodilates and diminishes airway reactivity; it allows for rapid induction and emergence; and, finally, it allows a high inspired oxygen concentration during OLA.

Prior to intubation, intravenous or intratracheal lidocaine may be administered to further blunt cardiovascular response to intubation. A DLET may be inserted at this time. After intubation, the patient is carefully turned to the LDP, with care taken to avoid pressure on the optic nerve, brachial plexus, and all other pressure points. Breath sounds should be rechecked to confirm proper placement of the DLET, which may be dislodged during turning.

Ventilation of the dependent lung alone causes right-to-left shunting in the upper lung, since the upper lung is perfused but not ventilated. Consequently, one-lung ventilation results in a much larger alveolar-to-arterial oxygen gradient and lower PaO_2 than does dual-lung ventilation. Carbon dioxide, however, is easily ventilated. Thus, although a single lung can easily eliminate enough CO_2, oxygen uptake is compromised because of the shunt caused by the unventilated lung.

Double-Lumen Endobronchial Tubes

Double-lumen endobronchial tubes allow selective ventilation of either lung during thoracic surgery, and protect a good lung from spillage of infected material or blood from the opposite lung. Both left- and right-sided endobronchial tubes are available (see Figure 9.2.). Many anesthesiologists use only left endobronchial tubes to avoid occlusion of the right upper lobe bronchus, which exits the right mainstem bronchus after only 1–2 cm. Indeed, National Catheter Corporation manufactures only double-lumen tubes for left endobronchial intubation.

However, some believe that only the bronchus of the dependent lung should be intubated, to avoid displacement by the surgeons of the endobronchial tube on the operative side.[11] Thus, tubes designed for intubation of the right bronchus for left thoracotomy must incorporate an additional right endobronchial opening to allow ventilation of the right upper lobe.

Double-lumen tubes are angled at their tips to facilitate placement. Some tubes employ a carinal hook to aid proper positioning; however, the carinal hook can be difficult to pass through the vocal cords. Isolation of the intubated lung is achieved by inflation of the endobronchial cuff, while an airtight seal for ventilation of the opposite lung is achieved by inflation of the tracheal cuff.

Proper placement of the DLET is initially ascertained by auscultation, and then confirmed either radiographically or with fiberoptic bronchoscopy, if necessary. Most DLETs are manufactured in 35, 37, 39, and 41 French sizes. The two smaller sizes are usually adequate for women and adolescents, while the two larger sizes are used for men.

Complications of DLETs include direct laryngeal trauma upon insertion, and tracheobronchial rupture. Insufficient ventilation, subcutaneous emphysema, airway hemorrhage, and cardiovascular instability are signs of possible airway injury. Tracheobronchial rupture is diagnosed by flexible or rigid bronchoscopy. Surgical repair of any laceration is essential at the time of injury.[11]

Improper positioning of the DLET is also a common problem. Often, the tube is not inserted far enough and never engages endobronchially. Ventilation will be difficult through the tracheal lumen, and both lungs are

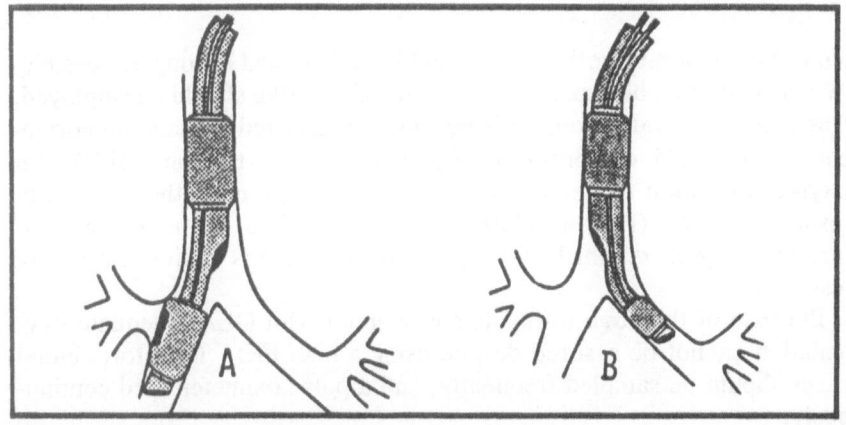

FIGURE 9.2. Schematic representation of right (A) and left (B) double-lumen endobronchial tubes (DLETs). Note the extra lumen in A, which provides ventilation to the right upper lobe.

inflated from ventilation through the bronchial lumen. If improperly placed, the right-sided DLET may obstruct the right upper lobe bronchus, leading to insufficient ventilation and atelectasis of the upper lobe. Also, the bronchial cuff may herniate over the endobronchial orifice, leading to difficulty in endobronchial ventilation.

Nevertheless, the most common abnormality associated with use of a DLET is hypoxemia.

Management of Hypoxemia

Because hypoxemia does tend to develop during OLA, several methods have been proposed to prevent and treat this problem (see Table 9.5.).

TABLE 9.5. Ventilatory management of one-lung anesthesia.

1. Maintain dual lung ventilation as long as possible.
2. Begin one-lung ventilation with a tidal volume of 10ml/kg.
3. Adjust the respiratory rate so that $PaCO_2$ = 40mmHg.
4. Use an FiO_2 as close to 1.0 as possible.
5. Monitor oxygen saturation continuously.
6. Monitor PaO_2 and $PaCO_2$ frequently.
7. If hypoxemia occurs:
   a. Add 5-10cmH_2O CPAP to nondependent lung.
   b. Consider adding 5-10cmH_2O PEEP to dependent lung.
   c. If necessary, use intermittent positive pressure ventilation to the nondependent lung.
8. Clamp the pulmonary artery to the nonventilated lung as soon as possible if a pneumonectomy is to be performed.

FiO_2 = fraction of inspired oxygen, CPAP = continuous positive airway pressure, PEEP = positive end-expiratory pressure.
Adapted from Ref. 15, (Benumof and Alfery, 1986).

First, ventilation to both lungs should be maintained as long as possible. When OLA must be used, a tidal volume of 10 ml/kg should be employed. The respiratory rate should subsequently be adjusted to maintain normocarbia, to avoid compromising hypoxic vasoconstriction (HPV). An oxygen-inhalation technique should be used to maintain the fraction of inspired oxygen (FiO) as close to 1.0 as possible. Although in vitro inhalation agents diminish HPV, their effect in vivo is minimal or greatly lessened.[12]

Because of the large intrapulmonary shunt with OLA, adequate oxygenation cannot be assured despite using a high FiO_2. Therefore, blood gases should be sampled frequently, and a pulse oximeter used continuously.

Should hypoxemia occur (PaO_2 <70 mmHg), 5–10 cm H_2O of continuous positive airway pressure (CPAP) should be added to the nondependent lung and arterial blood gases remeasured. Upper lung CPAP most reliably increases the PaO_2.[13,14] Next, 5–10 cm H_2O of positive end-expiratory pressure (PEEP) may be added to the dependent lung. This therapy may have variable effects on oxygenation, and the therapeutic window of PEEP seems to be very narrow.[15]

If severe hypoxemia still persists (which is very rare), the surgeon should be notified and the nondependent lung intermittently ventilated to minimize the shunt. Finally, ventilation-perfusion imbalances can be eliminated by clamping the pulmonary artery to the upper lung.

There are also several newer techniques, still under investigation, to avoid intraoperative hypoxemia, including selective nondependent-lung PEEP, high-frequency ventilation, differential lung PEEP, pulmonary artery balloon occlusion in the diseased, nonventilated lung, and apneic oxygenation.[15]

Postoperative Management

Several life-threatening complications can occur postoperatively. Massive hemorrhage is possible if a suture or clip around the pulmonary artery loosens. Exsanguination may be rapid, necessitating immediate thoracotomy in the recovery room to control the bleeding. Bronchopleural fistulas are possible if the bronchial closure is inadequate, or if airway pressures are excessive. If a chest tube is not inserted intraoperatively, a tension pneumothorax may result. With a chest tube in place, a persistent air leak will be present if there is a bronchopleural fistula. Herniation of the heart through a pericardial defect is also possible if the lingula was resected.

Finally, acute right-sided heart failure is possible, despite adequate screening. A pulmonary artery catheter should be inserted in any high-risk patient. The diagnosis is established if right atrial pressure exceeds left atrial pressure in the presence of a low cardiac output and pulmonary hypertension. Therapy consists of optimizing preload and inotropy with agents such as nitroglycerine and dobutamine.

The most common complications, however, are pulmonary, including atelectasis, hypoxia, pneumonia, and respiratory failure. During the first 18 hours after thoracic surgery, there is a 50%–75% reduction of vital capacity and other lung volumes that improves over the next few days. However, lung volumes may remain decreased for up to 2 weeks.[16] These lower lung volumes predispose the patient to atelectasis; they also cause much of tidal respiration to occur below the closing volume, resulting in transpulmonary shunting and hypoxemia.

Upright positioning, early ambulation, and hourly incentive spirometry will increase functional residual capacity (FRC) and restore a favorable FRC-to-closing-volume relationship.[15] Atelectasis may also lead to pneumonia via superimposed infection on collapsed lung tissue. Vigorous chest physiotherapy, frequent suctioning, and coughing may help loosen secretions and prevent postoperative infection.

Hypoxia may also occur secondary to atelectasis, and a trial of CPAP or PEEP may be helpful. Additionally, adequate analgesia will alleviate spinting and enable coughing, both of which can prevent atelectasis and pneumonia.

The trachea should be extubated as soon as possible after pulmonary operations to reduce the need for sedatives, to avoid further tracheal contamination and trauma, and to allow better humidification of inspired gases by the patient's natural airway.[17]

However, patients with severe chronic pulmonary disease may require postoperative ventilatory support. If mechanical ventilation is required, the DLET must be changed to a single-lumen endotracheal tube at the conclusion of the operation. Weaning is appropriate once the patient has achieved cardiovascular stability, has adequate hemoglobin levels and arterial blood gas values, and has no active lung pathology.

Postoperative Pain

Treatment of pain is important not only for patient comfort, but to enable the patient to cough and breathe deeply to minimize pulmonary complications. Systemic narcotics have traditionally been used to treat thoracotomy pain. Small doses of narcotics can be titrated in the recovery room to achieve analgesia. However, an overdose can cause diminished coughing and sighing that will promote atelectasis.[18] Systemic opioids have a narrow therapeutic margin between comfort and sedation.[15] Because of this, other techniques have been utilized.

Intercostal nerve blocks with 0.25% bupivacaine intra- or postoperatively will provide 6–8 hours of analgesia, and improve arterial blood gases and lung function.[19] Epidural local anesthetics work in a similar fashion, but have undesired side effects of sympathetic blockade and motor impairment.

Cryoanalgesia can provide 2–3 weeks of pain relief, but is associated with paresthesias that usually resolve by one month. Freezing the nerve causes local destruction, but apparently preserves the underlying neural elements.[20] Transcutaneous electrical nerve stimulation (TENS) has only a weak analgesic effect and is used as adjunctive therapy to narcotics.

Perhaps the most useful alternative method of analgesia is epidural narcotics. This has achieved widespread use because it provides a long duration of pain relief (up to 24 hours) without excess sedation, sympathetic block, or sensorimotor loss. Peridural opioids attach to receptors in the substantia gelatinosa in the dorsal horn, where they block pre- and postsynaptic neurons.[21]

Usually 5 mg of preservative-free morphine is diluted to a total volume of 10–20 ml with preservative-free saline. An epidural catheter may be placed in the lumbar region after thoracotomy, with the anesthetized patient in the lateral position. Side effects include early and later respiratory depression, urinary retention, pruritis, and nausea and vomiting, most of which can be treated easily with small doses of naloxone, which will not reverse the analgesia.

Finally, another recent technique uses intrapleural local anesthetics. Twenty milliliters of 0.5% bupivacaine can be instilled through an intrapleural catheter placed at the time of surgery or postoperatively. This provides good unilateral analgesia without respiratory depression, motor weakness, or significant sympathetic blockade.[22]

References

1. Miller JI, Mansour KA, Hatcher CR: Carcinoma of the lung: five-year experience in a university hospital. Am Surg 1980;46:147–50.

2. Miller JI, Grossman GD, Hatcher CR: Pulmonary function test: criteria for operability and pulmonary resection. Surg Gynecol Obstet 1981;153: 893–95.
3. Olsen GN, Block AJ, Swenson EW, et al: Pulmonary function evaluation of the lung resection candidate: a prospective study. Am Rev Respir Dis 1975;111:379–87.
4. Stein M, Koota GM, Simon M, et al: Pulmonary evaluation of surgical patients. JAMA 1962;181:765–70.
5. Stein M, Cassara EL: Preoperative pulmonary evaluation and therapy for surgery patients. JAMA 1970;211:787–90.
6. Miller JL: Thoracic Surgery, in JA Kaplan (ed): Thoracic Anesthesia. New York: Churchill Livingstone, 1983, pp 9–32.
7. Honig EG: Preoperative evaluation, in JA Kaplan (ed): Thoracic Anesthesia. New York: Churchill Livingstone, 1983, pp 121–70.
8. Van Nostrand D, Welsberg MO, Humphrey EW: Preresectional evaluation of risk from pneumonectomy. Surg Gynecol Obstet 1968;127:306–12.
9. Cander L: Physiologic assessment and management of the preoperative patient with emphysema. Am J Cardiol 1963;12:324–26.
10. Ali MK, Ewer MS: Preoperative cardiopulmonary evaluation of patients undergoing surgery for lung cancer. Cancer Bull 1980;32:100–4.
11. Wilson JF: Endobronchial Intubation, in JA Kaplan (ed): Thoracic Anesthesia. New York: Churchill Livingstone, 1983, pp 389–402.
12. Rogers SN, Benumof JL: Halothane and isoflurane do not impair arterial oxygenation during one-lung ventilation in patients undergoing thoracotomy. Anesthesiology, 1983;59:569–72.
13. Capan LM, Turndorf H, Chadrakant P, et al: Optimization of arterial oxygenation during one-lung anesthesia. Anesth Analg 1980;59:847–51.
14. Alfery DD, Benumof JL, Trousdale FR: Improving oxygenation during one-lung ventilation: the effects of PEEP and blood flow restriction to the nonventilated lung. Anesthesiology 1981;55:381–84.
15. Benumof JL, Alfery DD: Anesthesia for Thoracic Surgery, in RD Miller (ed): Anesthesia, 2nd ed. New York: Churchill Livingstone, 1986, pp 1371–462.
16. Hartwell P: Recovery room care after intrathoracic surgery, in EAM Frost (ed): Recovery Room Practice. Boston: Blackwell Scientific Publications, 1985, pp 199–209.
17. Downs JB: Postoperative Respiratory Care, in JA Kaplan (ed): Thoracic Anesthesia. New York: Churchill Livingstone, 1983, pp 635–63.
18. Egbert LD, Bendixen HH: Effect of morphine on breathing pattern: a possible factor in atelectasis. JAMA 1964;188:485–88.
19. Delilkan AE, Lee LK, Yong NK, et al: Postoperative local analgesia for thoracotomy with direct bupivacaine intercostal blocks. Anaesthesia 1973;28:561–67.
20. Myers RR, Powell HC, Heckman HM, et al: Biophysical and pathological effects of cryogenic nerve lesion. Ann Neurol 1981;10:478–85.
21. Cousins MJ, Mather LE, Wilson PR: Intrathecal and epidural administration of opioid analgesic. Anesthesiology 1984;61:276–310.
22. Reiestad F, Stomskag KE: Intrapleural catheter in the management of postoperative pain: a preliminary report, Reg Anaesth 1986;11:89–91.

CHAPTER 10

The Patient for Hepatic Transplantation*

Charles W. Whitten

Case History. *A 37-year-old woman was evaluated by the transplant service for acute necrotic hepatitis secondary to antimalarial prophylaxis with sulfadoxinelpyrimethamine (Fansidar®), which she had taken for one year while living in China. At the time of evaluation she was noticeably jaundiced and edematous and complained of nausea and vomiting. Her past history was unremarkable except for hypothyroidism diagnosed at the age of 18, and tonsillectomy performed the same year under general anesthesia. Family and social histories were unremarkable. The patient's only medication was prednisone 10 mg orally twice a day.*

Orthotropic hepatic transplantation was performed without technical complications. The patient did well until the sixth postoperative day, when her temperature rose to 106°F. Acute graft rejection was diagnosed and she was placed on a monoclonal antibody (OKT-3) directed against T lymphocytes. Her liver function continued to deteriorate despite aggressive medical therapy, necessitating a second transplant, which was scheduled for the twelfth postoperative day.

Preoperative evaluation revealed a disoriented, febrile, severely jaundiced woman, with a blood pressure of 150/100 mm Hg and a pulse of 112/min. Chest x-ray demonstrated bilateral basilar atelectasis and a right pleural effusion. Significant laboratory findings included: total bilirubin 41 mg%, prothrombin time (PT) 14.5 sec (normal 12), partial thromboplastin time (PTT) 33 sec (normal 30), blood urea nitrogen (BUN) 98 mg%, and creatinine 2.9 mg%.

Physical examination revealed developing encephalopathy, bilateral basilar râles, and progressive hepatorenal syndrome. Medications at the time of retransplantation included thyroid supplement, tobramycin, ampicillin, cefotaxime, clindamycin, OKT-3, prednisone, cyclosporine, and azathioprine.

---

* Reviewed by Dr. M. A. Ramsay, Directory of Transplant Anesthesiology, Baylor University Medical Center and The University of Texas Southwestern Medical School, Dallas, Texas.

Introduction

The patient with end-stage liver disease presents the anesthesiologist with a challenging combination of pathophysiologic alterations. Dysfunction of the liver changes cardiovascular, respiratory, renal, endocrine, and neurologic functions, as well as the coagulation cascade.

Liver transplantation, which began as a highly experimental surgical procedure over 20 years ago, became more commonly available in the early 1980s as a result of dramatic improvements in immunosuppression and anesthetic management, increased numbers of skilled surgeons, and improvements in organ procurement. Transplantation is now considered the therapy of choice for many patients with end-stage liver disease. At Baylor University Medical Center we have reported more than 83% survival after two years' experience. (See Figure 10.1.)

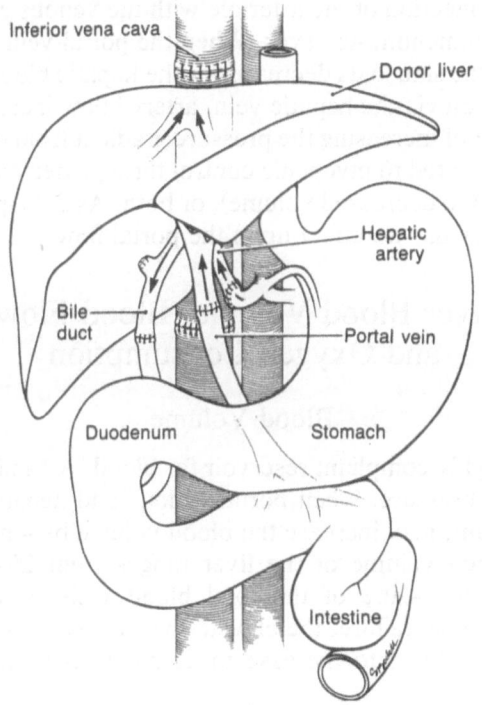

FIGURE 10.1. Completed Orthotopic Liver Transplantation.

Common indications for adult hepatic transplantation include cirrhosis, sclerosing cholangitis, primary liver tumors, Budd-Chiari syndrome, Wilson's disease, and acute liver necrosis.

Physiologic Anatomy of the Liver

The normal liver is a large organ that constitutes about 2% of the body weight. The liver, like the lungs, has two relatively independent blood supplies, from the hepatic cells, the space of Disse, communicates directly with terminal lymphatics in the septa.

Arterioles, which supply most of the oxygen to the liver, are located within the fibrinous septa, and have no specific capillary bed as in most other tissues but instead flow into the sinusoids close to the start of the hepatic plates. The arterioles are innervated by the sympathetic nervous system and by local tissue autoregulation since the cellular fluid that bathes the hepatocytes communicates directly with the smooth muscle of the arterioles in the septa via the space of Disse before it enters the terminal lymphatics. Thus, control of the arterial vasculature is analogous to control of most other arterial vascular beds, except that the discrete capillary network is absent.

The direct connection of the arteriole with the venous channel exhibits an unusual phenomenon, however. When the portal vein is clamped and the pressure in the sinusoids decreases as the hepatic blood volume shifts into the circulation via the hepatic vein, arterial flow increases. This may be a direct effect of increasing the pressure gradient from the artery to the sinusoid, or be related to myogenic control through decreased transmural pressure (related to decreased volume), or both. As anticipated, clamping the hepatic artery has no effect upon the portal flow.

Liver Blood Volume, Blood Flow, and Oxygen Consumption

Blood Volume

The liver is a highly compliant reservoir for blood. A 1 mmHg increase in hepatic venous pressure, when portal venous and hepatic arterial pressures are constant, may increase the blood volume by 4 ml/100 gm liver. The normal blood volume of the liver ranges from 25–30 ml/100 gm, accounting for 10%–20% of the total blood volume. Under extreme conditions of cardiac failure, the elevated vena cava pressure may cause the liver blood volume to increase to as much as 60 ml/100 gm liver weight.

While changes in liver blood volume occur mainly as a passive response to changes in hepatic vein pressure, sympathetic control of the capacitance vessels in this region may account for increased or diminished capacity of the normal hepatic blood reservoir. Carotid baroreceptors influence hepatic blood volume through the sympathetic nervous system. Systemic hypotension decreases hepatic blood volume, increasing circulating blood volume. Systemic hypertension has the opposite effect.

Normal portal vein pressures range from 7–12 mmHg but have been measured as high as 45 mmHg in severe liver disease. Hepatic vein pressure is slightly greater (1–2 mmHg) than central venous pressure, and fluctuates with respiration. Hepatic arterial pressure equals aortic pressure.

Blood Flow

Blood flow in the normal adult liver ranges from 1–1.5 L/min, or about 25% of the normal cardiac output. The hepatic artery carries 25%–33% of the total liver blood flow, demonstrates autoregulation of flow above a pressure of 80 mmHg, and is responsive to changes in portal flow. It is under sympathetic control and is responsive to alpha and beta$_2$ receptors.

Optimal electrical stimulation of sympathetic nerves in dogs resulted in decreased hepatic arterial flow and increased portal and hepatic venous pressure, without effect on portal vein flow. At constant flow, the portal venous pressure in response to alpha agonists was probably related to an effect upon capacitance vessels. There was no response to administration of beta agonists or antagonists.[1]

The portal flow exhibits no local autoregulation or control by alpha and beta receptors, but is regulated by prehepatic vasculature, namely the splenic and mesenteric circulations.

Respiration

Since hepatic blood volume and, therefore, hepatic vein flow, are affected by vena cava pressure, respiration alters the phasic nature of hepatic vein flow through changes in intrathoracic pressure, but not mean hepatic vein flow. Positive end-expiratory pressure (PEEP) transiently decreases hepatic vein flow as the liver blood volume rises in proportion to the increase in venous pressure. A decrease in cardiac output in response to PEEP proportionally decreases portal flow.

As demonstrated in critically ill patients,[2] the hepatic blood flow remained a constant fraction of output, and decreased as positive airway pressure increased. If, in addition, the systemic arterial pressure falls below the autoregulatory limit of the hepatic arterial vasculature, the hepatic arterial flow is reduced significantly.

Oxygen Consumption: The liver receives oxygen from both portal and arterial vessels. Under normal conditions about 50%–70% of the oxygen is provided by the hepatic artery. The oxygen content of the portal blood is variable and determined by the metabolic activity of the spleen and mesentery.

Oxygen consumption ranges from 2–6 ml/100 gm of tissue/min, ie, 15%–35% of the total oxygen consumption of the body. Unlike many other vascular beds, arterial blood flow does not appear to be regulated by oxygen requirements of the liver. Decreased oxygen delivery by hemodilution or lowered arterial pressure does not result in vasodilation but in an increase in oxygen extraction ratio.

Most anesthetic agents decrease hepatic blood flow. The effects are usually attributable to dose-related generalized cardiovascular depression and redistribution of cardiac output. In a recent study,[3] the effects of sodium thiopental, Althesin, and etomidate on hepatic blood flow and oxygen consumption were examined in the greyhound. The results indicated that while hepatic blood flow was decreased in all cases, oxygen consumption remained constant despite decreased oxygen delivery.

Except for extremes of cardiovascular depression, it is doubtful that the function of normal liver would be impaired by anesthetic-induced alterations in hepatic blood flow. However, the diseased liver may not exhibit the same safety factor, depending upon the stage of the disease, especially if the disease process involves hepatic arterial resistance. One review concluded that surgical trauma itself and the nearness of the operative site to the liver are the two most important determinants of the magnitude of perioperative decrease in hepatic blood flow.[4]

Metabolic Functions of the Liver

Among other important biochemical functions, the liver plays a vital role in glucose homeostasis. Patients with significant liver cell injury are given glucose to prevent the occurrence of hypoglycemia. The liver maintains the level of blood glucose by glycogenesis (storage of glucose as glycogen), glycogenolysis (conversion of glycogen into glucose), and gluconeogenesis (conversion of noncarbohydrates to glucose). Many hormones, including insulin, glucagon, epinephrine, glucocorticoids, and growth hormone, are involved in a complex interaction to maintain glucose homeostasis. The surgical patient with liver dysfunction may be susceptible to hypoglycemia as a result of the liver's inability to mobilize glucose. Hyperglycemia may also occur in patients with liver dysfunction, and is often associated with normal or elevated insulin levels, suggesting insulin resistance as the cause.

The liver synthesizes all proteins except gamma globulins and Factor VIII. Albumin, the major protein in human serum, is formed exclusively in the liver. The major functions of albumin include the regulation of oncotic pressure and the binding and transport of certain hormones, drugs, fatty acids, bilirubin, and toxic products. Albumin level is a useful index of the severity of hepatocellular dysfunction in chronic liver disease, with a serum albumin level of less than 3.5 gm/100 ml indicating liver disease. Hypoalbuminemia may lead to an increased drug sensitivity, as a result of decreased protein-binding capabilities and an increased fraction of unbound circulating drug. Proteins, because of their role as acid-base buffers, influence drug activity by altering the amount in the ionized or un-ionized form.

Hepatic dysfunction is unavoidably associated with alterations in coagulation resulting from decreased clearance of plasma activators of the fibrinolytic system leading to secondary fibrinolysis. Liver function, in general, must be depressed to a significant extent before disorders in coagulation occur, since many of the coagulation factors require only 20%–30% of normal levels to prevent excessive bleeding. The extent to which clotting occurs is dependent upon a fine balance between synthesis and utilization of coagulation factors. Fibrinogen (Factor I), prothrombin (Factor II), and Factors V, VII, IX, and X are synthesized in the liver. Factors II, VII, IX, and X are vitamin K-responsive and thus are dependent upon normal intestinal fat absorption. Antihemophilic factor (Factor VIII) is the only important procoagulant not synthesized in the liver. Prothrombin time (PT), which is dependent on the function of Factors II, V, VII, and X, and partial thromboplastin time (PTT), which requires factors II, IX, and X, are both prolonged in patients with parenchymal liver disease. PT is generally a more sensitive indicator of acute liver dysfunction, because of the short half-life of Factor VII (4 hours).

Patterns of Liver Disease

The types of liver disease can, in general, be divided into three categories: acute parenchymal, chronic parenchymal, and cholestatic.

Acute Parenchymal Disease

This category covers the majority of liver injuries commonly seen, including those caused by hepatitis A, hepatitis B, non-A, non-B hepatitis, and drugs. Less common etiologic factors are sepsis, congestive heart failure, and pregnancy.

Hepatitis A is highly infectious, with a mean incubation time of 30 days. It is transmitted almost exclusively via the fecal-oral route, normally has an acute onset, and occurs most commonly among children and young adults. Antibody of the immunoglobulin M (IgM) class is the earliest immunologic response and can persist for several months. During convalescence following hepatitis A infection, IgG antibody predominates. Diagnosis can be made by documenting a rising antibody titer.

Hepatitis B, which is more serious, has a mean incubation period of 60–90 days, frequently has an insidious onset, and shows no age preference. Transmission is primarily by percutaneous inoculation or sexual contact. Hepatitis B surface antigen (HBsAg) appears during the incubation phase and frequently is not present during the acute illness. Antibodies to HBsAg generally appear during convalescence. Hepatitis B e antigen (HBeAg) positivity is seen transiently early in the course of the disease in every patient suffering from acute hepatitis B. Persistent HBeAg positively correlates with ongoing viral replication, making this group of patients highly infective.

Non-A, non-B hepatitis is a designation given to a disease process caused by an as yet unidentified virus or viruses. The disease has a mean incubation period of 50 days, generally with an insidious onset, and occurs most often in adults, although any age group may be affected. Non-A, non-B hepatitis is now the most common cause of posttransfusion hepatitis, possibly responsible for over 80% of cases.[5] It is believed to be transmitted nonparenterally. Serologic tests to identify antigens and antibodies associated with this virus (or group of viruses) are still experimental, and details of the humoral response have yet to be elucidated.

Chronic Parenchymal Disease

Chronic parenchymal liver disease includes chronic hepatitis and cirrhosis.

Chronic hepatitis is an inflammatory process that persists for at least 24 weeks, with the cause generally known in only 10%–20% of cases. It may be further categorized as chronic persistent hepatitis and chronic active hepatitis. Chronic persistent hepatitis is a benign, nonprogressive disease characterized by little if any interruption of normal hepatic architecture. Chronic active hepatitis ultimately results in cirrhosis and/or hepatic failure. Multiple etiologic factors may initiate chronic active hepatitis, including hepatitis B, non-A, non-B hepatitis, drugs, inherited metabolic disorders, and poorly understood immunologic factors.

Cirrhosis is a generic term for a process resulting in extensive loss of liver cells, severe fibrosis, and nodular regeneration. The dominant characteristic is extensive disorganization of the lobular architecture of the liver. Alcohol may be linked to more than 50% of cases worldwide; other etiologic factors include primary biliary cirrhosis, hemochromatosis, and congestive heart failure. In many cases an etiology is never determined.

Cholestatia Disease

Causes of cholestatia liver disease may be intra- or extrahepatic. Intrahepatic diseases may be caused by viral hepatitis, synthetic estrogens, oral contraceptives, phenothiazines, diazepam, phenytoin, and numerous other drugs. Drug-induced cholestatic disease may be either a dose-related or a hypersensitivity response. Extrahepatic disease may be caused by biliary stricture, cancer, or gallstones. The diagnosis is usually made on the basis of history and physical findings, laboratory screening, and ultrasonography. It is imperative that the cause of cholestasis be determined in every patient, because there is an increased risk of anesthesia and surgery in patients with masked acute hepatocellular disease.[6]

All surgical candidates should undergo screening for hepatitis markers.

Systemic Pathyophysiologic Effects of Liver Disease

Cardiovascular Effects

Longstanding liver dysfunction leads to the development of a hyperdynamic circulation characterized by increased cardiac output, decreased systemic vascular resistance, flushed extremities, dilated veins, capillary pulsation, and a wide pulse pressure. Vascular shunting is a major factor in the development of this hyperdynamic state and has been demonstrated in the pulmonary and portal circulations and the extremities.[7,8] The etiology of these shunts is not well understood, but they may be due to an increase in degradation products liberated from damaged hepatocytes.[9] Chronically decreased systemic vascular resistance results in increased vascular volume and cardiac output.

Pulmonary Effects

Although pulmonary dysfunction related to gas exchange is seldom observed intraoperatively, characteristics commonly associated with end-stage liver disease include hypoxia, hyperventilation, and respiratory alkalosis. There is no demonstrable evidence, however, of consistent changes in lung mechanics or lung volumes in patients with severe liver disease, although the presence of ascites may moderately reduce the vital capacity and functional residual capacity. Hypoxia in the presence of hepatic compromise reflects a spectrum of pulmonary vascular disorders including intrapulmonary shunting, portopulmonary shunting, pulmonary hypertension, and ventilation-perfusion mismatching. Hypoxic pulmonary vasoconstriction is also impaired.

Renal Effects

The mechanisms responsible for hepatorenal syndrome (HRS) are not completely understood. In general, HRS is characterized by advancing azotemia, oliguria, and possibly intractable ascites. HRS is associated with diminished renal blood flow and glomerular filtration rate, leading to stimulation of the angiotensin-aldosterone system. Increased renal nerve activity, decreased mean arterial pressure, and increased intraabdominal pressure have been implicated as possible causes of decreased renal blood flow.

The restoration of normal renal function in kidneys from donors with hepatorenal syndrome, when such kidneys are transplanted into recipients without liver disease, suggests that the damaged liver may, directly or indirectly, significantly impair renal function.

Neurologic Effects

Dysfunction of the central nervous system often accompanies hepatic dysfunction. Hepatic encephalopathy is a reversible neuropsychiatric syndrome characterized by personality changes, asterixis, and alterations in the level of consciousness. Increased intracranial pressure and cerebral edema often accompany encephalopathy; herniation may occur in the terminal stages. Frequently, the onset of encephalopathy reflects a worsening of end-stage liver disease. (Other precipitating causes of increased portosystemic shunting—in addition to liver dysfunction—include infection, gastrointestinal tract hemorrhage, constipation, dietary excess of protein, or the administration of sedatives, opiates, or diuretics.)

No single biochemical or physiologic defect has been identified as the cause of hepatic encephalopathy. However, the underlying common denominator is that various toxic substances, including ammonia and nitrogenous compounds, accumulate in the brain as a result of impaired hepatic degradation.

Orthotopic Hepatic Transplantation

The patient who is a candidate for surgical replacement is evaluated by the transplant service on an outpatient basis weeks to months prior to transplantation. If the patient arrives in the hospital immediately prior to surgery, there is often insufficient time available for thorough preoperative evaluation.

History

The majority of patients presenting for hepatic transplantation have involved histories with complications arising from multisystem alterations. During the preoperative interview, patients should be questioned about neurologic difficulties, cardiorespiratory compromise, hepatitis exposure, gastrointestinal hemorrhage, bleeding disorders, renal dysfunction, allergies, medication ingestion, and surgical and anesthetic history. Some patients may have been discharged recently from the hospital following intensive therapy for gastrointestinal bleeding, renal dysfunction, or encephalopathy. Patient who have had recent upper gastrointestinal bleeding often present with alterations in coagulation secondary to anemia, thrombocytopenia, or factor deficiencies. Patients with a history of encephalopathy, in general, require little if any preoperative medication and seem to have less intraoperative anesthetic requirement.

Physical Examination

The routine preoperative physical examination should emphasize the cardiorespiratory system, vessel access ability, and coagulation status. Evaluation of the cardiovascular system is often confounded by the signs and symptoms of the underlying disease process of the liver. For example, the presence of the hepatomegaly, usually indicative of cardiac impairment, is caused by the hyperdynamic cardiovascular system. The patient should be examined for signs of respiratory embarrassment, which may be transient, resulting from ascites and/or pleural effusion, or longterm, such as pneumonia, pulmonary edema, or chronic ventilation-perfusion abnormalities. The clinical coagulation status can be judged by oozing or ecchymoses at recent puncture sites.

Laboratory Examination

Attention should be given to laboratory results reflecting the status of the kidneys, liver, and coagulation cascade. Unfortunately, recent laboratory data are rarely available at the time of induction, although arterial blood gas analyses, serum electrolytes, glucose, and hematocrit are readily obtainable.

Radiologic Examination

An upright chest x-ray, taken routinely prior to arrival in the operating room, should be examined for the presence of infiltrates, cardiac enlargement, increased intravascular markings, and pleural effusions. During the medical evaluation, prior to acceptance for transplantation, ultrasonography and CT scan of the abdomen are performed. Although primarily of medical and surgical interest, these two noninvasive examinations provide the anesthesiologist with clinically useful information.

Ultrasonography determines the patency of the hepatic blood supply and provides an assessment of spleen size. In our experience, if either the hepatic artery or portal vein is poorly visualized, the patient is at an increased risk for embolization. CT scan of the abdomen is performed to assess liver volume, although basilar pulmonary pathology including pleural effusions and atelectasis that might be unappreciated on chest film is often noted. Preoperative chest tubes should be placed for drainage of pleural effusions that may contribute to respiratory embarrassment.

Cardiopulmonary System

All patients undergo formal cardiology consultation, including a minimum history and physical examination, resting electrocardiogram, and a first-pass rest and stress test. ECGs often demonstrate axis shifts secondary to upward displacement of the diaphragm. Two-dimensional echocardiography is performed if a clinically unexplained murmer is appreciated or if there is clinical suspicion of left ventricular dysfunction. Coronary catheterization is performed if there is clinical evidence of coronary artery disease. Right heart catheterization is performed if pulmonary hypertension is suspected by echocardiography. The majority of patients have a hyperdynamic cardiovascular system. The presence of a normal or depressed cardiac index may indicate underlying cardiac dysfunction although transplantation is not contraindicated (unpublished data, Paulsen, Whitten, et al).

Pulmonary function tests should not be performed routinely but may be clinically indicated.

Fluid and Electrolyte Balance

Preoperative assessment of renal status should include determinations of serum electrolytes, BUN, creatinine levels, urinalysis, and glomerular filtration rate.

Alterations in fluid and electrolyte balance often occur in patients with liver dysfunction. Hyponatremia frequently accompanies liver dysfunction as a result of the kidney's inability to excrete free water or because of vigorous diuretic usage in an attempt to control ascites accumulation. Hypokalemia may result from secondary hyperaldosteronism or as a result of total body depletion of potassium stores secondary to diuresis.

Central Nervous System

Although hepatic encephalopathy occurs commonly in patients with end-stage liver disease, not all neurologic dysfunction in this group of patients is encephalopathy. It is important to suspect potentially treatable causes of neurologic dysfunction, including subdural hematoma or cerebral edema. Chronic subdural hematoma may be due to underlying coagulopathies, while cerebral edema may occur because of disruption of the blood-brain barrier.

Coagulation

Many patients have suffered gastrointestinal bleeding, leading to numerous hematologic alterations including anemia, thrombocytopenia, and dilutional coagulopathy. Microcytic hypochromic anemia results from gastrointestinal bleeding; macrocytic anemia is due to folic acid deficiency secondary to poor nutrition. Thrombocytopenia is caused by gastrointestional bleeding, folic acid deficiency, or splenic sequestration. Accumulation of the plasma activators of fibrinolysis, secondary to delayed removal, may also play a role in preoperative coagulopathies.

Preoperative Medical Therapy

Many patients presenting for hepatic transplantation receive medical therapy for problems associated with liver disease, including varices, encephalopathy, and ascites.

Sclerotherapy is the therapy of choice for acute variceal bleeding, although vasopressin and the placement of Sengstaken-Blakemore tubes continue to play a role. Vasopressin, which decreases portal venous pressure by constricting the splanchnic arteriolar bed and increasing the resistance of blood inflow to the gut, is usually administered to any patient with variceal bleeding and may lead to temporary control. Transient decreases in cardiac output, cardiac dysrhythmias, and ischemia secondary to coronary artery constriction and water retention are all complications.

Sengstaken-Blakemore tubes are considered the last line of medical therapy for variceal hemorrhage and are usually placed prior to the patient's arrival in the operating room for liver transplantation or portosystemic bypass. Improper placement or improper inflation of the balloons may lead to esophageal perforation. Airway obstruction and aspiration can also occur.

Specific treatment of hepatic encephalopathy is aimed at decreasing ammonia production in the colon and elimination or treatment of precipitating factors by restriction of dietary protein and control of gastrointestinal bleeding. Neomycin, a nonabsorbable antibiotic, decreases the bacterial population of the gastrointestinal tract, thereby reducing the amount of urea converted to ammonia by bacterial ureases. Lactulose, a nonabsorbable disaccharide, is effective in decreasing the concentration of ammonia via its ability to reduce the pH of the gastrointestinal tract. The presence of intraluminal acidosis favors the conversion of ammonia to ammonium (which is poorly soluble and not readily absorbed).

Ascites occurs frequently in patients with hepatic dysfunction. Intraabdominal factors contributing to ascites formation include portal hypertension and increased flow of hepatic lymph. Important systemic factors include a decreased plasma colloid oncotic pressure, hyperaldosteronism, and impaired water excretion. Initial therapy for patients with ascites includes bed rest and strict fluid and sodium restriction. If conservative management is not successful, diuretics such as spironolactone can be added to the therapeutic regimen. Diuretics are helpful if urinary sodium is low. Paracentesis is especially beneficial for acute control of respiratory embarrassment secondary to massive ascites.

Preanesthetic Management

Most patients undergoing transplantation have been evaluated medically on an elective, outpatient basis and remain outside the hospital while awaiting the transplant. The recipient arrives at the hospital and undergoes final evaluation as outlined. He receives initial immunosuppression, including oral cyclosporine or azathioprine and intavenous prednisolone.

Anesthetic preoperative medication, if indicated and if time allows, is administered prior to transfer to the operating room. Normally this consists of diazepam 5–10 mg orally or midazolam 0.05–0.07 mg/kg intramuscularly. Intramuscular injections are avoided in patients with severe coagulopathies and/or thrombocytopenia. Oral antacid medications are given. Patients with a history suggestive of encephalopathy are given little, if any, preanesthetic medication, as these patients frequently have an exaggerated response to pharmacologic sedation.

Anesthetic Plan

A standard operating room table covered with a warming blanket on top of an egg crate mattress with sacral padding is used. Padded boots are placed and extra padding is given to the head and bilaterally to the popliteal regions, elbows and wrists. The arms are placed on boards at less than 90° abduction to facilitate surgical access and are secured in mild anterior flexion with forearm supination. Reflective draping is placed on the lower and upper extremities, as well as the head, to minimize radiant heat loss.

Monitoring includes continuous arterial, pulmonary, and central venous pressures, ECG leads II & V, and esophageal, rectal, and blood temperatures; thermodilution cardiac output; mixed-venous oxygen saturation; end-tidal CO_2 and nitrogen extraction (the difference between end-tidal N_2 and inspired N_2); oxygen consumption and carbon dioxide production (mass spectrometry); arterial blood gas analyses, colloid oncotic pressure, serum and urine osmolarities, and electrolyte estimations (sodium, potassium, ionized calcium, and glucose).

Hemodynamic parameters are calculated from the measurements and include cardiac index, peripheral vascular resistance, and pulmonary vascular resistance. Urine output is measured every half-hour. PT, PTT, hematocrit, platelet count, fibrinogen, thrombin clot time, heparin assay, and thromboelastography are utilized to assess the patient's coagulation status.

After cannulation of the radial artery and an antecubital vein with a large-bore (8F) catheter, we use a rapid-sequence intravenous induction with diazepam 5–10 mg/kg, ketamine 2 mg/kg, succinylcholine 1.5 mg/kg, and gallamine 20 mg.

Theoretically, plasma cholinesterase (PCLE), which is synthesized by hepatocytes and is required to hydrolyze succinylcholine, may be reduced by end-stage liver disease. When PCLE levels are 20% of normal, the duration of apnea following succinylcholine administration is increased from 5 minutes to nearly 15 minutes.[10] Thus, in cases of total hepatic failure, atracurium may be the neuromuscular blocking agent of choice. Orthotopic liver transplantation may not only return PCLE levels to normal but may also revert abnormal genotypes of the enzyme, suggesting that determination of enzyme character is another liver function.[11]

Maintenance of anesthesia is with sufentanil and pancuronium and supplemental isoflurane in an air-oxygen mixture at an FiO_2, of 0.5–0.7.

Following induction, 8F catheters are placed bilaterally in the internal jugular veins. One of these is used for placement of an oximetric pulmonary artery catheter.

Ventilation is adjusted to maintain an end-tidal CO_2 of 35–40 mmHg. Positive end-expiratory pressure of 5 cm H_2O is routinely administered in an effort to prevent right lower atelectasis. Anesthetic gases are passed through a servocontrolled heated humidifier.

Maintenance intravenous fluid consists of Plasmalyte®, approximately 5–10 mg/kg/h, with the amount determined by individual patient requirements.

Management of Intraoperative Problems

Orthotopic hepatic transplantation can be divided into three distinct phases. The *preanhepatic phase* begins with induction of anesthesia and extends until the completion of the dissection of the liver to its vascular pedicle. The *anhepatic phase* begins when blood flow to the native liver is interrupted, and ends when the donor liver is reperfused. The *postanhepatic phase* constitutes the remainder of the procedure. Problems that can arise include: (1) massive fluid shifts and rapid blood loss; (2) coagulopathies; (3) hypocalcemia; (4) hyper- or hypokalemia; (5) air or particulate emboli; (6) severe acidosis; (7) alterations in serum glucose; (8) decreased urine output; (9) dramatic hemodynamic changes.

Although massive fluid shifts and rapid blood loss can occur at any time, the first large volume change occurs when the peritoneal cavity is opened and ascitic fluid is removed. Removal of several liters of ascitic fluid can result in acute enlargement of the intravascular space, leading to relative intravascular volume deficits and cardiovascular instability.

Our experience has shown that if careful fluid maintenance is administered prior to ascitic fluid removal, hemodynamics are improved with the release of elevated intraabdominal pressure. Intravenous fluids are given throughout the procedure, with therapy guided by urine output, central and pulmonary arterial pressure measurements, and urine and serum osmolarities.

Blood loss at the onset of the procedure may be of insidious nature, secondary to underlying coagulopathy or platelet dysfunction. As the procedure continues and the dissection becomes technically more difficult, rapid blood loss may occur from tearing of venous collaterals, the inferior vena cava, or the arterial supply to the liver.

Blood and blood-product therapy is guided by hourly thomboelas-tographs, coagulation profiles, and hemodynamic measurements. Each unit of packed red blood cells is mixed with one unit of fresh frozen plasma. If cell-saver blood is transfused, two units of fresh frozen plasma are given for each unit of cell-saver blood administered. A rapid-infusion device capable of delivering blood at a rate of approximately 2.5 L/min is always primed and available for emergency use.

Coagulation abnormalities are inherent to patients with end-stage liver disease. Our experience has shown that coagulopathies should be treated in the preanhepatic phase to minimize blood loss. Reperfusion of the donor liver is associated with a transient, severe coagulopathy, which is sometimes related in part to the release of sequestered heparin from the donor liver.[12]

The application of the thromboelastograph to the management of hemostasis during liver transplantation has recently been reviewed.[13] The thromboelastogram provides the clinician with a means of rapidly differ-entiating coagulopathy from surgical bleeding, as well as identifying specific coagulopathies (ie, presence of heparin or fibrinolysis), and testing the effectiveness of aminocaproic acid and/or protamine therapy ex vivo. Cryoprecipitate and platelet therapy are titrated to alterations in thromboelastograms and coagulation profiles.

Hypocalcemia occurs frequently, secondary to citrate overload from blood and blood-product therapy. Patients with liver dysfunction are more susceptible to citrate toxicity because of the diseased liver's inability to metabolize citrate. Calcium chloride is the therapy of choice for decreased serum ionized calcium in this setting. Calcium should be administered slowly, as transient hypercalcemia may cause ventricular dysrhythmias.

Hypokalemia is not usually a problem, but alterations in potassium metabolism occur secondary to hyperaldosteronism or may result from vigorous potassium-wasting-diuretic administration. Blood and blood-product administration should be considered for intraoperative potassium supplementation. Hyperkalemia occurs frequently following reperfusion of the donor liver[14] and may lead to bradycardia, hypotension, and possibly cardiac arrest.

Hypothermia often develops during any major intraabdominal proce-dure. Other factors exist in hepatic transplantation patients that make them more susceptible to temperature decreases. Patients with end-stage liver disease may have a decreased ability to generate heat because of metabolic impairment. During the anhepatic phase, O_2 consumption and CO_2 production decrease. The extracorporeal circuit utilized for ve-novenous bypass may also contribute to heat loss.[15]

Routinely, the operating room should be warmed prior to the arrival of the patient and maintained at 73–76°F until draping is completed. Heated and humidified gases, fluid warming, warming blanket, and placement of reflective drapes to the upper and lower extremities and head are routine. Irrigation of the abdominal cavity with warmed fluid and application of pediatric warming lights have been helpful in correcting hypothermia, although prevention is a primary goal.

Air or particulate emboli may occur most commonly during the late preanhepatic and anhepatic phases. Changes in nitrogen excretion, as well as O_2 consumption and CO_2 production, are closely monitored for early detection of embolic events. An increase in nitrogen excretion allows differentiation of air embolization from particulate embolization.

Metabolic acidosis, which occurs routinely particularly during the late anhepatic and early postanhepatic phases, may have multiple etiologies including hepatorenal syndrome, hemodynamic instability, massive transfusion, poor systemic perfusion during the anhepatic phase, or an acid bolus from a hypothermic, ischemic liver graft.

Hypoglycemia is typically not an intraoperative problem. Hyperglycemia, on the other hand, occurs frequently following reperfusion of the donor liver but seldom requires therapy.

Decreased urine output can occur during transplantation, associated with hepatorenal syndrome, cyclosporine nephrotoxicity, hypovolemia, decreased mean blood pressure, and activation of the renin-angiotensin system. Following a decrease in urine output (less than 0.5 ml/kg/h),

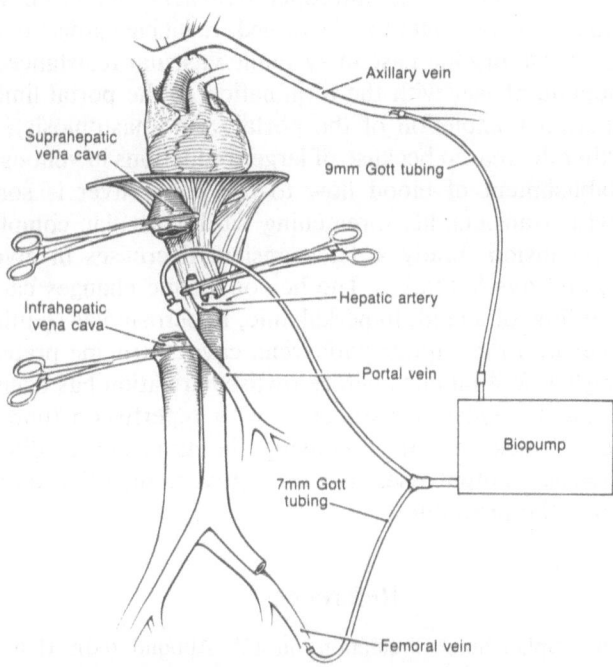

FIGURE 10.2. Venovenous Bypass.

preload is optimized and crystalloid is administered to improve free water clearance as indicated by changes in urine and plasma osmolalities. If urine output remains low, a low-dose dopamine infusion is started, followed by the administration of mannitol and/or loop diuretics, if required.

The hemodynamic changes associated with hepatic transplantation have been studied extensively.[14,16] The preservation of cardiovascular stability provides one of the greatest intraoperative challenges. The acute management of hypotension is complicated in the presence of chronically decreased systemic vascular resistance caused by intravascular shunts. Vasopressor administration may lead to a vascular steal that reduces blood flow to vital organs while enhancing shunt flow. The degree of hemodynamic instability during the preanhepatic phase is directly related to the difficulty of the surgical dissection and blood loss. Common causes of intraoperative hypotension during this phase are hypovolemia, cardiac dysfunction secondary to decreased ionized calcium, surgical manipulation that disturbs preload, and effective tamponade of the inferior vena cava.

Venovenous bypass (see Figure 10.2.) is utilized at many centers to enhance cardiovascular stability during the anhepatic phase. Other potential advantages of venovenous bypass include decompression of the gut leading to decreased intraoperative blood loss, improved perioperative renal function, and decreased intraoperative acidosis. Even with venovenous bypass, venous return is decreased, reducing cardiac output and causing a compensatory increase in systemic vascular resistance. During the late anhepatic phase, with the termination of the portal limb of the bypass (to permit completion of the portal vein anastomosis), cardiac output is further decreased because of larger reductions in venous return.

The reestablishment of blood flow to the donor liver is sometimes associated with transient life-threatening cardiovascular complications including hypotension, bradycardia, transient decreases in myocardial contractility, and dysrhythmias. The hemodynamic changes can be explained by the flow of a cold, hyperkalemic, hyperosmolar solution from the donor liver into the suprahepatic vena cava. Atropine pretreatment (0.02–0.04 mg/kg) 2–4 minutes before revascularization has been shown to minimize the bradycardia associated with reperfusion (unpublished data, Paulson, Valek, et al). Following the transient cardiovascular depression, cardiac output rises to a level greater than that obtained at any time during the procedure.

References

1. Donald DG: Splanchnic Circulation, in FA Abboud (ed): Handbook of Physiology, Volume III, Section 2, Part 1. Baltimore: Williams and Wilkins, 1983, pp 219–40.

2. Bonnet F, Richard C, Glaser P, et al: Changes in hepatic flow induced by continuous positive-pressure ventilation in critically ill patients. Crit Care Med 1982;10:703–5.

3. Thomson IA, Fitch W, Hughes RC, et al: Effects of certain intravenous anesthetics on liver blood flow and hepatic oxygen consumption in the greyhound. Br J Anaesth 1986;58:69–80.

4. Gelman SI: Disturbances in hepatic blood flow during anesthesia and surgery. Arch Surg 1976;111:881–83.

5. Seeff LB, Zimmerman HF, Wright EC, et al: A randomized double-blind controlled trial of the efficacy of immune serum globulin for the prevention of post-transfusion hepatitis. A Veterans Administration Cooperative Study. Gastroenterology 1977;72:111–21.

6. Harville DD, Summerskill WHJ: Surgery in acute hepatitis. Causes and effects. JAMA 1963;184:257–61.

7. Calabresi P, Belmann WH: Portacaval and portopulmonary anastomoses in Laennec's cirrhosis and in heart failure. J Clin Invest 1957;36:1257–65.

8. Bashour FĀ, Miller WF, Chapman CB: Pulmonary venoarterial shunting in hepatic cirrhosis. Am Heart J 1961;62:350–58.

9. Iber FL: Normal and Pathologic Physiology of the Liver in WA Soderman (ed): Pathologic Physiology Mechanisms and Disease. Philadelphia: WB Saunders, 1974, pp 790–817.

10. Vily-Mogensen J: Correlation of succinylcholine duration of action with plasma cholinesterase activity in subjects with the genotypically normal enzyme. Anesthesiology 1980;53:517–20.

11. Khoury GF, Brill J, Walts L, et al: Atypical serum cholinesterase eliminated by orthotopic liver transplantation. Anesthesiology 1987;67:273–74.

12. Belani KC, Estrin JA, Ascher NL, et al: Reperfusion coagulopathy during human liver transplantation. Anesth Analg 1987;66:S10.

13. Kang YG, Martin DJ, Marquez J, et al: Intraoperative changes in blood coagulation and thromboelastographic monitoring in liver transplantation. Anesth Analg 1985;64:888–96.

14. Paulsen AW, Valek TR, Blessing DD, et al: Hemodynamics during liver transplantation with venovenous bypass. Transplant Proc. Feb 1987;XI:no. 1, 2417–19.

15. Paulsen AW, Prater G, Whitten CW, et al: Cardiovascular effects of venovenous bypass during hepatic transplantation. J Extracorporeal Technol, 1987;19:268–73.

16. Carmichael FJ, Lindop MJ, Farman JV: Anesthesia for hepatic transplantation: Cardiovascular and metabolic alterations and their management. Anesth Analg 1985;64:108–16.

CHAPTER 11

The Patient for
Electroconvulsive Therapy*

Salvatore C. Scalafani

Case History. *A 68-year-old woman with a history of recurrent depression was scheduled for a course of electroconvulsive therapy (ECT), 3 treatments per week for at least 2 weeks, on an outpatient basis. She had received several courses of ECT in the past and her condition had improved significantly for 8–12 months. Her only current medication was lithium. She complained of not being able to attend to her usual daily activities. She had a history of hypertension with poor medication compliance attributed to episodes of orthostatic hypotension.*

Past hospital records indicated that the patient had moderate hypertension on no medication. In the ECT room she was always hypertensive. In addition, on two previous treatment occasions, her blood pressure (BP) was significantly increased after ECT. On another occasion, she developed hypotension after a hypertensive episode and required intravenous fluid resuscitation. Later, her husband recalled that she had refused to drink fluids for the previous two days.

The patient's most recent anesthetic and ECT records showed that the required dose of methohexital had been between 50 and 80 mg and the dose of succinylcholine was 40 mg; however, at that time she was not taking lithium.

Laboratory analyses and electrocardiogram (ECG) were within normal limits. X-rays of the cervical and thoracic spine showed generalized osteoporotic changes. Medical consult concluded that hypertension prior to ECT was related to anxiety.

Physical examination revealed an extremely anxious, slim woman weighing 58 kg. She had removable upper and lower dentures. The lungs were clear to auscultation, and no heart murmurs were present. Vital

* Reviewed by Dr. Anna Stanec, Chairman, Department of Anesthesiology, St. Joseph's Hospital and Medical Center, Paterson, New Jersey, and Clinical Professor, Department of Anesthesiology, University of Medicine and Dentistry of New Jersey, New Jersey Medical School, Newark, New Jersey.

signs were blood pressure 140/85 mmHg, heart rate 82/min, respiratory rate 16/min.

The anesthetic and ECT plans were discussed with the psychiatrist and internist. Use of nitroglycerin ointment in the ECT room was recommended to stabilize her BP. Close attention to maintenance of adequate fluid intake was emphasized to the patient and her family.

Introduction

Electroconvulsive therapy (ECT) has been used for almost a half century. During this time there have been significant improvements in ECT application methods and also in patient management including anesthetic technique. Central nervous system (CNS) seizure activity rather than electrical stimulus is responsible for the beneficial effect of ECT but the exact mechanism of the therapeutic effects is not yet understood. In the U.S., ECT is performed in approximately 100,000 psychiatric patients per year.[1] The overall psychiatric and anesthetic management of patients considered for ECT has been reviewed recently.[2,3] The aim of the anesthesiologist is to provide safe and effective anesthesia to these patients without interfering with the beneficial effects of ECT.

Historical Background

Convulsive therapies were introduced in the 1930s after psychiatrists observed that psychotic patients improved clinically after having spontaneous seizures and that the occurrence of schizophrenia and epilepsy in the same patient was a statistical rarity.[4] In addition, erroneous conclusions were made from pathologic studies of brains that showed CNS glial hyperplasia in epileptics and glial hypoplasia in schizophrenics. The two diseases appeared to be antagonistic. Based on this assumption, in 1934 Von Meduna first attempted to treat schizophrenia by inducing seizures with the pharmacologic agents camphor and pentylenetetrazol. Thus, the era of pharmacoconvulsive therapy was introduced primarily to treat schizophrenic patients.[4]

In 1938, Cerletti and Bini applied external electrical current to induce generalized seizures in man.[5] This idea originated from their involvement in epilepsy research, using electrical stimulation to produce seizures in animals. The type of electrical signal they used was the sine wave, the same type present in domestic electrical sockets.

In 1940, curare was introduced in ECT to modify the seizure-induced muscular response.[6] Later in the same decade galamine, another nondepolarizing muscle relaxant was used.[2] In 1951, succinylcholine was introduced, and because of its short duration of action, it became the drug of choice for producing muscle relaxation during ECT.[7]

Originally ECT was performed after administration of the relaxant to the awake patient. Although it was known that the patient became unconscious during application of the electrical current and had no recall of the treatment, the paralysis induced in the awake patient was a source of great discomfort, and the need to alleviate this problem became obvious. For this reason, short-acting barbiturates were introduced into ECT practice.[2] By the early 1960s, a simple and safe anesthetic regime was developed. This included a short-acting intravenous barbiturate, a depolarizing muscle relaxant, and oxygenation with controlled ventilation during the apneic phase.

ECT Apparatus

For ECT an electrical current is applied to the CNS. Originally, ECT devices used bilateral stimulation, which remains more popular than unilateral stimulation. The latter method can avoid post-ECT confusion and memory impairment, but its efficacy has been questioned.[4] In the equipment currently used, the stimulus frequency, pulse width, and duration can be adjusted to achieve optimal results.[2] Today the most commonly used device is the Monitored Electroconvulsive Therapy Apparatus (MECTA) introduced in the 1970s. This apparatus delivers 550-800 mA in brief, bidirectional square waves of 1–2 msec duration at 40–90 Hz to provoke a generalized seizure lasting for at least 20–25 sec. The electrical stimulus is delivered via electrodes fixed to the patient's forehead. Plate electrodes are used to provide a low impedance pathway after the skin has been prepared by cleansing, mild abrasion, and the application of electrode jelly. The new generation of MECTA devices developed in the 1980s is equipped with a two-channel recorder for simultaneous monitoring of the electroencephalogram (EEG) and the electrocardiogram (ECG).

Physiologic Changes and Clinical Manifestations

The purpose of ECT is to develop grand mal seizures, which must be of appropriate duration to have therapeutic benefits. It must be kept in mind that the barbiturates raise the seizure threshold and muscle relaxants abolish the classical clinical manifestations of grand mal seizures. Thus, EEG monitoring is a necessity and provides a guideline for achieving optimal therapeutic effects. The idea is to apply minimum electrical current necessary to produce adequate seizure activity in the brain, as documented by EEG changes.

ECT centrally activates the autonomic nervous system, which is responsible for the cardiovascular changes.[2,3] Upon application of electric current, a brief parasympathetic discharge is accompanied by a rise in circulating catecholamines.[8]

Upon awakening from ECT treatments, patients commonly are confused and may be in a state of excitement. Apart from the confusion, patients may demonstrate extremes of affect—euphoria, dullness, or amnesia. These changes, when they occur, are usually short-lived.

Immediately following ECT, the EEG corresponds to that of spontaneous seizure activity. Additional changes seen after the first ECT include a diffuse slowing in brain-wave activity that parallels cortical and subcortical impairment.[9] These changes revert after the cessation of treatments. The number of ECT treatments determines the severity and persistence of EEG changes.

Dysrhythmias or even brief periods of asystole frequently can occur during the seizures. The seizure itself, as well as controlled ventilation, increases intrathoracic pressure and decreases venous return to the heart, decreasing cardiac output. As a result of the massive sympathetic discharge, both systolic and diastolic blood pressures are consistently elevated. ECT candidates with essential hypertension may show more exaggerated responses than normotensive patients.[2] Severe post-ECT hypertension can be abolished by prior administration of alpha-adrenergic or beta-adrenergic blockers or nitroglycerin.[10,11]

Because of the significant autonomic changes produced by ECT, it is mandatory to monitor blood pressure and ECG regularly during the treatment and the recovery phase. The area where the ECT is to be performed should be equipped with cardiopulmonary resuscitative equipment including oxygen, suction, intubation equipment, a defibrillator, and appropriate medications. It is advisable that extremely high-risk patients have the ECT performed in the operating room area with elective intubation, until full recovery from anesthesia and ECT.

Clinical Indications

The indications for ECT have been reviewed.[2,3,12] (See Table 11.1.)

Major Depressive Disorders and Recurrent Depressive States

ECT is the prime mode of therapy for patients with endogenous depression who have failed pharmacologic treatment. ECT is superior to the tricyclic antidepressants and monoamine oxidase inhibitors (MAOIs). Patients who suffer from major depressive disorders such as melancholia or delusions are excellent candidates for ECT, and depression of old age not caused by arteriosclerotic or senile brain changes also responds. Neurotic or reactive depressions have less reliable results. It should be noted that patients who fail to respond to ECT also often fail to respond to drug therapy.

Should a patient be initially treated for his depression with medications or ECT? The answer lies in the severity of the depression or the risk of suicide. Pharmacotherapy is the first choice in early cases, usually being

TABLE 11.1. Indications for ECT.

Primary	Secondary
Major depressive disorders	Chronic schizophrenia
Recurrent depressive states	Psychosomatic disorders
Acute schizophrenia	Failure of pharmacologic therapy
Acute manic states	Chronic pain syndromes

prescribed by a patient's primary care physician before referral to a psychiatrist. With an outpatient who shows suicide potential, immediate ECT is strongly recommended.

The patient treated for depression should be started on lithium therapy if he suffers from a manic-depressive psychosis, or on tricyclic antidepressants if he suffers from a single major depression. Those patients who have difficulty with prophylactic medication for whatever reason should be considered for monthly follow-up ECT.

There are other factors to consider. Most pharmacotherapeutic regimens take considerable time to be effective, while ECT elicits a quicker response. This is an important consideration for a patient who risks losing his job if he undergoes slow therapy with an inherently higher failure rate. Hospitalized patients have shorter stays when ECT is a part of their treatment regimen.

Schizophrenia

ECT is quite effective in acute forms of schizophrenia, especially in catatonic and schizoaffective presentations, but it has not proved successful in chronic cases. When a patient presents with acute schizophrenia, the psychiatrist's preference determines whether ECT or drug therapy is tried first. External circumstances (hospital expense, time, degree of disturbance) can help to guide the decision.

ECT treatment of schizophrenia must be continued after the termination of symptoms, for a total of 10–15 treatments. Failure to do so results in a poor success rate. An acute onset of schizophrenia and a duration of illness of less than 12 months are two positive prognostic factors when considering ECT treatment.

Paranoid schizophrenia in the young patient has the best response of all the schizophrenias. Simple and hebephrenic subtypes show the least improvement. Chronic schizophrenics not responding to pharmacotherapy, patients with poor drug compliance, and those who suffer significant drug side effects are best managed with repeated ECT.

Manic States

Acute manic states can be treated successfully with ECT. Lithium, however, is the drug of first choice. Severely disturbed patients can be treated with ECT prior to starting the lithium treatment.

Other Conditions

The basic personality of a patient does not change after ECT, but some improvement is seen in patients with psychosomatic disorders such as neurodermatitis, ulcerative colitis, and anorexia nervosa,[12] and acute pain conditions such as trigeminal neuralgia and phantom limb pain also have occasionally shown good therapeutic results. Personality disorders are not improved with ECT.

Preanesthetic Assessment

Patients scheduled for ECT should undergo the same thorough preoperative evaluation as would any other patient who is to receive general anesthesia, including a detailed history, physical examination, and laboratory tests, as well as consultation with the patient's family and psychiatrist if necessary. Informed consent for ECT and anesthesia must be completed and its legal validity from the patient and/or his family verified.

The physical examination should pay particular attention to cardiopulmonary and neurologic functions. Symptoms of esophageal reflux, allergies, prior anesthetic experience, and spinal arthritic changes should be investigated. The condition of the patient's teeth (loose, missing, chipped) should be recorded and problems evaluated by a dentist. All loose teeth and bridges must be removed prior to administration of ECT.

Minimum laboratory investigation should include a complete blood count (CBC), urinalysis, serum electrolytes, glucose, blood urea nitrogen (BUN), creatinine, and liver enzymes. An ECG is also indicated, and in an older patient, cervical and thoracic spine x-rays should be reviewed. Discussion of the case among the primary care physician, the psychiatrist, and the anesthesiologist assures optimal conditions for ECT and patient safety.

Concurrent Disease

The patient's concurrent disease state may mandate consultation with a specialist prior to ECT. (See Table 11.2.) Certain disease processes are considered contraindications to ECT,[2,3] but opinion differs in regard to both relative and absolute contraindications. The latter category includes the presence of an intracranial space-occupying lesion (with or without changes in intracranial pressure), a recent cerebrovascular accident, presence of a large unstable aneurysm of a major vessel, and a recent myocardial infarction. Although there have been reports of successful ECT during the acute phase of a myocardial infarction and in the presence of a cerebral aneurysm,[2,10] in such patients ECT should be considered only when it is life-saving. (eg, suicidal attempts have occurred)

An even greater variation of opinion is seen when relative contrain-

TABLE 11.2. Contraindications for ETC.

Absolute	Relative
Intracranial mass lesion	Angina pectoris
Recent cerebrovascular accident	Congestive heart failure
Unstable aneurysm of a major vessel	Cardiac pacemakers
Recent myocardial infarction	Thyroid disease
MAOI therapy	Thrombophlebitis
	Severe pulmonary disease
	Pregnancy
	Severe osteoporosis
	Recent bone fractures
	Retinal detachment
	Glaucoma

dications are considered.[13] Frequently cited relative contraindications are angina pectoris, congestive heart failure, cardiac pacemakers, thyroid disease, glaucoma, retinal detachment, severe osteoporosis, major bone fractures, thrombophlebitis, severe pulmonary disease, and pregnancy. Safe application of ECT has been reported with all of these concurrent conditions.[2,14] The final decision concerning ECT should be made after careful consideration of associated risks and complications of chronic drug therapy or unchecked progression of the psychiatric illness.

Several medical problems present increased risk for ECT and anesthesia (see Table 11.3.), including hypertension, pulmonary, cardiac, and liver disease, malnutrition, a history of allergic reactions, a history of neuroleptic malignant syndrome, pseudocholinesterase deficiency, a family history of malignant hyperthermia, and the ongoing pharmacologic treatment of both medical and psychiatric conditions. The ECT-associated risk should be weighed against the risk of alternative treatment.

Concurrent Medication

Patients scheduled for ECT are frequently receiving multiple psychotropic medications, which may interact with anesthetics and muscle relaxants.[15]

Tricyclic antidepressants block the reuptake of norepinephrine by the presynaptic membrane. This leads to excess of circulating catecholamines and cardiotoxic effects such as tachycardia and dysrhythmias, even at therapeutic doses. Tricyclic therapy may also cause an exaggerated pressor response to direct-acting sympathomimetic amines. This can make treatment of unexpected hypotension during or after ECT hazardous or can produce hyperthermia, hypertensive crisis, and even death. Discontinuation of tricyclic antidepressant therapy two weeks before the scheduled general anesthesia has been recommended but may not be feasible in psychiatric patients. However, since many patients are sched-

TABLE 11.3. Conditions presenting increased anesthetic risk for ECT.

Hypertension	History of neuroleptic malignant syndrome
Pulmonary disease	Family history of malignant hyperthermia
Cardiac disease	Pseudocholinesterase deficiency
Unstable endocrine disease	Concurrent medication for medical and psychiatric
Liver disease	conditions
Malnutrition	
History of allergic reactions	

uled for ECT because of ineffectiveness of antidepressant therapy, discontinuation of their drugs is acceptable.

The mechanism of the antipsychotic effect of *phenothiazines* is not completely understood. These agents exert peripheral alpha-adrenergic blocking action and may diminish the hypertensive response to catecholamines. The also potentiate a hypotensive response and the sedative effect when bartiturates are given, presumably by a central action. Smaller doses of barbiturates given slowly minimize these interactions.

The *monoamine oxidase inhibitors (MAOIs)* are rarely used today as antidepressants or antihypertensives. These agents block intraneuronal metabolism of catecholamines and can interact with indirectly acting sympathomimetic amines to produce hypertensive crisis. Discontinuation of MAOI therapy at least two weeks before ECT to allow the regeneration of active monoamine oxidase minimizes this potential danger.[15] Because of the high risk associated with anesthesia and ECT in patients taking MAOIs, ECT should not be performed. If a patient is dependent on antidepressant therapy, a regimen of gradual replacement with some other appropriate drug must be considered prior to ECT.

Both MAOIs and tricyclic antidepressants interact with barbiturates to prolong sleep time and duration of anesthesia. Smaller doses of intravenous barbiturates should be used.

Lithium is commonly prescribed for psychiatric patients, especially for recurrent depression and manic states. The mechanism of its antipsychotic effect is not well understood. It is known, however, that lithium replaces sodium during depolarization and slows this process. As a result, lithium decreases the amount of released peripheral and central neurotransmitters. Lithium can interact with barbiturates to prolong recovery time.[16] The duration of action of both depolarizing and nondepolarizing muscle relaxants is prolonged in patients taking lithium.[17] In addition, patients on chronic lithium therapy may present with cardiac dysrhythmias.

Rauwolfia alkaloids, used for treatment of hypertension, produce their effects via intraneuronal catecholamine and 5-hydroxytryptophan depletion. Serious consequences of ECT reported in patients taking these alkaloids include prolonged apnea, profound hypotension, cardiac dysrhythmias, and death.[18] These medications should be discontinued two weeks before ECT and another antihypertensive agent substituted if required.

Psychiatric patients on medications for coronary artery disease or hypertension should continue to receive their normal medical regimens. Withholding beta-blocking agents could precipitate ischemic episodes, particularly under the stress of ECT. Local application of nitroglycerin ointment has been used as a supplement to antihypertensive therapy during ECT.[11] It is usually applied 15–45 minutes prior to the treatment and remains on the patient through the recovery period. Blood pressure and heart rate must be monitored when using topical nitroglycerin in the ECT area. Most other oral noncardiovascular medications can be withheld without complications until recovery from the ECT treatment. After the recovery period, a patient can be given all his regular medications.

Preanesthetic Management

Patients undergoing their first ECT have a high level of fear and anxiety. Both the psychiatric staff and the anesthesiologist must be as reassuring as possible. The brief nature of the anesthesiologist's contact with the patient precludes discussion of the patient's psychiatric illness during the preanesthetic visit. Inquiries into psychotropic therapy are best directed to the psychiatrist.

Pretreatment sedation is usually not required and may unnecessarily prolong the recovery period. The psychiatric staff is instrumental in reassuring patients. If necessary, a small oral dose of diazepam may be given 1–2 hours prior to ECT.

Patients must be fasted for 8 hours before ECT. Psychiatric patients need supervision to ensure compliance. ECT should be scheduled early in the morning to minimize the chance of breaking this order and to allow the patient to maintain as normal a daily schedule as possible. Dehydrated elderly patients may require intravenous hydration several days prior to ECT.

An area of controversy exists regarding pretreatment with anticholinergic agents.[2,3] Atropine was originally part of most protocols. Patients on phenothiazines or tricyclic antidepressants already have peripheral and central anticholinergic activity from their medication. If they require a drying agent, glycopyrrolate is the drug of choice. Many centers have eliminated routine anticholinergic premedication, reserving it for intravenous use on an individual basis before induction of anesthesia.

Anesthetic Management

The primary goal of anesthesia for ECT is to prevent complications of the procedure itself and to alleviate the fear and discomfort of the patient. The anesthetic plan is for a rapid, pleasant induction of anesthesia with a short-acting barbiturate and muscle relaxant, adequate oxygenation, protection of teeth and tongue, and rapid post-ECT recovery of consciousness and spontaneous respiration. The anesthetic plan must keep to a minimum the use of drugs with known antagonistic effect on seizure activity.

Anesthetic Agents and Muscle Relaxants

Of the intravenous agents available, thiopental, a short-acting barbiturate, was used first. Methohexital, an ultra-short-acting barbiturate, has become the most commonly used owing to its rapid onset and recovery. Barbiturates also raise the seizure threshold and may decrease the duration of seizures. Diazepam has been suggested as an alternative. Like the barbiturates, diazepam increases seizure threshold and shortens duration of seizure activity. Reports of longer induction and recovery times, as well as recollection of apnea, should restrict the use of diazepam to patients in whom barbiturates are contraindicated.[19]

The muscle relaxant most commonly used to modify ECT is succinylcholine. The rapid onset of paralysis and quick recovery make it highly suitable for this short procedure. Postparalysis muscle pains are rarely reported by ECT patients. Thus, routine pretreatment with a small dose of a nondepolarizing relaxant is unnecessary. The recommended dose of succinylcholine, 0.5 mg/kg, is adequate to produce skeletal muscle paralysis of short duration.[2,20] Alternatives to succinylcholine, when this agent is contraindicated, are the shorter-acting nondepolarizing muscle relaxants atracurium and vecuronium. For these situations, reversal agents such as edrophonium and neostigmine must be available but should be used with caution in patients on antidepressant drugs with anticholinergic properties.

Monitoring

All patients undergoing ECT must have their heart rate, blood pressure, and ECG continuously monitored. During ECT in the anesthetized patient, there is minimal or absent physical manifestation of a generalized seizure. Thus, EEG monitoring is also mandatory, to show the magnitude and duration of a seizure. Assessing the degree of neuromuscular blockade is facilitated by use of a peripheral nerve stimulator, which assures that the ECT is applied at the peak effect of the muscle relaxant. A temperature monitor should also be available, as should pulse oximetry, and fetal monitoring should be available for pregnant patients.

ECT must be performed in an area equipped for the immediate support and resuscitation of the unconscious patient. Venous access must be established prior to ECT. Blood pressure, ECG, and EEG monitors are applied to the patient and baseline values are obtained. At this time anticholinergic agents may be given intravenously, if indicated. An oral airway soft bite block is placed prior to induction of anesthesia.

The induction of agent is given intravenously, and, as soon as the patient is anesthetized, it is followed by the muscle relaxant. When the patient becomes apneic, controlled ventilation with a mask and 100% oxygen is instituted.

At the peak of muscle relaxation, the psychiatrist applies the current to induce the seizure. EEG monitoring will show seizure activity. The blood pressure should be monitored every minute to assess the degree of hypertensive response and guide antihypertenisve therapy as needed. Controlled or assisted ventilation is continued with 100% oxygen until adequate spontaneous respiration returns. When there is good spontaneous breathing and stable blood pressure and ECG, the patient may be transferred to the recovery area.

Post-ECT Recovery Room Care

The patient's vital signs should be monitored for 30–60 minutes. If nitroglycerin ointment was used to prevent significant increases in blood pressure, the ointment must be removed at least 15 minutes prior to discharge and the blood pressure followed after its removal. Once the patient is awake and stable, he may be discharged to the psychiatric floor or home (in the care of a friend or relative).

The recovery room personnel must be trained to deal with the post-ECT patient. Some patients exhibit a great deal of confusion and agitation upon recovery from ECT. Others find the amnesia extremely discomforting. The memory loss rarely lasts more than 24 hours. Reassurance and attentiveness by the ECT-room psychiatric staff are important in patient acceptance of ECT.[22]

Complications

Complications from ECT are extremely rare, being reported as approximately 1 in 1700 cases.[1] Before the introduction of modified ECT, fracture of thoracic vertebrae or long bones was the most common complication; the use of neuromuscular blocking agents has eliminated this problem. More common are patient complaints of headaches, muscle aches, and pretreatment anxiety. The most troublesome side effect is that of memory disturbance. Rare complications consist of skin burns from current passage at sites of patient contact with conductive surfaces, lacerations of the tongue and oral mucosa, and damage to the eyes and teeth. These complications can be minimized by careful vigilance of the attending personnel and with the use of modern ECT apparatus.

Mortality from ECT is rare.[21] During the 1940s, it was reported as 0.06%. Most often the cause of death involved the cardiovascular system. The latest available data, from four large studies over a 15-year period, report no deaths directly attributable to ECT.[22]

Case reports of mortality from ECT must be carefully reviewed to assess the actual contribution of ECT to the death. Many patients suffer from coexistent diseases and a death occurring during ECT treatments may be erroneously attributed to ECT. Cardiac arrest can develop from the anesthetic technique as well as from high levels of anxiety.

Summary

Today ECT is considered an accepted mode of treatment for selected psychiatric patients, especially those with severe depression. Carefully planned and executed anesthetic and ECT techniques are the best safeguards against morbidity or mortality during this procedure. Thorough investigation of the patient's medical conditions and concurrent medications is mandatory to assure the patient a safe and effective treatment. Communication among the anesthesiologists, psychiatrists, medical consultants, and the nursing staff is the most important factor in preventing complications from ECT.

References

1. Holden C: A guarded endorsement for electroshock therapy. Science 1985;228:1510–11.
2. Gaines GY, Rees DI: Electroconvulsive therapy and anesthetic considerations. Anesth Analg 1986;65:1345–56.
3. Marks RJ: Electroconvulsive therapy: physiological and anaesthetic considerations. Can Anaesth Soc J 1984;31:541–48.
4. Maletzky BM: Multiple-Monitored Electroconvulsive Therapy. Boca Raton: CRC Press, 1981, pp 1–12.
5. Cerletti V, Bini L: Un nuovo metodo di shockterapia "L'electro-shock." Bull Acad Med Roma 1938;64:136–38.
6. Bennett AE: Prevention of traumatic complications in convulsive shock therapy by curare. JAMA 1940;114:322–25.
7. Holmberg AG, Thesleff S: Succinylkolin jodid som muskelavslappande medel via elektroshock behandling. S Nor Med 1951;46:1567–70.
8. Gravenstein JS, Anton AH, Weiner SM, et al: Catecholamine and cardiovascular response to electroconvulsive therapy in man. Br J Anaesth 1965;37:833–39.
9. Weiner RD: The persistence of electroconvulsive therapy-induced changes in the electroencephalogram. J Nerv Ment Dis 1980;168(4):224–28.
10. Husum B, Vester-Andersen T, Buchmann G, et al: Electroconvulsive therapy and intracranial aneurysm. Anaesthesia 1983;38:1205–7.
11. Lee JT, Erbguth PH, Stevens WC, et al: Modification of electroconvulsive therapy—induced hypertension with nitroglycerin ointment. Anesthesiology 1985;62:793–96.
12. Kalinowski LB: Convulsive Therapies, in H Kaplan, A Freedman, B Sadock (eds): Comprehensive Textbook of Psychiatry/III. Baltimre: Williams & Wilkins, 1980, pp 2335–42.

13. Hurwitz TD: Electroconvulsive therapy: a review. Compr Psychiatry 1974;15:303–14.
14. Levine R, Frost EAM: Arterial blood-gas analyses during electroconvulsive therapy in a parturient. Anesth Analg 1975;54:203–5.
15. Cascorbi HF: Perianesthetic Problems With Nonanesthetic Drugs, in SG Hershey (ed): ASA Refresher Courses in Anesthesiology. Philadelphia: JB Lippincott Co., 1978, pp 15–30.
16. Jephcott G, Kerry RJ: Lithium: an anaesthetic risk. Br J Anaesth 1974;46:389–90.
17. Hill GE, Wong KC, Hodges MR: Lithium carbonate and neuromuscular blocking agents. Anesthesiology 1977;46:122–26.
18. Foster MW Jr, Gayle RF Jr: Dangers in combining reserpine with electroconvulsive therapy. JAMA 1955;154:257–60.
19. Allen RE, Pitts FN Jr: Drug modification of ECT: methohexital and diazepam. Biol Psychiatry 1979;14:69–76.
20. Pitts FN Jr, Woodruff Jr, Craig AG, et al: The drug modification of ECT. II. Succinylcholine dosage. Arch Gen Psychiatry 1968;19:595–98.
21. Rich CL, Ty Smith N: Anaesthesia for electroconvulsive therapy: a psychiatric viewpoint. Can Anaesth Soc J 1981;28:153–57.
22. Selvin BL: Electroconvulsive therapy 1987. Anesthesiology 1987;67:367–85.

Chapter 12

The Lithotriptor Patient*

Cathy Wall Thomas

Case History. *An 8-year-old white boy was admitted with a history of recurrent bouts of urinary tract infections and right flank pain. There was a strong family history of renal calculi on his father's side and the boy himself had undergone extracorporeal shock-wave lithotripsy (ESWL) six months earlier. His mother reported that on that occasion, when she first saw him in the recovery room, he had a tube in his mouth and was connected to a breathing machine. The doctor told her that the boy had "lung problems." Although he had been scheduled for the procedure as an outpatient, he remained in the hospital four days. He has had no further respiratory difficulties. Anesthesia at the time of cystoscopy was uneventful. The patient is currently taking chlorothiazide.*

Physical examination: weight 33 kg; height 54"; blood pressure 100/70 mmHg; pulse 86/min and regular; chest clear. All chemical analyses were within normal limits.

The previous anesthetic record revealed that after induction with atropine 0.3 mg, thiopental sodium 225 mg, and succinylcholine 40 mg, the trachea was intubated and anesthesia was continued with halothane. After 55 minutes, the anesthesiologist noted frequent ectopic beats with periods of bigeminy and tachycardia of 150 bpm. Initial therapy with lidocaine and carotid sinus massage was ineffective. Edrophonium 3 mg was given intravenously twice and isoflurane was substituted for halothane. The heart rate decreased to 130 bpm and normal sinus rhythm returned.

In the recovery room, signs and symptoms were consistent with pulmonary edema. Furosemide 40 mg was given and respiration supported for 40 minutes. Thereafter, the trachea was extubated and the respiratory changes subsided over 24 hours.

---

* Reviewed by Dr. Robert W. Vaughan, Chairman and Professor, Department of Anesthesiology, School of Medicine, The University of North Carolina at Chapel Hill, North Carolina Memorial Hospital, Chapel Hill.

TABLE 12.1. Indications for and contraindications to extracorporeal shock-wave lithotripsy.

Indications for ESWL
Stones in kidney
Stone in ureter (above iliac bone)

Contraindications to ESWL
Absolute:
Obstruction distal to the calculus
Untreated urinary tract infection
Relative:
Large stone in kidney
(opinion varies, but usually > 3cm in size)
Large cystine stone
(>1-2cm; a cystine stone is less readily disintegrated)
Bleeding disorders
Approximate height of patient <4' or >6'6"
Approximate weight of patient >300 pounds
Impacted ureteral stone, usually of >6 weeks' duration
Pregnancy (undesirable radiation exposure)
Comorbidity
Aortic aneurysm
Hemangioma in the vertebral canal
Orthopedic implants in the lumbar region
Cardiac dysrhythmias and cardiac pacemakers

Adapted with permission of the publisher from Jantzen JA, et al: Management of urolithiasis. *Tex Med* 1986; 82:37–43

Introduction

Extracorporeal shock-wave lithotripsy (ESWL) is a relatively new non-surgical technique for the removal of calculi in the kidney or upper two thirds of the ureter.[1] It involves the disintegration of renal calculi by a shock wave into fragments small enough to be carried from the body via a patent urinary tract system. When applied to suitably selected candidates (see Table 12.1.), it is more than 80% effective. Thus, ESWL has gained acceptance rapidly, and the availability of both stationary and mobile units has increased. There are some unique considerations for the anesthesiologist, who must be familiar with the options.

For example, one must be mindful of the hemodynamic alterations associated with immersion into a water bath up to the clavicles. It is also necessary to consider the positioning and monitoring problems inherent in placing a patient in a semi-Fowler's position in a hydraulic chair support, separated several feet from the anesthesiologist by a stainless steel tube and its fluoroscopy exposure.

Incidence of Urinary Calculi

Urolithiasis is a common disease in industrial countries. Each year approximately half a million people are affected; 250,000 will require

TABLE 12.2. Contributors to stone formation.

Primary hyperparathyroidism
Genetic diseases, eg, cystinuria
Gout
Immobility, eg, spinal cord injuries
Diet—high calcium, low in fiber
Medications
Dehydration
Renal tubular acidosis
Primary hyperoxaluria
Geographical—"stone belts" (Great Lakes area, Southeast, southern California)

hospitalization at a cost of $400 a day, for a total cost of $140 million a year. While the majority of patients are admitted for pain control, 15% have stones that are too large to pass spontaneously and another 7% have complicated stones that are often associated with infection or congenital anomalies.

The incidence of stones is 2–3 times greater for white men than women, and this discrepancy increases with age. The occurrence of calculi is 3–4 times less for American blacks and even rarer among African blacks.[2] It should be remembered, however, that the presence of urinary calculi is merely a reflection of an underlying disorder (see Table 12.2.).

Extracorporeal Shock-Wave Lithotripsy

ESWL was first introduced in 1980 as a result of the collaboration of aerospace engineers and urologists in Munich, West Germany. It developed from a study investigating shock-wave damage to satellites struck by micrometeorites and supersonic aircraft struck by raindrops. The question arose whether such energy could be used to disintegrate renal calculi.[3] ESWL received FDA approval in the United States in December 1984, by which time it was estimated that over 10,000 patients worldwide had been treated by this technique, and that number now exceeds 500,000.

Technical Aspects

The shock wave utilized in ESWL is generated by the electrical discharge of 18–22 kV from a capacitor through an underwater electrode to produce a spark (see Figure 12.1.).[4] The spark vaporizes the water within the electrode gap, causing a pressure wave of high velocity and energy—the shock wave. Ths shock waves are collected and focused by a metal reflector beneath the electrode onto a circular area 2 cm in diameter, located 24 cm above the electrode at the second focus. Materials of a different consistency, such as a renal calculus, when positioned into the

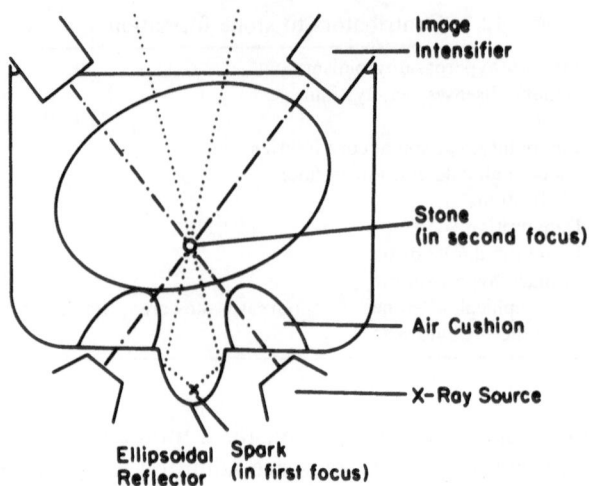

FIGURE 12.1. Cross-section of lithotriptor. (Reprinted with permission of Jantzen JA, et al: *Management of Urolithiasis*, Tex Med 1986; 82:37-43)

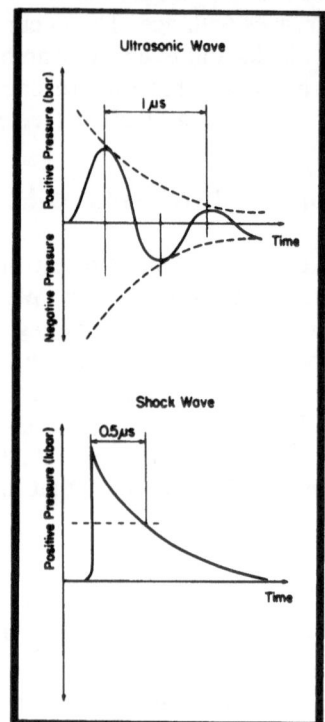

FIGURE 12.2. Characteristics of ultrasonic and shock waves. Note that there is no negative pressure phase in shock waves. (Reprinted with permission of Jantzen JA, et al: *Management of Urolithiasis*, Tex Med 1986; 82:37–43)

second focus absorb the shock wave energy. The change in acoustic impedance between the fluid medium and the solid-state stone causes shear and tear forces that destroy the stone.[3]

Frequently, the terms ultrasonic waves and shock waves are used interchangeably, but in fact these two energies have distinct and important differences. In contrast to ultrasonic waves, which have a sinusoidal pressure variation and a high frequency, shock waves have a single pressure spike and are a composite of both low and high frequencies (see Figure 12.2.).

In addition, biological tissue attenuates high frequencies more than low frequencies. Consequently, because shock waves are more powerful (1000×) and are of a mixed frequency, they can be generated outside the body and can be focused on a small area with less loss of power. Thus, shock waves have characteristics that make them uniquely suitable for their clinical application in ESWL as a noninvasive treatment.

Clinical Use

Biological tissue has the same acoustic density and properties as water. Thus, patients are immersed in a water bath because shock waves generated in water pass through biological tissue without change in acoustic impedance and therefore without tissue damage. If the shock wave strikes an air-containing tissue, however, a change in acoustic impedance occurs, which results in tissue destruction, particularly if it is localized in the second focus.[3] This can entail important considerations, especially for the lung and bowel. Shock waves should enter the body at an angle that ensures that the second focus is not closer than 4 cm to the lung tissue.[3]

It is more difficult to comply with such area restrictions in smaller patients. Therefore, the lower limit of the height specifications listed in Table 12.1. serves as a reminder not only of the increased difficulty of positioning children in the hydraulic support but also of the decreased margin of safety in avoiding air-containing structures.

The small stature of the patient in this case increases the likelihood of pulmonary injury from contact with the shock waves. Thus, positioning our patient for the repeat procedure is critical to avoid postoperative complications. In many institutions, shields (made of materials that impede shock waves) are placed on children to protect their lungs. Recently, attachment devices that facilitate positioning of these smaller patients have been introduced.

The second focal point remains stationary while the patient, immersed in a water bath, is moved by a hydraulic chair in order to position the stone. This precise aiming is accomplished by the use of two fluoroscopes set at right angles to each other, thereby yielding a three-dimensional localization of the stone.

The procedure usually takes about 45–60 minutes, depending upon the patient's heart rate (the R waves of the ECG trigger the shock wave) and the number of waves necessary to disintegrate the stone. The number of shock waves in turn depends upon the stone's size and its position and composition. Cystine stones, for instance, are less easily disintegrated than others.

In approximately 23% of cases, treatment is preceded by auxiliary cystoscopy and retrograde pyelogram or stent placement. At our institution, stents are routinely placed for stones larger than 1.5 cm in anticipation of the increased sand mass burden following ESWL, which can impede the successful spontaneous passage of the stone fragments.

Riehle and colleagues[5] include four indications for endoscopy: (1) delineation of distal ureteral anatomy; (2) manipulation of utereal stones retrograde; (3) better localization of poorly calcified or radiolucent renal calculi; (4) injection of contrast medium during ESWL to visualize ureteral or renal fragments.

Preoperative Plan

The preoperative evaluation should include a medical history, physical examination, electrocardiogram (ECG), intravenous pyelogram, chest x-ray, and hemoglobin, electrolyte, and coagulation studies.

Patient Selection

During the initial clinical trials of ESWL, patient selection criteria were stringent. Thus the first patients to undergo ESWL were primarily ASA I or II. However, as experience has been gained, more ASA III and IV patients have been treated. As a result, many contraindications (see Table 12.1.) have now been relegated to the relative-contraindication category.

For instance, cardiac pacemakers were once considered an absolute contraindication to ESWL because of the concern over mechanical failure caused by the shock wave discharge. Now, pacemaker patients are successfully treated with a team approach by the anesthesiologist, cardiologist, and urologist.[6] It is now more appropriate, therefore, to evaluate each patient individually, taking into account the specific medical history. It is important to remember that although ESWL is a safe technique, several complications have been associated with the procedure (see Table 12.3.).

Anesthetic Selection

Only one or two shock waves can be tolerated by an unanesthetized patient. Repeated bombardment of shock waves, averaging 800–1200 shocks per treatment, requires anesthesia. Local anesthesia is not adequate for the lithotriptor equipment commonly used today.

Regional Anesthesia

The renal tract innervation is T10 to L2. A sensory block from T6 to L2 segments provides adequate anesthesia without causing a high incidence of postural hypotension.[7] Occasionally, however, a level up to T5 may be necessary to block the pain sensation thought to be transmitted by the autonomic nervous system via the celiac plexus.[1]

At our institution we utilize regional anesthesia for most cases. General anesthesia is administered for those who refuse this technique or if contraindications to regional anesthesia exist.

Advantages of Regional Anesthesia:

● Monitoring during transportation to and from the lithotriptor is easier.
● The patient can assist with positioning and tell the operator of malpositions (see Table 12.3.).
● The combined effects of immersion and general anesthesia, which at this time are poorly understood and difficult to assess, are avoided.[1]
● Postoperatively, there is improved pain relief, especially if a catheter is maintained for postoperative analgesia; fewer constitutional disturbances; quicker recovery, which hastens ambulation and thereby fragment passage.

TABLE 12.3. Complications associated with the use of ESWL.

Fluid/air transition zone injury
  Pulmonary damage
  Abdominal viscera contusion
Mild hematuria
  Microscopic, after as few as 18 shocks*
  Macroscopic, after as few as 200 shocks
Cardiac arrhythmias
  Cardiac pacemaker patient
  Iatrogenically induced
Subcapsular/perinephric hematoma
  0.9% incidence by ultrasound and CT, greater incidence by magnetic resonance imaging (MRI)
Hemodynamic alterations
  Associated with water immersion
  Vasodilation iatrogenically induced by anesthetics or warm water
Infection
  Post-ESWL, 5% will develop an infection, 1.7% will develop urosepsis
Pain
  Colic
  Obstruction
Positioning
  Patient size—obesity; children; amputees
  Anatomic abnormalities—scoliosis; contractures; spinal fusion; hip joint replacement
  Result of malpositioning, eg, brachial plexus palsy
Hypothermia
  Allergic reaction, eg, to contrast medium

Disadvantages of Regional Anesthesia:

• A longer preparation time is required.
• Potential exists for the development of hypotension and possibly bradycardia. This is usually associated with a high level of blockade where both the cardiac and the peripheral sympathetic outflow are compromised. The compensatory changes, which prevent a fall in cardiac output when the patient is placed in a head-up position, are lessened.

General Anesthesia

General anesthesia requires intubation. Anesthesia may be maintained with a balance of a narcotic low-dose inhalational agent (such as fentanyl) and a muscle relaxant that is intermediate in duration.

General anesthesia is preferred by some because it is more predictable, patient acceptance is better, and the control of patient movement and respiratory excursion during treatment is more predictable.[8]

The use of high-frequency jet ventilation (HFJV) has become increasingly advocated. Compared to regional anesthesia or conventional ventilation, HFJV causes less diaphragmatic displacement, which in return minimizes abdominal movement and, consequently, renal stone movement. More-precise localization and fixation of the calculus in the focus of the incoming shock waves is probably more efficient—thus, the number of impulses is reduced, fewer electrodes for spark discharges are used, shock waves are of lower intensity, radiation-exposure time is decreased, and there is less trauma to adjacent organs.[9,10]

Although theoretically a reduction in stone movement should allow more efficient lithotripsy, we await the definitive study. In a comparison of techniques using conventional ventilation versus HFJV, there were no statistically significant differences with regard to the average number of shocks per treatment, the regression of stone burden on shock numbers, or the numbers of patients requiring fragment manipulation after ESWL.[12,13]

Intraoperative Considerations

Monitoring

Monitoring should include the modalities used with any general anesthetic, specifically, ECG (benzoin may be necessary to secure the patches to the skin); BP monitoring (preferably automated); a ventilator disconnect alarm; esophageal or precordial stethoscope; and oxygen monitor. Also highly recommended are pulse oximetry and capnography.[9] This suggestion is especially pertinent because of the factors that separate the anesthesiologist from the patient, such as the size of the tube or fluoroscope. Those patients at risk for congestive heart failure may require invasive monitoring such as arterial cannulation or pulmonary artery catheterization.

Intravenous Fluid

Intravenous fluid (500–1000 ml) may be given before the patient enters the bath, to compensate for postural hypotensive effects and to maintain a high urinary output to flush out stone fragments. Occasionally a diuretic agent may also be necessary.

Cardiovascular Effects

Dysrhythmias: Early in the use of ESWL, dysrhythmias triggered by the shock wave were observed in 80% of patients.[14] Extrasystolic beats have been decreased by programming from the ECG to deliver the shock wave 20 msec after the R wave. Thus, the shock waves strike at a time when the ventricles are refractory to stimulation. While this has significantly reduced the occurrence of premature ventricular contractions, dysrhythmias may still develop, especially when attempts are made to manually trigger the delivery of shock waves. Artifacts produced by electrode movement, defective wires, or signals from other electrical equipment (eg, a nerve stimulator) can also trigger the delivery of shock waves.[13]

Dysrhythmias may occur in healthy patients; premature supraventricular contractions have been reported in 10% of patients during ESWL.[15] These abnormalities may be caused by rapid changes in right atrial and ventricular wall tension associated with immersion or emersion. In addition, the mechanical energy associated with ESWL can induce reentrant atrial tachyarrhythmias, including paroxysmal supreventricular tachycardia (PSVT).[15] The tachycardia experienced by the patient in our case history during previous ESWL may have been due to either of these factors.

Treatment should initially include maneuvers or drugs to increase vagal tone or intravenous drugs to slow the heart rate, such as verapamil or the new short-acting beta blocker, esmolol. If unsuccessful, the possibility of applying DC cardioversion must be available. However, this introduces the necessity of removing the patient from the bath. Atropine should not be used, as it can also induce dysrhythmias.

Ventilatory and Hemodynamic Alterations: With the patient in the semisitting position in the hydraulic support, the right heart and arterial pressures may decrease secondary to venous pooling. At immersion, the arterial BP may initially further decrease, presumably secondary to vasodilation in the warm water bath, while an increase in hydrostatic pressure affects ventilation and hemodynamics. With continued immersion the BP increases. (See Tables 12.4. and 12.5.).

The hydrostatic pressure change displaces venous blood from the capacitance vessels in the abdomen and periphery and thereby increases the intrathoracic blood volume bv several hundred milliliters. There is, in

TABLE 12.4. Effects of immersion on Respiration and circulation.

		Respiration			Circulation
(−10%)	→	Vital capacity	(−10%)	→	Heart rate
(−30 to −60%)	→	Functional residual capacity	(+5%)	←	Systolic arterial blood pressure
(+15%)	←	Closing volume		↑	Diastolic arterial blood pressure
	→	Compliance	(+100%)	⇈	Central venous pressure
	←	Respiratory work	(+80%)	⇈	Pulmonary artery pressure
	←	Airway impedance	(+110%)	⇈	Pulmonary cap, wedge pressure
(−12 to −15%)	→	Maximum voluntary ventilation	(+50%)	→	Cardiac output, cardiac index
(−10%)	→	Diffusion capacity		←	Stroke volume
(+15%)	←	Alveolar arterial oxygen gradient (A_2PO_2)		→	Total peripheral resistance
	←	CO_2 response	(+50%)	←	Cardiac blood volume
(−5 to −10%)	→	PO_2	(+80%)	⇈	Pulmonary blood volume

BLE 12.5. Circulatory effects of immersion.

	Before immersion	Immersion 10min	Immersion 30min	Immersion 50min	After removal
\P (mmHg)	85.0	80.5	81.5	87.0	92.5
P (mmHg)	3.0	15.0	16.5	16.5	8.5
WP (mmHg)	6.5	16.5	16.0	17.5	10.0
L/min/m²	2.05	2.51	2.58	2.48	2.15

ɔrinted from Weber W, et al: Circulatory changes during anesthesia for extracorporeal shock-wave otripsy. *J Urol* 1984; 13:246A.

\P = mean atrial pressure; RAP = right atrial pressure; PCWP = pulmonary capillary wedge ssure; CI = cardiac index

turn, a reduction in functional residual capacity (FRC) by 30% and alteration in the ventilation-perfusion relationship. The work of breathing is increased by approximately 50%, which may destabilize small airways and increase the closing volume and the airway resistance.[1,16]

The redistribution of blood volume to the central compartment causes a 32%–50% increase in cardiac output and a 35% increase in stroke volume. Pulmonary capillary blood flow also increases. Right atrial and pulmonary capillary wedge pressures increase by about 10–13 mmHg.[16,17] Consequently, there is increased risk of adverse hemodynamic changes if the patient has a history of ischemic heart disease, valvular disease, or cardiomyopathy. Such patients may not be able to compensate for the increased preload associated with immersion and may develop heart failure.

Specific management should include: (1) a preoperative cardiac evaluation; (2) a slow rate of immersion and emersion to allow time to adapt to the changing preload; (3) fluid restriction; and (4) the pharmacologic manipulation of drugs with positive inotropic and peripheral vasodilator effect, to maintain cardiac output. Invasive monitoring, such as arterial and central venous cannulations, are indicated. Also because of the ventilatory changes encountered with immersion (see Table 12.4.), such patients are usually better managed under general anesthesia.

Hypothermia

Despite attempts to maintain the water bath at approximately 35°–37°C, patients lose heat. They must be dried thoroughly upon emersion, with ambient temperatures kept high enough to prevent shivering. The increased oxygen demand that otherwise may occur, combined with increased intrapulmonary shunting and respiratory depression due to residual anesthetic effect, may lead to hypoxia. These events may also precipitate myocardial ischemia in the susceptible patient, hence the need for perioperative administration of oxygen to all patients under regional or general anesthesia who are at risk for myocardial ischemia.

Postoperative Management

Pain during the first few postoperative hours is believed to be due to colic, sand mass obstruction, or bladder irritation by the urinary catheter. Most patients do not require any analgesics in the first 24 hours. Another 25%–30% of patients can be managed with oral pain medicines, and 12%–15% will require intramuscular narcotics, usually for less than 24 hours.

Though pain occurs with less frequency and severity after ESWL than following a surgical procedure, it is the most common postoperative complication of ESWL and is a major consideration when assessing these patients for ambulatory procedures. It is difficult to predict which patient is likely to suffer colic, and therefore oral pain medication should be made available to all.

Most patients begin to pass stone fragments within 12 hours of treatment. Increased levels of physical activity are associated with more-rapid and more-complete stone passage, and thus patients are encouraged to resume their normal activities.

On average, adjunctive endourological procedures are performed in approximately 13% of patients, including basket extraction, nephrostomy tube drainage, or percutaneous nephrolithotomy. Ten percent to 12% will require additional ESWL.[18]

The majority of sand mass is passed over an average of 3–4 weeks, at which time the patient is seen again for x-ray. In 3-month follow-up studies, 70%–80% were shown to be stone-free.[5,8] In approximately 20% of patients, residual fragments—most of which were small (less than 5 mm) and asymptomatic—remained. The longterm significance or potential risk of these fragments is not known, but it has been speculated that they may, in fact, serve as centers for further stone formation, depending upon the patient's metabolism.

Conclusion

ESWL can be the primary form of treatment for up to 80% of all patients with urinary calculi and is expected to become the preferred mode of treatment because of its effectiveness, lower morbidity, and potentially lower expense when compared to an invasive renal procedure. Thus, anesthetic involvement in yet another area outside the operating room will increase, and the anesthesiologist will be called upon frequently to administer safe anesthesia, given the unique considerations of ESWL.

References

1. Jantzen JA, Erdmann K, Wilbert DM, et al: Management of urolithiasis: an analysis of 1,293 lithotriptor procedures. Tex Med 1986;82:37–43.

2. Sarmina I, Spirnak JP, Resnick MI: Urinary lithiasis in the Black population: an epidemiological study and review of the literature. J Urol 1987;138:14–17.
3. Brendel W: Shock waves: a new physical principle in medicine. Eur Surg Res 1986;18(3–4):177–86.
4. Frank M, McAteer EJ, Cohen DG, et al: One hundred cases of anesthesia for extracorporeal shock wave lithotripsy. Ann R Coll Surg Engl 1985;67:341–3.
5. Riehle RA, Fair WR, Vaughan D: Extracorporeal shock-wave lithotripsy for upper urinary tract calculi. JAMA 1986;255:2043–48.
6. Lazica M, Gleibner J, Albert KF, et al: Experimental and clinical experience with pacemaker function during ESWL. The First International Symposium on Anesthesia and Extracorporeal Shock Wave Lithotripsy. Urologische Klinik, Klinikum Barmen, Wupertal, West Germany, June 1986.
7. Abbott MA, Samuel JR, Webb DR: Anesthesia for extracorporeal shock wave lithotripsy. Anesthesia 1985;40:1065–72.
8. Lingeman JE, Newman D, Mertz J, et al: Extracorporeal shock wave lithotripsy: The Methodist Hospital in Indiana experience. J Urol 1986;135:1134–37.
9. Carlson CA, Gravenstein JS, Banner MJ, et al: Monitoring techniques during anesthesia and HFJV for extracorporeal shock-wave lithotripsy. Anesthesiology 1985;63:A178.
0. Schulte J, Kochs E, Meyer WH: Improved efficiency of extracorporeal shock wave lithotripsy during high frequency jet ventilation. Anesthesiology 1985;63:A177.
1. Perel A, Hoffman B, Podeh D, et al: High frequency positive pressure ventilation during general anesthesia for extracorporeal shock wave lithotripsy. Anesth Analg 1986;65:1231–34.
2. Finlayson B, Thomas WC Jr: Extracorporeal shock-wave lithotripsy. Ann Intern Med 1984;101:387–89.
3. Gravenstein JS, Peter K: Extracorporeal shock wave lithotripsy for renal stone disease. In JS Gravenstein, K Peter (eds): Technical and Clinical Aspects. Boston: Butterworth, 1986, pp 78–86, 119–24.
4. Chaussy C, Schmeidt E, Jochman D, et al: Extracorporeal shock-wave lithotripsy for treatment of urolithiasis. Urology 1984;23:59–66.
5. Walts LF, Atlee JL: Supreventricular tachycardia associated with extracorporeal shock wave lithotripsy. Anesthesiology 1986;65:521–23.
6. Gissen D: Anesthesia for extracorporeal shock wave lithotripsy. Semin Anesth 1987;6(1):57–60.
7. Weber W, Chaussy C, Madler C, et al: Circulatory changes during anesthesia for extracorporeal shock-wave lithotripsy. J Urol 1984;13:246A.
8. Report of American Urological Association ad hoc committee to study the safety and clinical efficacy of current technology of percutaneous lithotripsy and non-invasive lithotripsy. Baltimore: American Urological Association, Inc., 1985.

CHAPTER 13

The Patient for Cervical Cerclage

Robert Rosenlund

Case History. *A 29-year-old woman, para 1041, was admitted from the prenatal center in the 13th week of gestation, with the diagnosis of incompetent cervix.*

Past gynecologic history included a normal spontaneous vaginal delivery 10 years ago, two elective terminations of pregnancy under general anesthesia, and two subsequent spontaneous abortions. During the first pregnancy, she had mild hypertension that was not treated.

This pregnancy was uncomplicated except for mild nausea and vomiting in the 2nd month. Weight gain was normal. The patient complained of mild dyspnea after climbing two flights of stairs. She denied back pain or other neuromuscular disorders, easy bruisability, or bleeding. The patient's last oral intake was breakfast 7 hours earlier.

Physical examination was normal; the chest was clear; there were no murmurs. Blood studies from the prenatal center included hematocrit 33%, platelets 220,000, and glucose 68 mg/dl.

The patient was scheduled for a McDonald procedure. During the preanesthesia assessment, she inquired as to which anesthetic technique had the least risk of affecting the baby.

Introduction

A cervical cerclage (circumferential suture around the cervix) is performed for cervical incompetence and is one of the most common surgical procedures undertaken in the pregnant woman. The operation presents two specific problems: first, the need for administration of anesthetic drugs at a time close to the period of maximal teratogenicity; and second, the risk of initiating premature labor and spontaneous abortion. Furthermore, attention should be paid to the maintenance of adequate utero-

---

Reviewed by Dr. Gertie F. Marx, Professor of Anesthesiology, Albert Einstein College of Medicine, Bronx, NY.

TABLE 13.1. Maternal causes for
habitual abortion

Hormonal abnormalities
Nutritional disorders
Infection
Blood group incompatibility
Psychiatric disorders
Uterine anatomic defects
Incompetent cervix

placental perfusion. Proper anesthetic management must involve a careful preoperative evaluation, knowledge of the physiology of pregnancy, and good rapport with the expectant mother.

Definition

Threatened abortion occurs in 1 of 4 to 5 pregnancies and is presumed when bloody discharge with or without cramping pain develops in the first 20 weeks of gestation. Approximately one half of these pregnancies terminate at this time.[1] The mean incidence of spontaneous abortion is 15%.

After three or more consecutive spontaneous abortions, the diagnosis of habitual abortion is made and a cause is sought. Spontaneous abortions occurring in the first few weeks are usually due to cytogenetic abnormalities. Those manifesting themselves during the second trimester are likely to be the result of maternal causes, as outlined in Table 13.1: hormonal abnormalities; severe nutritional disorders; infection such as mycoplasmosis, brucellosis, or toxoplasmosis; psychiatric disorders; uterine anatomic defects; and cervical incompetence.[1]

The diagnosis of cervical incompetence is made when evacuation of the uterine contents in the second trimester follows acute painless rupture of membranes not accompanied by bleeding or contractions. This sequence is often repeated in each pregnancy. Possible causes for incompetent cervix include previous cervical trauma, such as dilation and curettage or conization, and abnormal cervical development.[2]

In a pregnant woman with a history of habitual abortion in whom cervical incompetence is suspected, weekly cervical examinations are recommended. If significant dilation or effacement is noted on examination, cervical cerclage should be performed. Results are best if undertaken after the 12th week of pregnancy and before the cervix is 4 cm dilated. If uterine contractions or bleeding has occurred, cerclage is contraindicated, as it is when membranes are ruptured or chorioamnionitis is suspected.

Pathophysiology

Lash published in 1950 the first paper in the American literature that described a procedure, to be performed before conception, aimed at preventing habitual abortion.[3] Currently, two procedures are directed at treating an incompetent cervix, the McDonald and the Shirodkar procedures. The McDonald procedure, described in 1963, involves simple encirclement of the cervix with a minimum of sutures; it results in less trauma and a low incidence of scarring and dystocia.[4] Suture removal is easily performed electively at 37 weeks' gestation.

The Shirodkar suture, described in 1955, is the more complicated operation; it involves incision of the vaginal mucosa and advancement of the bladder.[5] A purse-string suture is then placed so as to close the upper part of the cervical canal. Removal is more difficult, and if the patient desires more children, the suture may be left in place and the baby delivered by cesarean section.

The diagnosis of cervical incompetence is usually made in an outpatient setting. The patient is admitted directly to the hospital for bed rest, possibly in a slightly head-down position, and placement of a cerclage on an urgent basis. Thus, frequently an anxious, unprepared patient is scheduled for emergency surgery.

Preanesthetic Considerations

Teratogenicity

The period of human organogenesis, from the 13th through the 60th postconceptual day, is the critical period in which a teratogenic agent can cause major congenital malformations or even embryonic demise. After the 8th week of gestation, organ growth begins. Fetuses exposed to teratogenic agents in this period can develop minor morphologic and/or functional malformations. Patients presenting for cerclage procedures belong to the second group, in which fetal organ growth has begun.

In animal experiments, all agents used in anesthesia have been shown to be teratogenic.[6] No investigation has as yet presented conclusive evidence linking exposure to anesthetic agents to human malformations.[6] Even more complicated is the relationship between the use of anesthetic agents and fetal death or abortion. Animal studies again have implicated inhalation anesthetics in an increased incidence of fetal loss, while retrospective reviews disagree as to whether a significant rise in premature termination of pregnancy occurs in gravidas undergoing surgery.[7-9] Therefore, spontaneous abortion may be attributed to surgical manipulation or to direct effects of the disorder for which surgery was performed. Because of the nature of surgery for incompetent cervix, the incidence of fetal loss is expectedly higher than in the gravida with a competent cervix who is not undergoing surgery.

Recently much attention has been paid to the use of nitrous oxide (N_2O) during the first two trimesters of pregnancy. In laboratory animals, N_2O irreversibly inactivates vitamin B_{12}, a cofactor for the enzyme methionine synthase.[10] This enzyme is necessary for the resynthesis of methionine and important in DNA formation. However, in humans, hematopoietic changes have been found only after prolonged (ie, greater than 5 hours) exposure.

In rats, N_2O increases fetal deformities after considerable exposure, but these changes can be prevented by pretreatment with folinic acid.[10] Pretreatment with folinic acid 30 mg prior to administration of N_2O during pregnancy, with a second dose 12 hours later, has been recommended.[11] However, enzyme inhibition of methionine synthase is much slower in humans, and no evidence of fetal abnormalities has been demonstrated in large retrospective studies. Also, cerclage is performed after the critical period of organogenesis, and the exposure time is limited to less than 2 hours, the critical level under which no human effects have been seen.

A recent review of 375 cases of cerclage under general anesthesia revealed no neonatal abnormalities that could be attributed to N_2O.[12] Also, there was no difference in the incidence of abortion between these patients and 96 cases of cerclage performed under regional block. Therefore, it appears that N_2O is safe to use for cerclage procedures, and pretreatment with folinic acid is now regarded as probably unnecessary.

Halothane has been shown to be teratogenic in rats and to increase the number of abortions in hamsters, but no such effects have been recorded in humans.[6] Therefore, its use is justified during cerclage surgery.

Benzodiazepines should be avoided because of suspicion linking their use during early pregnancy with the development of cleft lip or cleft palate.[13,14]

Uterine Activity

Cerclage is performed only when there is no evidence of contractions. Every effort should be made to avoid stimulating the uterus in the perioperative period to limit the incidence of premature labor and to allow the fetal membranes to recede from the cervical canal into the uterus. A beneficial maneuver includes positioning the patient in a slightly head-down position both pre- and postoperatively. Ketamine is not recommended, since it produces a dose-related increase in uterine resting tone. In contrast, halogenated agents may be of advantage because of their potential for relaxing the uterus.

Uteroplacental Perfusion

As the placental vessels are normally maximally dilated, uterine blood flow is mainly determined by the perfusion pressure. During anesthesia, therefore, any changes limiting the perfusion pressure should be prevented. These include maternal hypotension during regional or general anesthesia, as well as the use of alpha-adrenergic agents such as methoxamine and phenylephrine. Ephedrine remains the drug of choice in treating maternal hypotension. Hyperventilation and hypocarbia cause uterine vascular constriction and should be avoided. Aortocaval compression is first encountered after 24 weeks' gestation and thus is not problematic.

Aspiration Prophylaxis

As the enlarging uterus rises out of the pelvis, abdominal contents are increasingly compressed, and intragastric pressure rises. This effect begins at about 20–24 weeks. Gastric emptying is significantly delayed after 34 weeks. Since cerclages are performed on an urgent rather than emergent basis, it is prudent to wait 6–8 hours after the last ingestion of food before administering anesthesia. Under these circumstances, the patient in early pregnancy is probably not at higher risk for aspiration than a nonpregnant patient would be. Weighing the disastrous effects of aspiration against the relatively harmless nature of antacid prophylaxis, ranitidine and intubation with cricoid pressure should be routine.

Preanesthetic Assessment

Troubled by past fetal losses and faced with the prospect of unexpected urgent surgery, the gravida confronting a cerclage procedure is most often extremely anxious. A thorough evaluation carried out in a relaxed and compassionate manner is a necessity. A history of multiple spontaneous abortions requires a thorough medical evaluation, including nutritional assessment and thyroid function assays. Past surgical, gynecologic, and anesthetic history must be taken, with special inquiry about terminations of pregnancy, dilation and curettage procedures, and conization.

Particular attention must be paid to the cardiac system and the presence of any new murmurs or dyspnea, as cardiac output begins to increase at about 8–10 weeks of gestation and valvular lesions become detectable. One must search for the presence of infections such as hepatitis, herpes, or AIDS for protection of mother and personnel.

The last food intake should be determined. Only minimal laboratory work is necessary, consisting of hemoglobin or hematocrit determinations and blood glucose level. The concentration of glucose should be maintained between 90 and 120 mg/dl, as evidence links maternal hypoglycemia with fetal abnormalities.[15]

Chest x-ray is unwarranted if no previous pulmonary pathology is suspected.

Anesthetic Plan

There is no single correct method of anesthesia for a cerclage procedure. Rather, the choice of anesthetic is based on the preoperative assessment and any significant findings made therein. The preference of the mother should be considered.

Regional Anesthesia

Regional anesthesia is most frequently employed because it avoids use of multiple systemic medication during the period of possible development of minor morphologic or physiologic abnormalities. Only one agent is necessary if a local anesthetic of the ester group is chosen; the concentration reaching the fetal circulation is negligible. Also, the risk of regurgitation and aspiration is negated.

Hypotension, a potential problem, is mostly preventable by adequate prehydration with approximately 20 ml/kg of an electrolyte-containing solution. Should hypotension develop, circulating blood volume can be improved by placing the patient in the lithotomy position; circulation to the brain can be improved by using a steeper Trendelenburg position.

Spinal or Epidural Block

The sympathomimetic agent of choice is ephedrine because it does not appear to decrease uterine perfusion while increasing blood pressure. Either spinal or epidural block can be chosen.

Spinal anesthesia to a T10 level has the advantage of requiring minimal dosages, and it exposes the fetus to the least amount of pharmacologic agents. The intrathecal dose may already be slightly reduced toward the end of the first trimester, but not to the extent that it is at term. No definitive recommendations have been made as to the dose requirements in early pregnancy.

Hyperbaric tetracaine 6–8 mg, in the sitting position, is usually adequate to achieve a level to T10. Because the level achieved by subarachnoid block is somewhat variable, some recommend choosing epidural anesthesia for cerclage.[16] The optimal agent is chloroprocaine 3%, an ester-type drug with rapid metabolism; an initial dose of 10 ml can be given with the patient in the sitting position and can be supplemented if analgesia is inadequate.

Epidural anesthesia with insertion of a catheter has the advantage of postoperative pain relief and improved comfort for the patient, who usually remains in bed for 24 hours.[17] In addition, the problem of postdural puncture headache is avoided. One disadvantage of epidural anesthesia is that it takes slightly longer to place. In a patient with cervical incompetence, prolonged sitting may cause the membranes to bulge and could theoretically precipitate rupture, although this has not been described.

General Anesthesia

General anesthesia should be considered: (1) if the patient, aware of her options, requests this technique and there is no contraindication; (2) if there is a contraindication to regional anesthesia; and (3) if membrane rupture appears imminent and the sitting position is deemed undesirable.

In choosing agents for general anesthesia, one should rely on those with a long history of proven safety, such as sodium thiopental, meperidine, curare, succinylcholine, and the halogenated inhalational agents. The newer agents such as the recently introduced narcotics and muscle relaxants should be avoided. Nitrous oxide may be used, and pretreatment with folinic acid can be withheld at the discretion of the anesthesiologist.

To prevent regurgitation and pulmonary inhalation of gastric contents, all women undergoing general anesthesia for cerclage should be intubated, with Sellick's maneuver applied until placement of the endotracheal tube is verified and the cuff has been inflated. Hyperventilation is to be avoided to maintain uteroplacental perfusion.

Summary

The patient with cervical incompetence presents certain unique problems for the anesthesiologist. As cerclage is one of the procedures most frequently performed on pregnant women, the anesthesiologist should be well acquainted with the anesthetic requirements. The final choice of anesthetic method depends on the preoperative findings, the stage of gestation, the level of anxiety of the patient, the degree of cervical incompetence, and patient preference. No single technique is to be recommended for all patients; rather, the choice of anesthetic must be tailored specifically to each patient.

References

1. Pritchard JA, MacDonald PC, Gant NF: Williams Obstetrics, 175th ed. Norwalk, Conn, Appleton Century Crofts, 1987; pp 472–77.
2. Cousins L: Cervical incompetence 1980: a time for reappraisal. Clin Obstet Gynecol 1980;23(2):467–77.
3. Lash AF, Lash SR: Habitual abortion: the incompetent internal os of the cervix. Am J Obstet Gynecol 1950;59:68–76.
4. McDonald IA: Incompetent cervix as a cause of recurrent abortion. J Obstet Gynecol British Commonwealth 1963;70:105.

5. Shirodkar VN: A new method of operative treatment for habitual abortion in the second trimester of pregnancy. Antiseptic 1955;52:299.
6. Pedersen H, Finster M: Anesthesia for surgery during pregnancy, in James FM, Wheeler A (eds): Obstetric Anesthesia: The Complicated Patient. Philadelphia, FA Davis Co, 1982; pp 333–46.
7. Levine W, Diamond B: Surgical procedures during pregnancy. Am J Obstet Gynecol 1962;81:1046–51.
8. Smith BE: Fetal prognosis after anesthetic during gestation. Anesth Analg 1963;42:521–26.
9. Shnider SM, Webster GM: Maternal and fetal hazards of surgery during pregnancy. Am J Obstet Gynecol 1965;92:891–900.
10. Ninn JF: Clinical aspects of the interaction between nitrous oxide and vitamin B_{12}. Br J Anaesth 1987;59:3–13.
11. Keeling PA, et al: Folinic acid protection against nitrous oxide: teratogenicity in the rat. Br J Anaesth 1986;58:528.
12. Crawford JS, Lewis M: Nitrous oxide in early human pregnancy. Anaesthesia 1986;41:900–5.
13. Saxen I, Saxen L: Association between maternal intake of diazepam and oral clefts. Lancet 1975;2:498.
14. Safra MJ, Oakley GP: Association between cleft lip with or without cleft palate and prenatal exposure to diazepam. Lancet 1975;2:478.
15. Hannah RS, Moore KL: Effects of fasting and insulin on skeletal development in rats. Teratology 1971;4:135–40.
16. Albright GA, et al: Anesthesia in Obstetrics; Maternal, Fetal and Neonatal Aspects. Boston, Butterworth, 1986; pp 490–501.
17. Crawford JS: Obstetric Analgesia and Anaesthesia. New York, Churchill Livingstone, 1984; p 133.

CHAPTER 14

The Patient with an Intracranial Tumor

Efrem Miller

Case History. *A 49-year-old right-handed man came to the hospital complaining of right-sided weakness and dysphagia. There were no sensory changes and no weight loss. He gave a long history of hypertension. Past surgical history was significant for left thoracotomy and upper lobectomy for carcinoma 1 year previously. Medications consisted of hydrochlorothiazide, dexamethasone, cimetidine, and acetaminophen. He had no allergies and had smoked two packs of cigarettes daily for 30 years. He had continued to smoke since his surgery last year.*

Physical examination revealed a well-developed male with a mild right facial palsy; blood pressure was 130/70 mmHg; pulse, 80/min; respiratory rate, 12/min; height, 5ft 8in; weight, 176 lb. Examination results for the heart and lungs were normal. Neurologic examination showed 4/5 hemiparesis, no sensory deficits, and brisk reflexes with no clonus on the right side.

Laboratory data: hematocrit, 42%; SMA-12, normal; ECG, nonspecific ST-, T-wave changes; chest x-ray, inflation of the left upper lung fields, surgical clips noted. CT scan showed a left frontal ring enhancing lesion with much surrounding edema and mass effect. He was scheduled for left frontoparietal craniotomy.

Introduction

The frequency of intracranial tumors is estimated to be about 5 per 100,000 population. Almost 10% of all benign and malignant tumors requiring hospitalization for surgical removal are intracranial. They account for just under 1% of deaths from all causes.[1] Primary tumors occur most often in patients between 40 and 60 years of age. Seventy percent arise in the middle or anterior fossa (ie, supratentorial).

Reviewed by Dr. Paul Kornblith, Professor and Chairman Department of Neurosurgery Albert Einstein College of Medicine, Bronx, NY.

Classification

Glioblastoma is a highly malignant and infiltrative intracranial tumor most often arising in a cerebral hemisphere and surrounded by cerebral edema. The prognosis is poor, the average survival being less than 6 months after diagnosis.

Astrocytoma begins as a slowly growing lesion in a cerebral hemisphere, leading to symptoms of intracranial hypertension. These tumors are more frequent in children than in adults and tend to recur following excision. They do not metastasize to distant sites.

Medulloblastoma arises most commonly in the cerebellum in children. Combination therapy with surgical excision, radiation, and chemotherapy has improved survival.

Meningioma is a slowly growing, benign, highly vascular tumor that often infiltrates the skull. It is most frequently found in middle-aged women. Treatment is surgical excision, and prognosis is good. However, as total extirpation is often impossible, the tumor may recur.

Pituitary adenoma: Eighty percent of pituitary adenomas can be classified as chromophobe adenomas, which rarely secrete hormones. These tumors result in panhypopituitarism. Suprasellar expansion produces bitemporal hemianopia due to compression of the optic chiasm. Surgical excision and radiotherapy are the most common modalities of treatment.

Acoustic neuroma is a benign neurofibroma of the eighth cranial nerve. The tumor produces progressive unilateral deafness and ataxia as it exerts pressure on the cerebellum. Prognosis is good following surgical excision.

Metastatic intracranial tumors are not uncommon, the lung and breast being the most common primary sites. Other common primary neoplasms associated with intracranial metastases are melanomas, renal cell carcinoma, and intestinal carcinoma. Excision of accessible intracranial metastases can reduce symptoms and prolong life. Frequently these tumors are well demarcated, and removal is relatively simple.

Clinical Presentation

Signs and symptoms of intracranial tumors are most commonly related to raised intracranial pressure (ICP). Classic symptoms are headache, nausea, vomiting, and mental changes progressing to disturbances of consciousness. Characteristically, the patient has a headache on awaking, presumably due to hypercarbia during sleep and decreased venous drainage in the supine position. This improves as the patient ambulates, only to recur the next morning. Papilledema and abducens paralysis can contribute to visual disturbances. As ICP rises, systemic hypertension develops in an attempt to maintain cerebral perfusion pressure (CPP).

Compression, invasion, and altered blood supply may affect neuronal excitability, causing generalized or focal seizures. Direct local tissue destruction may produce progressive focal neurologic deficits, which are usually partial rather than complete. With a parietal lesion, hemiparesis develops, rather than hemiplegia, and partial rather than total sensory deficit occurs.

Mental and behavioral changes predominate in patients with neoplasm in the frontal cortex. Perineoplastic vasogenic cerebral edema may contribute to loss of neurologic function. This is probably due to altered capillary permeability, hence giving the impression that the tumor is larger than its actual size.

A further mechanism for the production of symptoms is displacement of brain and compression of tissue at distant sites. Herniation of the uncus of the temporal lobe through the incisura of the tentorium can lead to oculomotor paralysis. Midbrain compression causes apnea and unconsciousness. Contralateral hemiplegia is due to compression of the cerebral peduncle. Posterior fossa tumors obstruct normal cerebrospinal fluid (CSF) drainage, and herniation of the cerebellar tonsils through the foramen magnum manifests as decreased consciousness and a slowed respiratory rate.

Diagnosis is aided by isotope brain scan, magnetic resonance imaging (MRI), CT scanning, radiography of the skull, angiography, pneumoencephalography (rarely required nowadays), and electroencephalography.

Intracranial Dynamics

The cranium may be regarded as a partly closed, nondistensible box. The contents include brain matter, which represents 80%–85% of intracranial contents (1000–1200 gm); CSF, which comprises 8%–12% (120–150 ml); and blood in the intracranial vessels, which constitutes 3%–7% (75–100 ml).[2] The total volume of these factors is constant, and an increase in one necessitates a decrease in another to prevent an increase in ICP (Monro-Kellie doctrine).

As an intracranial tumor surrounded by edema expands, well-defined events result. Compensation for increased brain bulk is initially via translocation of CSF from the cranium to the distensible spinal space through the foramen magnum. Increased venous reabsorption is an additional route of compensation.[3] Normal ICP is 10 mmHg; moderate elevation is 20 mmHg; severe intracranial hypertension is 35 mmHg. Ordinarily, CSF production is independent of ICP and ranges between 0.3 and 0.35 ml/min. The total CSF volume is exchanged three times a day. Once CSF volume accommodation is exceeded, ICP begins to rise.

There is some further compensation by reduction of cerebral blood volume (CBV) as a result of compression of the venous system or capillary collapse leading to cerebral ischemia. However, the collapsed draining veins impede venous return, which further increases ICP.

The relation of incremental increases of volume to resultant alteration of ICP is depicted in Figure 14.1. This curve was generated by gradually expanding a balloon in the supratentorial cavity.[4] Points 1–2 represent the compensatory capabilities of the system. Points 2–3 represent exhaustion of the compensatory mechanisms. Between points 2 and 3, the classical signs and symptoms of intracranial hypertension, including nausea, vomiting, headache, decreased mentation, and papilledema, are manifest.

Any patient with a lesion larger than 100 ml is at risk of intracranial hypertension if stressed. The significance of the compliance curve shown in Figure 14.1 is that appropriate selection of anesthetic technique, drugs, and monitoring can favorably affect the system dynamics, an effect that is more apparent than with any other system in the body.

The significance of controlling and decreasing the level of ICP is to maintain CPP (CPP = MAP − ICP, ie, mean arterial pressure minus intracranial pressure). The critical level of CPP is about 50 mmHg. Ideally, it should be about 70-100 mmHg. The cardiovascular response to a decreased perfusion pressure is a rise in systemic pressure. Once hypertension exceeds cerebral blood flow (CBF) autoregulation, or if autoregulation is impaired, the progressive increase in CBV will further increase ICP, thereby decreasing CPP. The increased ICP will lead to ischemia as well as potentially dangerous brain shifts and possible herniation.

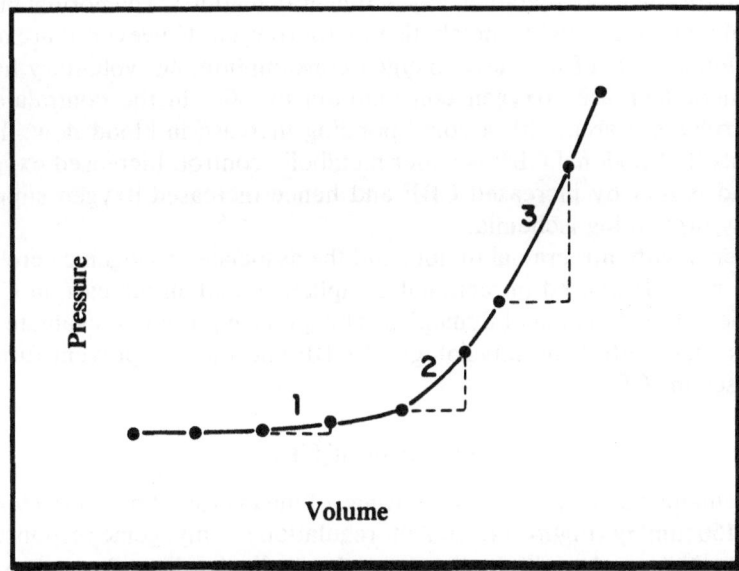

FIGURE 14.1. Intracranial pressure-volume curve. (1) On the flat portion of the curve an increase in volume causes little change in pressure. (2) Later, small increases in volume produce a rise in ICP. (3) Compensatory mechanisms exhausted with large pressure increases are associated with added volume.

A manifestation of autoregulation occasionally seen is Lundberg's plateau, or A waves.[5] They are characterized by a sudden increase in ICP to 80–100 mmHg, which lasts for 10–20 min. Following the wave, ICP rapidly decreases to below baseline. Plateau waves coincide with increases in regional CBV and paradoxical decreases in CBF. It has been hypothesized that plateau waves are set off by a stimulus to vasodilatation or by nonspecific stimuli such as pain, aroused mental activity, hypoventilation, or hyperventilation. As patients are already on the steep ascending limb of the elastance curve, it is postulated that vasodilatation rapidly increases ICP, with obstruction of venous drainage resulting in the combination of increased CBV and decreased CBF[5].

As the pathophysiologic process of intracranial hypertension nears the terminal stages, progressively more areas of the brain become ischemic. The number of areas of nonautoregulating brain and cerebrovascular paralysis increases, which may manifest as Cushing's triad—intracranial hypertension, systemic arterial hypertension, and reflex bradycardia.

Physiology of Cerebral Blood Flow

About 20% of the cardiac output is directed to the brain, which accounts for only 2% of body weight. Overall CBF is about 50 ml/100 gm/min globally and ranges from 20 ml/100 gm/min for white matter to 80 ml/100 gm/min for the more metabolically active gray matter.[12] The normal brain has a globally high, stable metabolic rate for oxygen. However, there may be regional areas of increased oxygen consumption; eg, voluntary hand movement increases oxygen consumption by 30% in the contralateral hand (rolandic) area with a corresponding increase in blood flow. This suggests that regional CBF is under metabolic control. Increased oxygen demand is met by increased CBF and hence increased oxygen supply, thereby preventing ischemia.

Patients with intracranial tumors and the associated vasogenic cerebral edema have decreased intracranial compliance, and an increase in CBV could lead to worsening of dynamics. Thus, it is important to evaluate the factors that control the physiology of CBF and thereby prevent further increases in ICP.

Regulation of CBF

CBF remains constant over a wide range of mean arterial pressure (MAP) at 50–150 mmHg (Figure 14.2.). Autoregulation is a myogenic response of the smooth muscle cells in the arteriolar wall. As distending pressure increases, vasoconstriction occurs. At lower levels of MAP the response is one of vasodilatation. Perivascular sympathetic innervation modifies the response by about 5%–10%, explaining a slight rightward shift of the curve in hypertensive patients. Below the lower limit of autoregulation, CBF decreases, and symptoms of cerebral ischemia appear in the form of dizziness, slow cerebration, and eventually syncope. Above the level of autoregulation, the constrictor response is overcome with an increase in CBF.

ICP Monitoring

Intracranial pressure is measured by the epidural, subdural, or intraventricular route.[6] Each method has advantages and limitations. Use in the appropriate clinical condition can yield valuable information and allow calculation of CPP.

Epidural Pressure Monitoring

Epidural monitoring is performed either by placing a transducer directly in contact with the dural surface or by pressure sensor implantation and telemetric recording.[7] The principal advantage is the avoidance of ventricular puncture. However, values obtained by epidural recording are commonly higher than those obtained from the ventricles, and the divergence increases as ICP increases. The usefulness of epidural pressure monitoring is that trends are more easily documented.

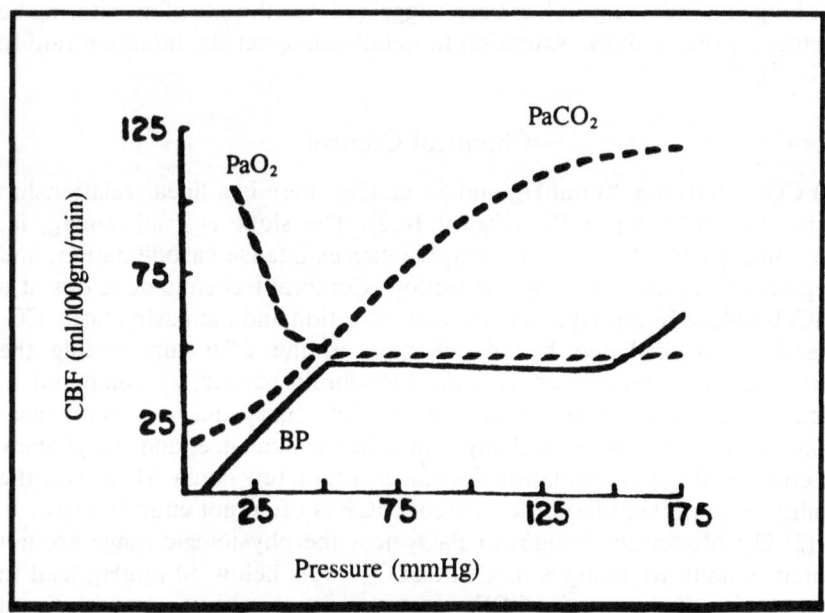

FIGURE 14.2. Schematic control of cerebral blood flow.

Subdural Pressure Monitoring

A burr hole is performed just anterior to the coronal suture and 5 cm from the midline. A hollow screw is then inserted into the subdural space.[8] The disadvantages of this system include dampening of the waveform and frequent clogging of the tubing, especially after severe brain contusion when ICP is raised.

Ventricular Pressure Monitoring

The advantage of ventricular puncture is easy removal of CSF, which reduces ICP promptly and hence improves CPP.[9] The success of ventricular puncture is increased by using CT scanning to localize and determine the size of the ventricles. If the lateral ventricles are collapsed, then subdural monitoring is performed, as ventricular pressure monitoring is not technically possible. If the ventricles are visualized, the contralateral displaced ventricle is catheterized. The catheter is connected to a strain-gauge pressure transducer via fluid-filled plastic tubing. Ventricular catheterization makes it possible to compute cerebral compliance, CSF production, and outflow resistance by injecting or withdrawing small amounts of fluid.[10]

The major potential risks of ventricular pressure monitoring relate to intracranial hemorrhage and infection. Infection can be minimized by attention to sterile technique at the time of insertion and by avoidance of prolonged monitoring. It has been suggested that the site of monitoring be changed every 3 days. Attention to detail can lower the infection rate to 1%–3%.[11]

Chemical Control

(1) CO_2: Between 20 mmHg and 80 mmHg there is a linear relationship between $PaCO_2$ and CBF (Figure 14.2). The slope is 2 ml/mmHg, ie, 4%/mmHg CO_2 change. Hypercapnia causes intense vasodilatation, and hypocapnia results in vasoconstriction. Cerebral ischemia develops at a $PaCO_2$ below 20 mmHg, causing vasodilatation and increasing flow. CO_2 reactivity is mediated by pH changes in the CSF surrounding the arterioles. CO_2 readily crosses the bloodbrain barrier, as compared to bicarbonate, which moves more slowly. Pulmonary and renal compensation follow in response to changes in acid-base balance, and the efficacy of controlled hyperventilation decreases after a few hours. However, the ability of hyperventilation to decrease ICP is often not entirely lost.

(2) O_2: Moderate changes in PaO_2 near the physiologic range are not potent stimuli to changes in CBF. PaO_2 levels below 50 mmHg lead to progressive increases in CBF. At these levels there is a significant increase in glucose uptake, with a 16% reduction in aerobic metabolism

and a 14% increase in anaerobic metabolism.[13] This is the probable stimulus to increasing CBF.

Intracranial Pressure

A rise in ICP decreases CPP in a similar manner to a decrease in MAP and results in compensatory vasodilatation. However, patients with intracranial hypertension have increased cerebrovascular resistance.[14] Hemodynamic responses are further complicated by a compensatory increase in MAP. There is usually little change in CBF until ICP reaches 35 mmHg, although autoregulation may be impaired at lower levels of ICP.

Preanesthetic Management

Knowledge of preexisting disease or system malfunction will aid planning and appropriate decision making to ensure a smooth anesthetic and postoperative course. Intracranial hypertension is recognized by the classic signs and symptoms of nausea, vomiting, altered sensorium, mydriasis, hypertension, and (in the late stages) bradycardia, papilledema, and disturbances in respiratory pattern. Evidence of a midline shift on CT scanning or obliteration of the lateral ventricles is confirmatory evidence of raised intracranial pressure.

Patients with brain tumors may present with various ECG changes that are possibly due to increased sympathetic tone. The most common ECG changes are tachycardia, prolonged QT interval, large U waves, and T- and ST-wave changes.[15] Preexisting cardiac disease should be optimized, recognizing that patients with the highest risk are those with evidence of left ventricular failure and those with a history suggesting myocardial ischemia. Hypertensive patients have a shift to the right in the cerebral autoregulatory curve, with a higher lower limit for adequate cerebral perfusion and decreased tolerance to hypotensive episodes.

A history of pulmonary dysfunction or heavy cigarette smoking may necessitate pulmonary function testing, especially if the intracranial tumor represents metastasis, most commonly from the lung. The patient may have had a lobectomy, further decreasing pulmonary reserve. A previous history of radiation therapy for breast carcinoma may have caused lung damage and fibrosis.

Tests for serum electrolytes, blood urea nitrogen (BUN), and creatinine are useful for assessing renal function, state of hydration, and any water and electrolyte imbalance that may be present in neurosurgical patients. The picture may be complicated by high-dose steroid administration, a therapy often employed to decrease the edema surrounding a tumor.

Patients with pituitary tumors may have increased ACTH secretion. The resultant Cushing's disease has classic morphologic changes and is associated with a hypokalemic alkalosis and elevated serum glucose levels. Panhypopituitarism is associated with diabetes insipidus and hypernatremia. Hepatic dysfunction is rarely a source of neurosurgical morbidity with the not infrequent exception of coagulopathies. A preoperative coagulation profile is required and preoperative correction made if necessary. A thorough assessment of the airway must be performed, especially in the acromegalic patient with macroglossia and a large epiglottis.

Many medications interact with anesthetic agents. Thorough knowledge of possible drug interactions is important. Most neurosurgeons electively treat patients undergoing supratentorial intracranial surgery with prophylactic phenytoin. Hyperglycemia and glycosuria may develop from phenytoin induced inhibition of insulin secretion.

Most neurosurgical patients requiring intraoperative brain manipulation are given steroids to minimize postoperative edema formation. The drug of choice is usually dexamethasone, which is started either preoperatively if there is evidence of raised ICP or the night before surgery. It is continued throughout the perioperative period. Steroid administration leads to an increase in intravascular volume resulting in hypertension and hyperglycemia.

Hyperglycemia can be potentially harmful, with a poor outcome in the neurosurgical patient if incomplete ischemia develops as a result of hypotension, intracranial hypertension, hypoxia, or excessive brain retraction.[16] The most accepted hypothesis is that in the presence of ischemia, the oxidative metabolism of glucose fails, and glycolysis, which has lactate as the end product, increases; this leads to a decrease in tissue pH, triggering the biochemical chain of events leading to cell death.

There is a direct association between cerebral malignancies and thromboembolic complications (TEC).[17] Patients with suprasellar tumors have a higher incidence of TEC than those with tumors in other locations, suggesting that the tumor interferes with the hypothalamopituitary axis as a "center" for the control of blood coagulation. In a retrospective study, TEC occurred frequently in young, fully ambulatory, nonparetic patients. Meningiomas and glioblastomas have also been associated with TEC. In one study, 66% of patients with meningiomas had deep venous thrombosis in their calves postoperatively, detected prospectively by ^{125}I fibrinogen scans. Production of procoagulants by brain tumors has been demonstrated, and some tumors contain substances capable of inhibiting the fibrinolytic enzyme system.[18]

Prophylactic measures, including early ambulation, leg wrapping, and possibly intraoperative electrical stimulation of the leg muscles, should be actively sought for patients undergoing craniotomy for tumors. The use of heparin prophylaxis is controversial when intracranial surgery is contemplated.[19]

Thrombocytopenia and disseminated intravascular coagulopathy have also been identified preoperatively in patients with malignancies. Platelet transfusion and possibly heparin therapy are indicated before surgical extirpation.[20] Thus, careful hematologic evaluation is essential in all patients with brain lesions.

Recently, interleukin 2 (IL2) and lymphokine-activated killer (LAK) cells have been used in the treatment of malignant gliomas.[21] Lymphocytes from the patient's blood are cultured with IL2 over 72 hours. LAK cells with the capacity to lyse autologous and allogenic glioblastoma are produced. During craniotomy as much as possible of the tumor is removed and the cells are injected into the tumor bed. Unlike the profound toxic effects experienced when IL2 is given intravenously,[22] early observations following LAK-cell placement indicate that it is a safe technique. However, if brain compliance is severely reduced, instillation of an 8–10 ml volume may cause brain herniation.

Other techniques in the treatment of brain tumors have involved therapeutic disruption of the blood-brain barrier. Under general anesthesia, mannitol in a flow sufficient to totally replace internal carotid or vertebral flow for 20–30 sec is injected intraarterially.[23] After the verification of disruption by intravenous injection of a radionucleotide, methotrexate is infused through the arterial catheter. Complications have included blanching of the ipsilateral face and dilatation of the pupil, seizures in almost 50% of patients, and bradycardia and hypotension followed by tachycardia and hypertension. Atropine and phenytoin or barbiturates should be given prior to the injection of mannitol.

Preoperative Medication

Preoperative medication that produces sedation and ventilatory depression should be avoided in patients with intracranial tumors and decreased compliance. Narcotic-induced hypoventilation can lead to increased CBF and ICP. It is difficult to distinguish nausea and vomiting following administration of preoperative narcotics from that caused by progressive rise in ICP. Likewise, drug-induced sedation can mask decreasing levels of consciousness that accompany progressive increases in ICP. No preoperative medication should be administered to a patient manifesting a decreased sensorium.

In an alert adult patient 0.1–0.15 mg/kg of diazepam may be given orally 1.5–2 hr preoperatively. The decision to administer an anticholinergic drug or cimetidine is independent of ICP. Perhaps most important, it should be remembered that physician-patient rapport is most useful in allaying anxiety and decreasing a preoperative hypertensive response to stress.

Anesthetic Plan

Monitoring

Beat-to-beat monitoring of heart rate and blood pressure is essential to rapidly detect changes in CPP. Direct intraarterial blood pressure monitoring affords the ability to intermittently measure arterial blood gases, hematocrit, and serum electrolytes. The continuous beat-to-beat monitoring of blood pressure by means of the recently available finger plethysmography monitor permits one to perform a hemodynamically stable induction without performing an invasive maneuver in the awake patient. ECG monitoring is essential to detect myocardial ischemia and dysrhythmias related to the presence of an intracranial tumor (surgical manipulation of vital medullary centers may trigger dysrhythmias).

Temperature can conveniently be monitored through the esophageal stethoscope. Pulse oximeters and mass spectrometers or capnographs are now utilized as routine monitors in most centers. CVP monitoring is performed if the patient's general medical condition warrants it or if the patient is in the sitting position. If employed, cannulation of an antecubital vein is preferred to prevent any impediment of cerebral venous drainage. Venous air embolism is detected most sensitively by a precordial Doppler (0.02 ml/kg/min)[24] and reasonably early by capnography and transesophageal echocardiography. Alternatively, an increasing end-tidal nitrogen level as measured by mass spectrometry is a reliable indicator that air is being entrained intravascularly.

A urinary catheter is inserted to aid management of fluid balance, especially if hyperosmotic diuretic agents are used. A peripheral nerve stimulator is useful for monitoring the state of skeletal muscle relaxation. It is important to realize that if a supratentorial tumor has caused hemiparesis, the affected side will be relatively resistant to nondepolarizing muscle relaxants, and monitoring should be done on the normal extremity. Visual- and brainstem-evoked responses are being utilized in the operating room to guide the surgeon in certain circumstances.

Craniotomy for supratentorial tumor resection is usually performed in the supine position with the head elevated 10–15° to facilitate venous drainage. Care must be taken to avoid excessive rotation to the long axis of the body, as this may impede venous drainage. During posterior fossa explorations, positions include sitting, parkbench, "concorde," or a three-fourths prone position. The principal advantage of the sitting position is excellent surgical exposure due to facilitated gravitational drainage of CSF and blood. Disadvantages of the sitting position include hypotension and venous air embolism.[25] The incidence of venous air embolism is about 25%. Paradoxical air embolism through a probe-patent foramen ovale is a much rarer complication but could theoretically occur in about 20%–30% of patients.

Fluid Therapy

Hypotonic solutions should be avoided, as the extravascular extravasation may lead to cerebral edema. Stress, steroids, and phenytoin all tend to increase blood glucose, which has been shown to worsen neurologic outcome after a period of incomplete ischemia.[16] Dextrose-containing solutions should be avoided, and blood glucose levels are checked intermittently and maintained below 200 mg/dl. Lactated Ringer's solution or any of the other non-dextrose-containing maintenance and replacement solutions may be used. Fluid administration should not exceed 1–3 ml/kg/hr in the perioperative period to minimize cerebral extravascular fluid sequestration.

Anesthetic Agents

All anesthetic agents affect intracranial dynamics. It is vital to establish a comprehensive pharmacologic understanding of the effects of available anesthetic agents on cerebral circulation and metabolism. The agent selected should decrease or have little or no effect on increased ICP. Systemic homeostasis and physiologic function for the patient must be maintained. Possibly as important, and probably more so in neuroanesthesia than in any other discipline, is technical skill in the administration of anesthesia. Wide swings in blood pressure are poorly tolerated, as patients commonly have pathologic brain regions with loss of autoregulation.

A guide to the relative changes in CBF with various anesthetic agents is shown in Figure 14.3. A smooth induction is essential and can be achieved with intravenous agents (except ketamine, which increases CBF). A combination of a barbiturate, in a small dose prior to muscle relaxation, and lidocaine is effective in maintaining hemodynamic stability and providing sufficient anesthetic depth to allow a relatively smooth intubation, which is attempted only after total paralysis is achieved. Any bucking on the tube can lead to dangerous elevation of ICP.

Hyperventilation is begun by mask as soon as consciousness is lost. Nondepolarizing muscle relaxants are preferred, as the effects of succinylcholine on ICP are inconsistent. Marked tolerance to vecuronium is induced by dilantin. As a few minutes will have elapsed between induction and total muscle paralysis, a further small dose of barbiturate or lidocaine is given just prior to intubation to prevent a catecholamine surge on laryngoscopy.

Alternatively, isoflurane may be administered from the time of induction. Although all inhalation agents increase CBF, isoflurane has the least effect. At concentrations of 0.6–1.1 MAC isoflurane does not cause a significant increase in CBF.[26] Isoflurane will depress cerebral metabolic rate for oxygen ($CMRO_2$) more than the other agents and will also decrease the level of critical blood flow.[27] A further advantage of

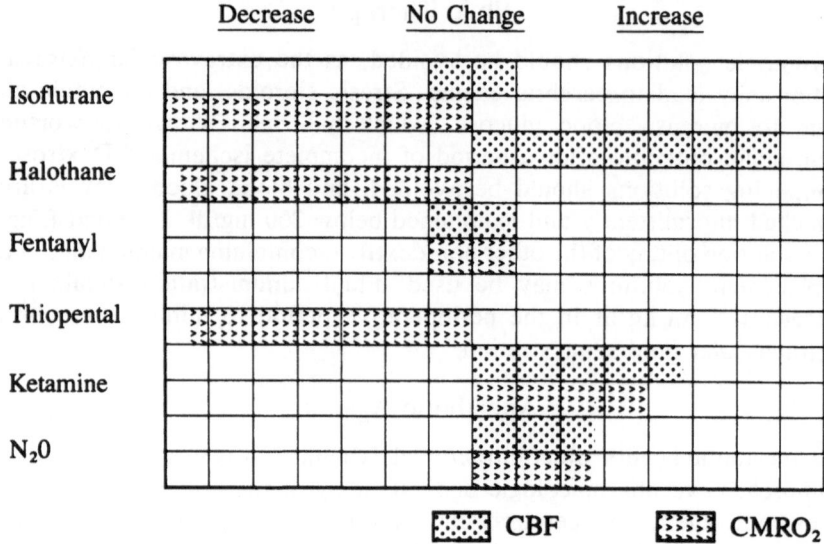

FIGURE 14.3. Schematic representation of effects of anesthetic agents on intra-cranial dynamics.

isoflurane is that prior establishment of hypocarbia is not necessary to prevent increases in CBF.[28] Enflurane, which causes more cerebral vasodilation than isoflurane but less than halothane, has been associated with dose-related seizure-type activity especially associated with hypocarbia.

If hemodynamic stability is not achieved below 1.1 MAC, narcotics or vasoactive agents such as labetalol may be supplemented. Nitrous oxide causes cerebral vasodilatation, increases the size and/or pressure of air spaces, and has been associated with convulsive activity on EEG[29]; for these reasons it is avoided in neuroanesthesia. Narcotics are often used as the primary anesthetic agent in patients with intracranial tumors. Advantages are a decrease in CBF and possibly more-stable hemodynamics. If nitrous oxide is avoided, low concentrations of inhalational agents are added to complete anesthesia and provide amnesia. The principal disadvantages of narcotics are prolonged recovery and possible postoperative need for controlled ventilation. Ventilation is controlled intraoperatively to a $PaCO_2$ of 25–30 mmHg.

Lidocaine and small doses of barbiturates are useful adjuncts to a smooth emergence. Endotracheal and pharyngeal suctioning is done prior to reversal of muscle relaxants. Hemodynamic stability is achieved with titrated boluses or an infusion of labetalol or any other appropriate vasoactive agent with minimal effect on cerebral circulation. Most patients will exhibit some sympathetic stimulation on emergence, which is also a stressful period during which hemodynamic stability must be maintained.

Adjuvants to Decrease ICP

Even though appropriate measures are taken to prevent an increase in ICP, the brain may remain noncompliant, making dural opening and exposure of deeper layers technically difficult. Various adjuvants are available to further decrease ICP. The neck must not be excessively rotated on the long axis of the body, torquing veins and impeding venous drainage. A slight head-up position may aid drainage, bearing in mind the increased incidence of venous air embolism with the elevated cranium.

The postulated membrane-stabilizing effect of steroids to decrease vasogenic cerebral edema has been discussed. Dexamethasone is continued throughout the perioperative period. Patients with metastatic tumors and glioblastomas respond best to these agents.[30]

An intraoperative dose of barbiturates can acutely decrease ICP. Hyperosmotic agents and diuretics are commonly employed to rapidly decrease ICP. Mannitol is the preferred hyperosmotic agent. The disadvantages of urea are that it is reabsorbed by the kidneys, it eventually crosses the blood-brain barrier causing rebound intracranial hypertension, and it has a high incidence of venoirritation.[31] Mannitol is usually administered as a 20% solution at a dose of 0.25–1 gm/kg intravenously. Disadvantages of mannitol are volume loading, with fluid and electrolyte abnormalities, and rebound intracranial hypertension. The latter is avoided if volume replacement is no more than two thirds of urine volume. Furosemide may be added to mannitol to further reduce ICP. An effective protocol is to administer 0.5 gm/kg mannitol at the time of skin incision. Fifteen minutes after the mannitol has been infused, 0.5 mg/kg furosemide is administered intravenously, resulting in an excellent diuresis and consistently good operating conditions.

Lumbar CSF drainage is commonly used for tumors that are technically difficult to expose, eg, pituitary or base-of-skull tumors. One must take care to control the rate of CSF drainage, as rapid drainage may cause tonsillar herniation. Excessive negative pressure on the catheter may draw a nerve root into the catheter, causing damage.

Conclusion

A clear understanding of intracranial dynamics and the physiology of CBF is the background required for the anesthesiologist. After understanding the patient's underlying medical condition, the anesthesiologist can utilize a pharmacologic armamentarium and technical skill to deliver an anesthetic that will maximally benefit the unfortunate patient with an intracranial mass.

References

1. Cutler RWP, Neurology, in E Rubinstein, DD Federman (eds): Scientific American Medicine. 1981;1:1–7.
2. Koht AH. Neurosurgical Anesthesia, in RD Dripps, JE Eckenhoff, LD Vandam (eds): Introduction to Anesthesia. Philadelphia: WB Saunders, 1982, pp 333–40.
3. Shapiro HM. Neurosurgical Anesthesia and Intracranial Hypertension, in RD Miller (ed): Anesthesia. New York: Churchill Livingstone, 1986, pp 1563–68.
4. Langfitt TW, Weinstein JD, Kassel NF. Vascular factors in head injury contribution to brainswelling and intracranial hypertension, in WF Caveness, AE Walker (eds): Head Injury Conference Proceeding. Philadelphia: Lippincott, 1966, pp 172–94.
5. Lundberg N. Crongvist K, Jallquist A. Clinical investigation on interrelations between intracranial pressure and intracranial hemodynamics, in W. Luyendijk (ed): Progress in Brain Research. Amsterdam: Elsevier, 1968, pp 69–75.
6. Tabaddor K. Physiology of intracranial pressure, in EAM Frost (ed): Clinical Anesthesia in Neurosurgery. Boston: Butterworth, 1984, pp 45–9.
7. McGraw CP. Epidural intracranial pressure monitoring, in N Lundberg, U Ponten, M Brock (eds): Intracranial Pressure, vol. 2. New York: Springer-Verlag, 1975, pp 394–96.
8. Vries JK, Becker DP, Young HF. A subarachnoid screw for monitoring intracranial pressure. J Neurosurg 1973;39:416–19.
9. Lundberg N. Continuous recording and control of ventricular fluid pressure in neurosurgical practice. Acta Psychiatr Neurol Scand 1960;36(Suppl):149.
10. Marmarou A, Shulman K, LaMorgese J. Compartmental analysis of compliance and outflow resistance of the cerebrospinal fluid system. J Neurosurg 1975;43:523–34.
11. Grucer G, Viernstein LS, Chubuck JG, et al. Clinical evaluation of long-term epidural monitoring of intracranial pressure. Surg Neurol 1979;12:373–77.
12. Siesjo BK. Cerebral circulation and metabolism. J Neurosurg 1984;60:883.
13. Cohen PJ, Alexander SC, Smith TC, et al. Effects of hypoxia and normocapnia on cerebral blood flow and metabolism in conscious man. J Appl Physiol 1967;23:183–89.
14. Kety SS, Shenkin HA, Schmidt CF. The effects of increased intracranial pressure on cerebral circulatory functions in man. J Clin Invest 1948;27:493–99.
15. Graf CJ, Rossi NP. Catecholamine response to intracranial hypertension. J Neurosurg 1978;49:862–68.
16. Sieber FE, Smith DS, Traystman RJ, Wollman H. Glucose: A reevaluation of its intraoperative use. Anesthesiology 1987;67:72–81.
17. Kitchens CS. Concept of hypercoagulability. A review of its development, clinical application and recent progress. Semin Thromb Hemost 1985;11:293–315.
18. Sawoya R, Cummins CJ, Kornblith PL. Brain tumors and plasmin inhibitors. Neurosurgery 1984;15:795–800.
19. Roberts HR, Adel S, Bernstein EF. Prevention of venous thrombosis and pulmonary embolism. National Institutes of Health Consensus Development Conference Statements, 1986;6(2).

20. Sawoya R, Donlon JA. Chronic disseminated intravascular coagulation and metastatic brain tumor: A case report and review of the literature. Neurosurgery 1983;12:580–84.
21. Jacobs SK, Wilson DJ, Melin G, et al. Interleukin-2 lymphokine activated killer (LAK) cells in the treatment of malignant glioma: Clinical and experimental studies. Neurol Res 1986;8:81–7.
22. Lotze MT, Matory YL, Etlinghausen SE. In vivo administration of purified human interleukin 2. J Immunol 1985;135:2865–75.
23. Williams WT, Lowry RL, Eggers BWN. Anesthetic management during therapeutic disruption of the blood brain barrier. Anesth Analg 1986;65:188–90.
24. Edmunds-Seal J, Prys-Roberts C, Adams AP. Air embolism. A comparison of various methods of detection. Anaesthesia 1971;26:202–98.
25. Albin NS, Babinski M, Maroon JC, et al. Anesthetic management of posterior fossa surgery in the sitting position. Acta Anaesthesiol Scand 1976;20:117–28.
26. Murphy FL, Jr, Kennel EM, Jober DR, et al. The effects of Forane on cerebral blood flow and metabolism in man. New Drug Application, Ohio Medical Products, Madison, WI, 1975; pp 2386–95.
27. Smith AI, Wollman H. Cerebral blood flow and metabolism: Effects of anesthetic drugs and techniques. Anesthesiology 1972;36:378.
28. Isoflurane: A compendium. Madison, WI: Ohio Medical Products, 1981, p 59.
29. Kitahata LM, Katz JD. Tension pneumocephalus after posterior fossa craniotomy: A complication of the sitting position. Anesthesiology 1976;44:448–50.
30. Maxwell RE, Lang DM, French LA. The clinical effects of a synthetic glucocorticoid used for brain edema in the practice of neurosurgery, in HJ Reulin, K Schurrman (eds): Steroids and Brain Edema. Berlin: Springer-Verlag, 1972, p 219.
31. Stoelting RK. Diuretics, in RK Stoelting (ed): Pharmacology and Physiology in Anesthetic Practice. Philadelphia: Lippincott, 1987, p 430.

CHAPTER 15

The Child with an Open Eye Injury

Jonathan S. Daitch

Case History. *An 8-year-old boy was struck over the right eye with a stick. The incident occurred at midnight. Cursory examination in the emergency room revealed a cut right upper eyelid and a corneal laceration. Skull films showed an intact orbit. The patient had no significant past medical or surgical history. He had last eaten at 11 PM. The operating room staff was notified of the pending procedure at 2 AM. After discussion with the anesthesiologist, the operation was postponed until 6 AM to allow time for gastric emptying.*

The child arrived in the holding area accompanied by his mother. He had patches on both eyes, and an intravenous line was in place. He was crying and resisting all attempts at examination. Diazepam 1.5 mg was administered intravenously, and good sedation was achieved. The remainder of the physical examination was unremarkable except for a loose upper incisor.

Introduction

In spite of the excellent protection afforded by the bony orbit and cushioning by the retrobulbar fat and eyelids, the incidence of ocular injuries is high. There has been some decrease since the introduction of better safety measures and goggles in certain sports and workplaces. Childhood eye injuries commonly occur as a result of trauma, slingshots, fireworks, and sports injuries.

Eye injuries can be penetrating or nonpenetrating. Nonpenetrating injuries comprise corneal abrasions and contusions and foreign bodies in the cornea or sclera. Penetrating injuries include intraocular foreign bodies in the anterior and posterior chambers, the lens, or the vitreous humor, as well as lacerations of the cornea or sclera. The latter injuries

Reviewed by Dr. Deryck Duncalf, Professor of Anesthesiology Albert Einstein College of Medicine, Montefiore Medical Center, Bronx, NY.

can result in extrusion of intraocular contents. The main anesthetic goal in such cases is to prevent further increases in intraocular pressure (IOP), which can result in additional prolapse and loss of intraocular contents.

Intraocular Physiology

Intraocular pressure is normally 16 ± 5 mmHg[1] and is maintained within this normal range to ensure a constant corneal curvature and refractive index. IOP is the sum of internal and external forces on the eye. Choroidal blood volume, aqueous humor (AH), and vitreous humor exert an outward pressure within the eye, while the scleral capsule and extraocular muscles exert an opposing inward pressure. IOP is mainly influenced by the volume of AH and choroidal blood, as well as by extraocular muscle tone.

Aqueous Humor

The balance between production and elimination of AH is the main determinant of normal IOP. AH occupies the anterior and posterior chambers of the eye (Figure 15.1.). The total volume of AH is only 0.3 ml; about 80% of it is located in the anterior chamber. Two thirds of the AH is produced in the posterior chamber by epithelial cells in the ciliary body. This entails an active secretory process involving carbonic anhydrase. The remaining third is formed by simple filtration through the surface of the iris in the anterior chamber.

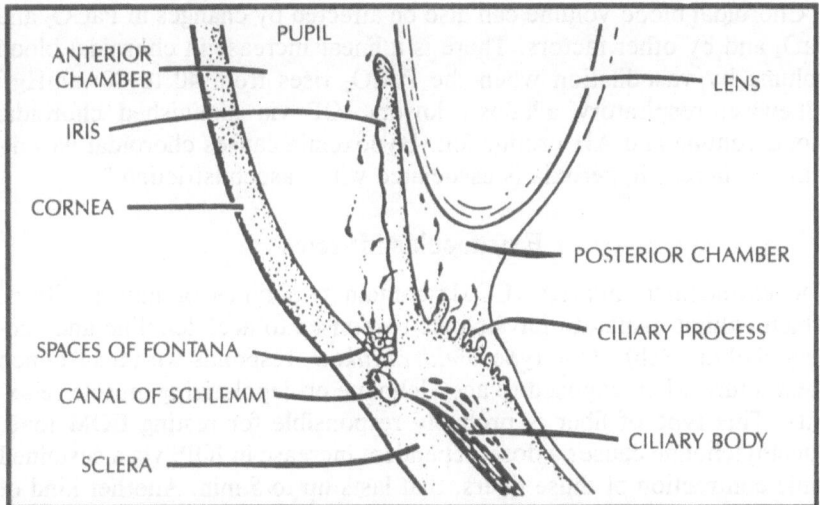

FIGURE 15.1. Diagram of ocular anatomy showing the areas of production, circulation, and drainage of aqueous humor.

AH circulates from the posterior chamber through the pupil into the anterior chamber, where it bathes the lens and cornea and supplies them with oxygen, glucose, and proteins. AH exits the eye though the trabecular mesh, located in the angle of the anterior chamber, into the canal of Schlemm; from there it drains into the episcleral veins.

Choroidal Blood Flow

The choroid is a highly vascular layer on the inner surface of the eye that can vary considerably in blood volume. This layer autoregulates to maintain a constant perfusion pressure despite wide fluctuations in systolic blood pressure.[2] However, a sudden increase in blood pressure transiently increases IOP. Below a mean arterial pressure of 90 mmHg, IOP falls.[3] At a systolic blood pressure of 50–60 mmHg, IOP approaches zero owing to diminished choroidal blood flow and decreased AH production.

Venous drainage of the choroid joins the eliminated AH in the episcleral veins. Choroidal blood then passes from the cavernous sinus to the internal jugular veins and finally into the right atrium. There is also venous drainage from anterior eye structures through the external jugular veins. Obstruction of blood return by a tight neck collar or circumferential taping of the endotracheal tube may raise episcleral venous pressure and IOP. Similarly, elevations in the central venous pressure caused by a Valsalva maneuver or by bucking or straining on the endotracheal tube will increase resistance to venous blood return and elevate IOP. In fact, a cough can increase IOP by 30–40 mmHg.[4]

Choroidal blood volume can also be affected by changes in $PaCO_2$ and PaO_2 and by other factors. There is a linear increase in choroidal blood volume by vasodilation when the $PaCO_2$ rises from 40 to 80 mmHg.[5] Likewise, respiratory alkalosis lowers IOP via diminished choroidal blood volume and AH production. Hypoxemia causes choroidal vasodilation, whereas hyperoxia is associated with vasoconstriction.[6]

Extraocular Muscles

The extraocular muscles (EOM) contain two types of muscle fibers, which exhibit disparate physiologic responses to acetylcholine and succinylcholine (Sch).[7] One type, *Felderstruktur,* responds with a sustained contracture when exposed to acetylcholine or depolarizing muscle relaxants. This type of fiber is probably responsible for resting EOM tone. Succinylcholine causes a dose-dependent increase in IOP, via a sustained tonic contraction of these fibers, that lasts up to 5 min. Another kind of muscle fiber, the *Fibrillenstruktur,* responds to acetylcholine and depolarizing muscle relaxants with a twitch response. This type of fiber is mainly responsible for ocular movements.

Small doses of Sch increase resting muscle tension but do not depress the twitch response.[8] Larger doses of Sch continue to elevate EOM tone while depressing the twitch response. The dosage needed to depress the twitch response of the EOM is greater than that needed for skeletal muscle. Nevertheless, section of the recti muscles still results in an increase in IOP after administration of Sch; this may be mediated by choroidal vasodilation or contracture of smooth muscle in the eye.[9]

Movement of the eye into extreme positions elevates IOP slightly because of traction by the EOM.[10] Voluntarily opening the eyelids widely also increases IOP because it forces the globe forward against the restraining EOM.[11] Forcibly closing the eyelids will profoundly elevate IOP.[12]

CNS Mediation

Although a negative feedback system has never been conclusively demonstrated, the CNS performs a role in controlling IOP. In stereotactic experiments, electrical stimulation of numerous areas in the cat diencephalon caused changes in IOP.[13] Some responses were mediated by contraction of ocular smooth muscle and striated EOM, and other responses were neurovascular. Additionally, stimulation of the ventral zone of the hypothalamus increased sympathetic nervous system outflow, resulting in elevated mean arterial blood pressures and increased IOP. It is believed that general anesthesia lowers IOP by depressing these cerebral centers. Laryngoscopy may increase IOP by stimulating the same centers.

Miscellaneous Factors

Other factors that affect IOP are diurnal variation (2–3 mmHg higher in the morning), arterial blood pressure changes (1–2 mmHg changes in IOP), changes in body position, plasma oncotic pressure, and pupillary size. Pupillary dilation causes narrowed trabecular channels and diminished AH outflow from the eye.

Measurement of IOP

Intraocular pressure can be measured directly by manometry or indirectly by tonometry. Direct manometric measurements involve cannulation of the anterior chamber and are therefore limited to experimental use. Indirect clinical measurements use applanation and indentation tonometry. In applanation tonometry, the force needed to flatten an area of spherical cornea is measured. The IOP is then calculated from the equation: Pressure = Force/Area.

Pneumatic applanation tonometers, which flatten the cornea by an air jet, have been employed more recently. Corneal flattening is detected photoelectrically, and IOP is then calculated. The Schiotz indentation tonometer (Figure 15.2.) utilizes a weighted plunger that indents the anesthetized cornea. A nomogram is used to convert the amount of indentation to IOP. A newer technique uses noninvasive radiotelemetry to measure IOP continuously.

Pharmacology

Drugs can directly affect IOP by actions on AH production and elimination, EOM, orbicularis muscles, and the diencephalic and hypothalamic centers, or indirectly by effects on $PaCO_2$ or central venous and arterial pressure.

Many studies have confirmed that inhalation agents promptly decrease IOP. The same decrease occurs with the onset of nighttime sleep. In both conditions EOM tone is lost and AH production fails. In conjunction with nitrous oxide, halothane 0.5%[14] and enflurane 1%[15] lower IOP by 50% and 35%, respectively. Isoflurane also diminishes IOP significantly in children.[16]

Other CNS depressants lower IOP, including barbiturates, etomidate, diazepam, droperidol, and narcotics. The reported effects of ketamine on IOP, however, are controversial. In any case, the nystagmus caused by ketamine renders it unsuitable for ophthalmologic surgery.

Carbonic anhydrase inhibitors diminish the rate of AH formation because carbonic anhydrase is involved in transport across the ciliary epithelium. Acetazolamide (Diamox®) 250–500 mg can be given intravenously to lower IOP acutely.

IOP also can be lowered rapidly by increasing blood osmolarity with intravenous mannitol or urea; these agents cause dehydration of the aqueous and vitreous humors. Conversely, administration of 1L of free water can raise IOP by 8 mmHg or more if AH outflow is obstructed.[12]

Topically administered agents also have significant effects. Miotic drugs produce constriction of the ciliary muscle, which opens up the trabecular mesh, facilitating outflow of AH. Mi-

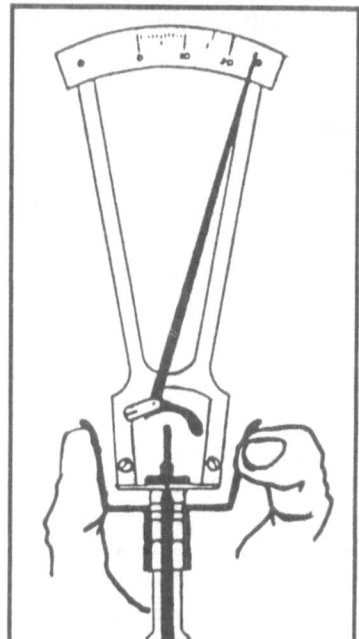

FIGURE 15.2. Schiotz tonometer.

otic agents act either directly (eg, pilocarpine) or indirectly (eg, cholines-terase inhibitors such as physostigmine or echothiophate). Topical epi-nephrine can increase IOP because of increased AH production, whereas timolol, a beta-adrenergic blocking agent, decreases AH production and lowers IOP.

Muscle Relaxants

Succinylcholine significantly increases IOP and has led to loss of vitreous humor on many occasions. IOP can increase 18 mmHg in unanesthetized patients[17] and 6–8 mmHg in anesthetized patients.[18] The peak increase is after 2–4 min; return to baseline occurs in 6 minutes. Endotracheal intubation after Sch exaggerates the increase but does not lengthen the duration. The lighter the anesthetic plane, the greater the increase in IOP after Sch.

Many methods of attenuating this rise in IOP after Sch have been studied, but no reported method consistently prevents the increase. A 10 mg self-taming dose of Sch prevented the rise in IOP after the full dose in one study,[19] but this result could not be duplicated in another.[20] Despite some evidence to the contrary,[21] Miller et al[22] and others have shown that pretreatment with a nondepolarizing muscle relaxant will not increase IOP. Libonati et al[23] reviewed the course of 63 patients who received Sch after a pretreatment dose of curare 3–6 mg or gallamine 10–15 mg. In none of these cases was any extrusion of intraocular contents noted by the surgeons. Indeed, there are no published reports of any loss of intraocular contents after inductions utilizing Sch with pretreatment doses of nondepolarizers.

Nondepolarizing muscle relaxants, on the other hand, either reduce IOP or have no effect. Administration of curare results in the greatest decrease in IOP, probably secondary to its hypotensive effect.[24] Pancu-ronium also lowers IOP, whereas atracurium[25,26] and vecuronium[26] appear to have no significant effect on IOP.

Most recently, a rapid-sequence technique with high-dose vecuronium (0.2 mg/kg) showed adequate intubating conditions after 60 sec without coughing or bucking.[27] No increase in IOP occurred in 70% of the patients, and the highest increase in any patient was 5 mmHg, which lasted only 1–2 min. However, the mean time until return of the third twitch in the train of four was 70 min. The same study showed that, with preoxygenation, even after 3 min of apnea there was no significant fall in oxygenation saturation from preinduction levels.

In summary, it would seem prudent to employ mainly nondepolarizing muscle relaxants for rapid-sequence inductions in penetrating eye inju-ries. Sch, when used with a pretreatment dose of a nondepolarizing muscle relaxant, should be reserved for situations involving a difficult airway.

Surgical Considerations

Open eye injuries consist of intraocular foreign bodies and corneal lacerations. On rare occasions blunt trauma can rupture the eye by a sudden increase in IOP. Foreign bodies usually imbed in the cornea and can often be removed under topical anesthesia. However, small foreign bodies can penetrate the cornea or sclera and lodge intraocularly. These small fragments must be removed, for they can cause subsequent infection, cataract formation, or loss of visual acuity.

Foreign bodies can be detected by direct visualization, ophthalmoscopy, ultrasonography, radiography, or CT scan. Foreign bodies in the anterior and posterior chambers are removed through an incision at the corneoscleral limbus. Foreign bodies in the vitreal compartment are removed via scleral incision. Metal fragments can be removed with a magnet; nonmetallic objects are removed either by a combination of vitrectomy and suction or with a forceps.

Sometimes intralenticular foreign bodies are not removed initially but later, when a cataract forms. In general, early removal is desirable because foreign bodies may become enmeshed in fibrin and will be more difficult to remove later. Large foreign bodies can destroy ocular structures, often necessitating enucleation.

Aside from foreign bodies, lacerations account for the remainder of penetrating injuries. Simple lacerations of the cornea are sutured closed; the anterior chamber is then re-formed with normal saline or air. With larger lacerations, the iris usually prolapses to close the wound. Exposed iris is usually excised, and the remaining iris is returned to its normal position when the anterior chamber is re-formed. Ocular lacerations with more severe prolapse require enucleation.

Preanesthetic Considerations

Most cases of intraocular injury are not truly emergent; nevertheless, they are considered urgent if sight is to be preserved. The operation can often be delayed several hours if the patient has recently eaten. Because of the everpresent risk of aspiration, these patients should receive antacid aspiration prophylaxis. If an intravenous line is present, the child may also receive an H_2-receptor antagonist or metoclopramide. No attempt should be made to pass a nasogastric tube.

Associated injuries must be sought, such as skull and orbital fractures, as well as intracranial injuries. If the ocular injury is the result of child abuse, an associated subdural hematoma may be present.

Both eyes should be patched preoperatively to minimize eye movements. Such patches are very frightening to a child, and the assurance of a parent is most comforting. Otherwise, small amounts of sedation can be given. Acetaminophen should be given initially to treat any pain. Narcotics are best avoided since associated nausea and vomiting may raise IOP. If the child has severe pain and narcotics are required, an antiemetic should be included. The child's weight must be known for accurate dosing regimens. In addition, the child's teeth must be inspected; children over 6 years old are likely to have loose or missing teeth.

Preoperatively, it is important that the child not cry, since this straining can raise IOP. If possible, the parents should remain with the child to comfort him. If the child is healthy, no preoperative blood work is necessary, nor should an intravenous cannula be placed preoperatively if doing so elicits crying. If preexisting medical conditions outweigh the risk of worsening the open eye injury, then the need for an intravenous line and preoperative laboratory analyses should be discussed among the pediatrician, ophthalmologist, anesthesiologist, and parents.

Pain or photophobia caused by the ocular injury may produce severe blepharospasm that can interfere with adequate examination of the eye. Usually, only topical anesthesia is required to examine the eye. Nevertheless, it may not be possible to examine adequately a small child with severe blepharospasm under topical anesthesia. If rupture or laceration of the eye is suspected in this circumstance, it is prudent to examine the child under general anesthesia.

Anesthetic Plan

Attempting to separate the child from his parents at the time of surgery will frequently instigate crying. It may be beneficial to have a parent present during the induction to minimize crying and concomitant increases in IOP, if the anesthesiologist is comfortable with this arrangement. After the child is unconscious, the parents are escorted out of the operating room. If any difficulty arises, the parents must leave immediately. This arrangement should be documented in the chart.

Since a retrobulbar block is tolerated poorly in this age group and may increase IOP from the volume injected, general anesthesia is preferred. Rectal methohexital 30 mg/kg can be administered to an uncooperative child under continuous supervision by the anesthesiologist. If the child is more cooperative and is without an intravenous line, then a gentle inhalation induction can be performed, while minimizing positive pressure ventilation. Once the child has lost consciousness, an intravenous apparatus is procured.

For the child who already has an intravenous line, a rapid-sequence induction must be performed after preoxygenation, using cricoid pressure and a peripheral nerve stimulator, to expedite securement of the airway. Care must be taken to avoid ocular pressure by the mask. The patient must be completely paralyzed before intubation to avoid bucking, which can lead to additional prolapse of the injured eye.

A large dose of an intermediate-acting muscle relaxant (vecuronium

0.15 mg/kg or atracurium 0.8 mg/kg) can achieve good intubating conditions in about 90 sec when a priming dose is used. Pharmacologic reversal should be possible after 45–70 min. Intravenous lidocaine
1.5 mg/kg can be given to further blunt tracheal responses to intubation. If
swiftly performed, laryngotracheal anesthesia can also be used to
anesthetize the trachea to facilitate a smooth extubation.

When Sch is used with a pretreatment dose of a nondepolarizing muscle
relaxant, it probably does increase IOP; however, it is generally not
needed for routine ocular emergencies. Succinylcholine certainly has a
place in cases in which a difficult intubation is anticipated, though its
effect on intragastric pressure also needs to be considered. Awake
intubations should be avoided. Either an inhalation or a nitrous oxide–
narcotic technique can be used for maintenance anesthesia.

Consideration must also be given to an appropriate extubation. The
stomach should be emptied while the patient is deeply anesthetized and
paralyzed. The trachea can be safely extubated when the protective
reflexes have returned. These reflexes are present when the patient has
purposeful movements and responds to commands. This is most easily
attained with a nitrous oxide–narcotic technique. If an inhalation technique is used, it can be converted to a nitrous oxide–narcotic technique
over the last 30 min with the titration of a small amount of fentanyl
(1–2 μg/kg) as the inhalation agent is discontinued. A small amount of
droperidol (0.075 mg/kg) given 20 min before the end of the case should
prevent nausea and vomiting in response to the narcotic.

Muscle relaxation is maintained until the surgery is completed and the
dressing has been applied. After reversal of the neuromuscular blockade,
the nitrous oxide can be discontinued, and the patient should tolerate the
endotracheal tube because of the residual narcotic. The patient should
then be able to open his eyes on command and can be safely extubated.
Any bucking can again raise IOP to critical levels and place the surgical
repair in jeopardy.

Alternatively, an inhalation technique may be utilized. However, the
child may react to the endotracheal tube at the end of the procedure
before he is awake enough to protect his airway. Intravenous lidocaine
1.5 mg/kg diminishes airway reactivity and allows the patient to tolerate
the endotracheal tube until he is more fully awake. This dose may be
repeated. Alternatively, a small dose of Sch will prevent further bucking,
and the patient can be ventilated until more anesthetic is removed. If
there is no risk of aspiration, extubation at a deep level of anesthesia can
be performed once adequate spontaneous respirations have returned.

Summary

Understanding the principles of intraocular physiology makes it possible
to provide safe preoperative, intraoperative, and postoperative conditions
for the child with an open eye injury. Of paramount importance are the

avoidance of preoperative crying, as well as bucking on the endotracheal tube during intubation and extubation, to avoid major increases in IOP and loss of ocular contents. Such a task requires preoperative discussion with the other physicians involved and much planning to conduct a safe anesthesia.

References

1. Donlon JV: Anesthesia for eye, ear, nose, and throat, in Miller RD (ed): Anesthesia. New York, Churchill Livingstone, 1986; pp 1837–94.
2. Jay JL: Functional organization of the human eye. Br J Anaesth 1980;52: 649–54.
3. Schroeder M, Linssen GH: Intraocular pressure and anaesthesia. Anaesthesia 1972;27:165–70.
4. Macri FJ: Vascular pressure relationship and intraocular pressure. Arch Ophthalmol 1961;65:571–74.
5. Wilson TM, Stang R, McKenzie FT: The response of the choroidal and cerebral circulation to changing arterial PCO_2 and acetazolamide in the baboon. Invest Ophthalmol Vis Sci 1977;16:576–82.
6. Saltzman HA, Anderson B, Hart L, et al: The retinal vascular functional response to hyperbaric oxygenation, in Hyperbaric Oxygenation. Proceedings of the Second International Congress. London, Churchill Livingstone, 1965; p 202.
7. Hess A, Pilar G: Slow fibers in the extraocular muscles of the cat. J Physiol 1963;169:780–98.
8. Katz RL, Eakins KE: The effects of succinylcholine, decamethonium, hexacarbacholine, gallamine, and dimethyltubocurarine on the twitch and tonic neuromuscular systems of the cat. J Pharmacol Exp Ther 1966;154: 303–8.
9. Bjork A, Halldin M, Wahlin A: Enophthalmos elicited by succinylcholine. Acta Anaesthesiol Scand 1957;1:41–53.
10. Moses RA, Lurie P, Wette R: Horizontal gaze: position effect on intraocular pressure. Invest Ophthalmol Vis Sci 1982;22:551.
11. Moses RA: Proptosis and increase of intraocular pressure in voluntary lid fissure widening. Invest Ophthalmol Vis Sci 1984;25:989.
12. Moses RA: Intraocular pressure, in Moses RA, Hart WM (eds): Adler's Physiology of the Eye: Clinical Applications. St. Louis, C.V. Mosby Co, 1987; pp 223–45.
13. Von Sallmann L, Lowenstein O: Responses of intraocular pressure, blood pressure, and cutaneous vessels to electrical stimulation in the diencephalon. Am J Ophthalmol 1955;39:11–29.
14. Adams AP, Freedman A, Henville JD: Normocapnic anaesthesia for intraocular surgery. Br J Ophthalmol 1979;63:204–10.
15. Rose NM, Adams AP: Normocapnic anaesthesia with enflurane for intraocular surgery. Anaesthesia 1980;35:569–75.
16. Ausinch B, Graves SA, Munson ES, et al: Intraocular pressure in children during isoflurane and halothane anesthesia. Anesthesiology 1975;42:167–72.
17. Hoffman H, Holzer H: Die Wirkung von Muskelrelaxantien auf dem Intraokularen Druck. Klin Monatsbl Augenheilk 1953;123:1–16.

186 Jonathan S. Daitch

18. Pandley K, Badola RP, Kumar S: Time course of intraocular hypertension produced by suxamethonium. Br J Anaesth 1972;44:191–96.
19. Verma RS: "Self-taming" of succinylcholine-induced fasciculations and intraocular pressure. Anesthesiology 1979;50:245–47.
20. Myers EF, Singer P, Otto A: A controlled study of the effect of succinylcholine self-taming on intraocular pressure. Anesthesiology 1980;53:72–4.
21. Myers E, Krupin T, Johnson M, et al: Failure of nondepolarizing neuromuscular blockers to inhibit succinylcholine-induced increased intraocular pressure. Anesthesiology 1978;48:149–51.
22. Miller RD, Way WL, Hickey RF: Inhibition of succinylcholine-induced increased intraocular pressure by non-depolarizing muscle relaxants. Anesthesiology 1968;29:123–26.
23. Libonati MM, Leahy JJ, Ellison N: The use of succinylcholine in open eye surgery. Anesthesiology 1985;62:637–40.
24. Al-Abrak MH, Samuel JR: Effects of general anaesthesia on the intraocular pressure in man. Comparison of tubocurarine and pancuronium in nitrous oxide and oxygen. Br J Ophthalmol 1974;58:806–10.
25. Badrinath S, Vazeery AK, Ivankovich AD: Effects of atracurium on intraocular pressure. ASA abstract. Anesthesiology 1985;63:A362.
26. Schneider MJ, Stirt JA, Finholt DA: Atracurium, vecuronium, and intraocular pressure in man. ASA abstract. Anesthesiology 1985;63:A334.
27. Abbott MA: The control of intraocular pressure during the induction of anaesthesia for emergency eye surgery. A high dose vecuronium technique. Anaesthesia 1987;42:1008–12.

CHAPTER 16

The Patient with Maxillofacial Injury

Jonathan S. Daitch

Case History. *A 38-year-old man was hit by a car while riding his bicycle. According to witnesses, his head struck the hood of the car, and he was unconscious for approximately 5 min after the injury. On arrival in the emergency room, he was arousable and complaining of abdominal pain. His vital signs were: pulse 120/min, blood pressure 110/90 mmHg, respiratory rate 28/min, temperature 37°C. Physical examination showed marked facial edema, bilateral raccoon eyes, trismus, and jaw misalignment. His airway was unobstructed, and examination showed normal heart and lung function. He had diffuse abdominal tenderness, and abdominal lavage was positive for blood.*

Other laboratory studies were unremarkable. Skull and facial x-rays revealed basilar and frontal bone fractures and multiple mandibular fractures, as well as left-sided LeFort III and right-sided LeFort II fractures. Cervical films showed no fractures or dislocations of the spine. In addition, no fractured ribs or pneumothorax was noted on chest x-ray.

The patient was taken to the operating room for an exploratory laparotomy. An oral fiberoptic intubation was attempted but was unsuccessful because of intraoral bleeding. Therefore, the airway was secured via tracheostomy under local anesthesia. Subsequently, a laparotomy was performed under general anesthesia, and a ruptured spleen was removed. Arch bars were also placed at this time to stabilize the fractured lower jaw. A postoperative CT scan of the head revealed a left frontal contusion, a depressed frontal bone fracture, and air in the left temporal lobe. One week later the patient was scheduled for an open reduction and internal fixation of his skull and facial fractures.

Reviewed by Dr. Joel M. Friedman, Director of Oral and Maxillofacial Surgery. Albert Einstein College of Medicine/Bronx Municipal Hospital Center, Bronx, NY.

Introduction

Maxillofacial injuries, although rare, pose many challenges in airway management for the anesthesiologist. Many factors that concern the airway must be assessed, including the presence of airway obstruction, a full stomach, airway bleeding, possible cervical and skull fractures, and associated injuries, as well as the timing and type of surgical repair contemplated. Only then can an educated decision be made as to whether a tracheostomy, an oral/nasal intubation, an oronasopharyngeal airway placement, or simply observation is indicated.

In a study of 1042 cases of major facial injury,[1] more than 50% of the injuries were the result of automobile accidents. Other causes included accidents at home and at work, athletic injuries, animal bites, and fights. The most commonly fractured facial bones were the nasal bones (37%), followed by the zygoma and its arch (15%), mandible (11%), orbital floor (11%), and maxilla (8%).

Mandibular Fractures

Because the mandible occupies a prominent position on the face, it is easily fractured. In rural areas motor vehicle accidents account for most mandibular injuries, whereas in indigent urban populations physical violence is the most likely etiology.

Mandibular fractures occur in well-defined areas (Figure 16.1.). The most common sites are the condylar neck and the angle of the mandible. The condylar neck is often fractured because it is relatively thin. In fact, a fracture here may actually avert more serious injury by preventing the condyle from being driven into the base of the brain.[2] Coronoid fractures are uncommon because of protection by the zygomatic arch, and ramus fractures are rare because this strong part of the bone transmits force to other areas of the mandible.

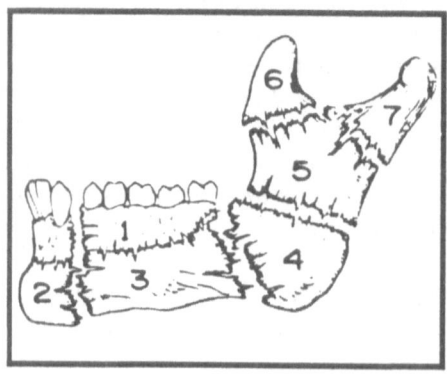

FIGURE 16.1. Common sites of mandibular fractures: (1) alveolar process, (2) symphysis, (3) body, (4) angle, (5) ramus, (6) coronoid process, (7) condylar neck.

Multiple mandibular fractures are very common; the average number of jaw fractures per trauma patient is 1.8.[3] Frequently, the body of the mandible is directly broken, and the opposite angle or condylar neck is fractured indirectly from transmitted forces. A symphyseal impact may lead to a parasymphyseal or bilateral condylar neck fracture. High-velocity blows will often cause compound or comminuted fractures at the point of impact. Three or more fractures are not uncommon.

After mandibular injury the muscles of the lower jaw distract the mandibular fragments. Traction must be applied to return the mandibular fragments to their proper anatomic positions. When a full complement of teeth is present, upper and lower jaw arch bars are placed, and the mandible is wired to the maxilla to provide proper apposition. A broken edentulous mandible, however, requires direct wiring or plating. Alternatively, an external fixator may be applied to achieve proper alignment of the separated bones.

Following bilateral mandibular angle or body fractures (Andy Gump fractures), respiratory obstruction may occur. The tongue is normally tethered anteriorly by attachments to the mandible and hyoid bone. After bilateral mandibular fractures, the tongue and mandible are displaced posteriorly by the suprahyoid muscles, often occluding the pharynx (Figure 16.2.). This type of respiratory obstruction can be relieved by forward traction of the tongue or by placement of an oropharyngeal airway.

Maxillary Fractures

René LeFort studied maxillary fractures in cadavers almost 90 years ago. He delivered powerful blows to cadaver heads and found reproducible relationships between the area of impact and the nature of the fractures produced. LeFort noted that, depending on the type of fracture, different fragments would be freely mobile from the rest of the face and cranium (Figure 16.3.). His classification was published in 1901[4] and is still used today.

Airway obstruction in LeFort injuries can occur from several causes. Pharyngeal obstruction can ensue if the soft palate sags against the tongue or the posterior pharynx or against a hematoma or edema of the pharyngeal wall (Figure 16.4.). Airway obstruction also can occur from foreign material in the mouth. Nasal obstruction may occur from septal dislocation or swelling or, less often, from clots or foreign bodies in the nose.

Isolated LeFort injuries are rare because the impact needed to cause such fractures is usually severe enough to break other facial bones. Depending on the type of LeFort injury, there is a 20%–55% chance of an associated mandibular fracture.[5] LeFort fractures are often associated with skull fractures and other traumatic injuries.

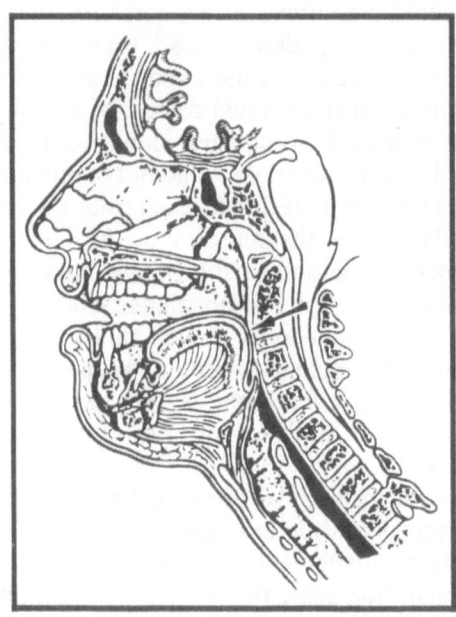

FIGURE 16.2. Airway obstruction from prolapse of the tongue after bilateral mandibular fractures. (Reprinted with permission from Rowe NL, Killey HC: *Fractures of the Facial Skeleton*, Edinburgh, Churchill Livingstone, 1968.)

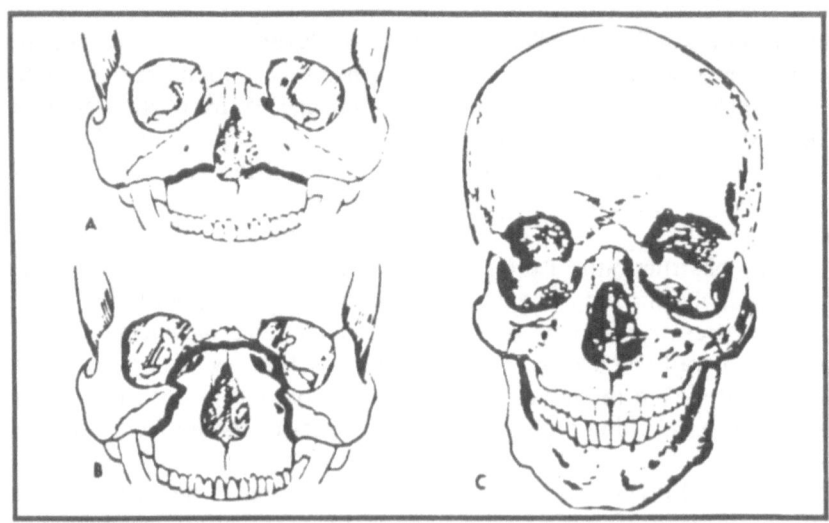

FIGURE 16.3. The LeFort fractures: (A) LeFort I (dental alveolar fracture), (B) LeFort II (pyramidal fracture), (C) LeFort III (craniofacial dysjunction). (Reprinted with permission from Kazanjian and Converse: *The Surgical Treatment of Facial Injuries,* 3rd ed. Baltimore, Williams and Wilkins, 1974.)

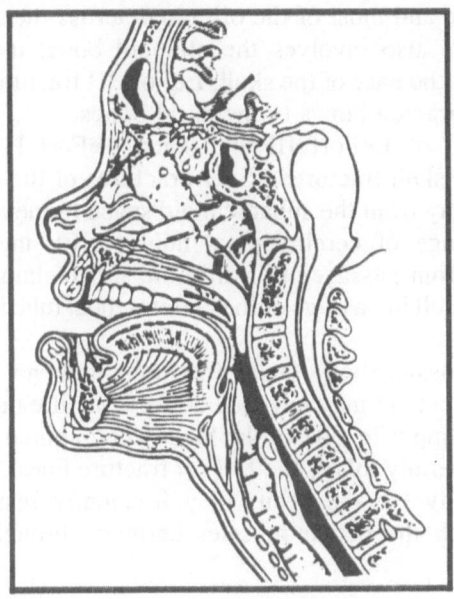

FIGURE 16.4. Airway obstruction caused by fracture of the maxilla with occlusion of the oropharynx by the soft palate. Note the basilar skull fracture with resultant cerebrospinal fluid leakage. (Reprinted with permission from Rowe NL, Killey HC: *Fractures of the Facial Skeleton,* Edinburgh, Churchill Livingstone, 1968.)

LeFort I Fractures

The least severe maxillary fracture is the LeFort I (Guerin's) fracture. It is a dental-alveolar fracture that follows a horizontal plane above the floor of the nose. LeFort I fractures separate the palate from the rest of the facial skeleton. They are caused by direct low-maxillary blows or by lateral impacts to the maxilla.

LeFort II Fractures

Also referred to as pyramidal fractures, LeFort II fractures are the most common of the LeFort injuries. They extend from the lower nasal bridge through the medial wall of the orbit and cross the zygomaticomaxillary process. The freely mobile fragment consists of a pyramid-shaped portion of the maxilla. LeFort II fractures are caused by direct middle-alveolar blows, lateral impacts, and inferior blows to the mandible when the mouth is open.

LeFort III Fractures

LeFort III fractures, also known as craniofacial dysjunctions, completely separate the midfacial skeleton from the base of the cranium, resulting in a characteristic "dish face" deformity. The fracture extends through the upper nasal bridge and most of the orbit and across the zygomatic arch. Since the fracture also involves the ethmoid bone, it may affect the cribriform plate at the base of the skull. LeFort III fractures usually result from superiorly directed blows to the nasal bones.

Twenty percent of LeFort III and some LeFort II fractures have associated basilar skull fractures.[6] Such fractures of the cribriform plate create a passageway from the subarachnoid space to the nasal cavity that can lead to leakage of cerebrospinal fluid (CSF), meningitis, and a pneumocranium from passage of air into the subarachnoid space. Nasal intubations can result in passage of the endotracheal tube into the cranium itself.

Despite this classification, facial fractures may not be distributed symmetrically. A patient may have a LeFort I fracture on one side and a LeFort II on the opposite side of the face. Comminuted facial fractures also occur but generally follow the LeFort fracture lines. Since LeFort II and III injuries involve the orbit, they frequently result in blow-out fractures, in which the ocular muscles herniate through the fractured orbital floor.

Initial Therapy

Despite the often appalling appearance of severe cases of maxillofacial trauma, maxillofacial injuries themselves are rarely life-threatening unless airway obstruction occurs. Patients with maxillofacial injuries are usually most comfortable in a 30° head-up, sitting, or lateral position, all of which allow drainage of blood, saliva, and CSF from the airway while preventing obstruction by avulsed tissues.

Signs of airway obstruction should be sought—for example, suprasternal retractions, labored respirations, use of accessory muscles of respiration, and paradoxical movement of the chest. Obstruction may be due to pharyngeal blood clots, vomitus, loose teeth, dentures, or posterior displacement of either the maxillary fragment in LeFort fractures or the tongue in bilateral mandibular fractures. Therefore, the first step is to clear the oropharynx of all foreign matter with a sweep of the index finger and gentle suctioning. Second, obstruction from a prolapsed tongue can be alleviated by pulling the tongue and fractured mandible forward.

A suture can be placed through the posterior portion of the tongue to pull the tongue anteriorly. Next, if the maxilla is causing pharyngeal obstruction, it can be brought forward by manipulation with forceps. A more secure airway can be achieved by gentle insertion of a well-lubricated nasopharyngeal tube, which serves to lift the soft palate away from the posterior pharyngeal wall. Before insertion of the airway, the nasopharynx should be sprayed with a combination of local anesthetic and vasoconstrictor drugs to anesthetize the area and minimize bleeding.

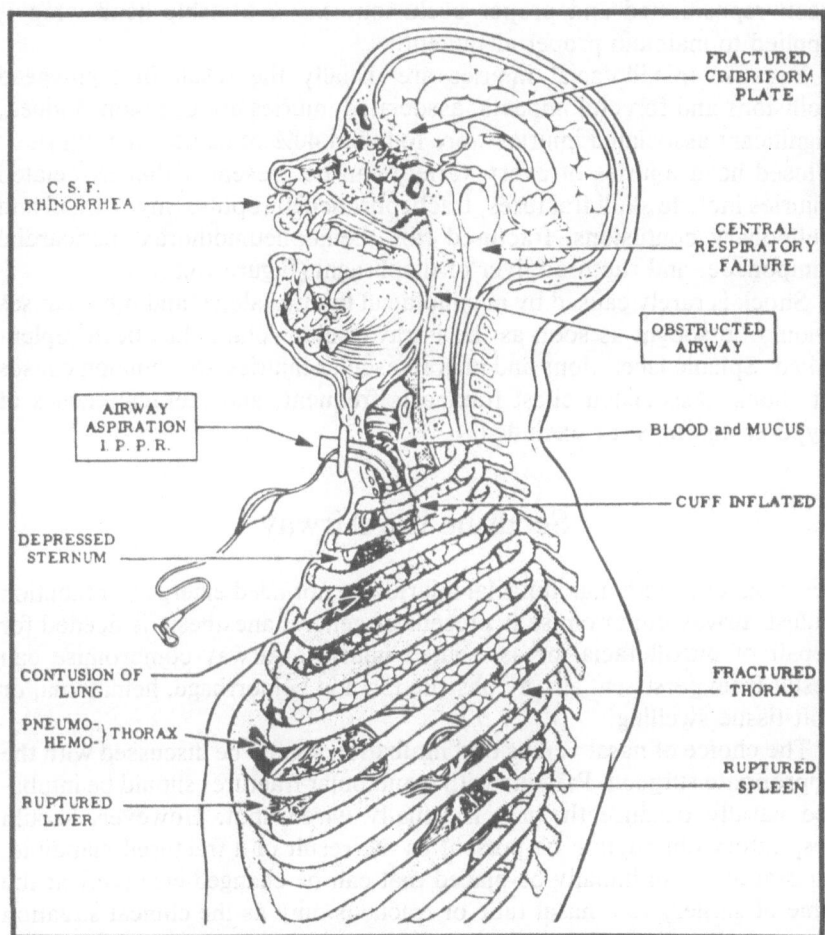

FIGURE 16.5. Some of the associated injuries after trauma, resulting in maxillofacial injuries. After basilar skull and bilateral mandibular fractures, a cricothyrotomy or tracheostomy may be necessary if oral intubation is unsuccessful. (Reprinted with permission from Rowe NL, Killey HC: *Fractures of the Facial Skeleton,* Edinburgh, Churchill Livingstone, 1968.)

Nevertheless, placement of a nasopharyngeal tube does have significant risks. It may cause further bleeding in the nasopharynx or infection. The airway may kink or become completely occluded with mucus or blood. Thus, the patency of nasopharyngeal airways must be ensured via frequent suctioning. Once the maxillary and mandibular fragments have been repositioned and proper occlusion exists, a stable head wrap is applied to maintain proper alignment.

Because maxillofacial injuries are usually the result of high-speed collisions and forceful impacts, associated injuries are common. Indeed, significant associated injuries were found in 40% of mandibular injuries.[7] Closed head injuries of every variety can be present. Other associated injuries include skull fractures, tracheobronchial rupture, myocardial and pulmonary contusions, fractured ribs, hemopneumothorax, pericardial tamponade, and ruptured liver or diaphragm (Figure 16.5.).

Shock is rarely caused by maxillofacial injuries alone, and other causes should be sought as soon as the intravascular volume has been replenished. Splenic lacerations and major vascular injuries are common causes of shock. Associated chest trauma is frequent, and thoracic causes of hypotension must be excluded.

Securing the Airway

Most patients with maxillofacial injuries do not need emergent intubation unless airway compromise is present or general anesthesia is needed for repair of maxillofacial or associated injuries. Airway compromise can result from persistent airway obstruction and hemorrhage, hematoma, or soft-tissue swelling.

The choice of nasal versus oral intubation should be discussed with the appropriate surgeon. Patients with mandibular fractures should be intubated nasally because the jaw is usually wired shut. However, should respiratory obstruction be present as the result of a fractured mandible, an oral tube can initially be placed that can be changed electively at the time of surgery to a nasal tube or tracheostomy as the clinical situation dictates. A nasotracheal tube should be used in patients with LeFort fractures in which there is no radiographic evidence of a basilar skull fracture, since intermaxillary fixation is necessary. Physical signs of a basilar skull fracture include raccoon eyes (orbital hematomas), battle signs (retroaural hematomas), CSF rhinorrhea or otorrhea, and anosmia (loss of the sense of smell).

All patients with maxillofacial trauma are presumed to have a full stomach. Thus, sedation should be minimized and administration of muscle relaxants avoided unless the ability to visualize the vocal cords has been demonstrated. The presence of spontaneous respirations will facilitate awake orotracheal or nasotracheal intubation. It is preferable to insert the endotracheal tubes under direct vision or with fiberoptic endoscopy to avoid advancing foreign material into the airway. In cases where there is extensive airway hemorrhage that cannot be controlled by packing alone, intubation should be performed to prevent aspiration of blood into the trachea. All comatose patients should be intubated.

Emergent tracheostomy is rarely needed for facial fractures alone. Indeed, of 1042 patients with maxillofacial trauma, only 8 required tracheostomy.[1] Indications were always associated injuries of the larynx, trachea, neck, or spine. Absolute indications for tracheostomy include (1) a fractured larynx or trachea, (2) associated neurologic or thoracic injuries that will require prolonged intubation, (3) inability to intubate a patient with respiratory obstruction, and (4) basilar skull fracture or severe nasal deformity requiring intermaxillary fixation. A fiberoptic intubation can sometimes be used to avoid a tracheostomy or at least allow the tracheostomy to be performed under general anesthesia after the airway has been secured. Thus, oral fiberoptic intubation should be attempted in the case of (1) a basilar skull fracture with an associated mandibular fracture or (2) a maxillary fracture with a cervical spine injury.

In the emergency room, if an airway is emergently needed and oral/nasal intubations are either unsuccessful or contraindicated, then a cricothyrotomy should be performed. Tracheostomies for maxillofacial injuries should be done electively in the operating room when the appropriate staff and equipment are available.

Definitive Repair

Fortunately, many maxillofacial injuries can be repaired under local anesthesia provided there is no degree of airway obstruction. Repair under local anesthesia alleviates the need for intubation and general anesthesia. Local anesthesia also allows the surgeon greater ease in operating since there will be no interference from an endotracheal tube. Patients must be psychologically well prepared and cooperative for such repairs to be successful. Repairs of facial lacerations are often undertaken in the emergency room. However, since large amounts of local anesthetic and sedative agents are needed in patients with compromised airways, these repairs are best performed in the operating room with an anesthesiologist present.

Nerve blocks for repair of facial lacerations include supraorbital, nasal, infraorbital, maxillary, and mandibular blocks. The addition of epinephrine improves hemostasis, prolongs the anesthetic effect, and decreases the rate of absorption. Cocaine is ideal for anesthetizing mucous membranes because of its vasoconstrictive effect.

Local anesthesia can also be used to apply arch bars for intermaxillary fixation. After a topical anesthetic has been applied to the mucosa, bilateral inferior alveolar nerve blocks are placed to anesthetize the fracture sites. Bilateral greater palatine nerve blocks are performed, along with infiltration at the buccal-labial surface of the gingiva to anesthetize the maxillary dental arch.

Definitive treatment of maxillary and mandibular fractures entails intermaxillary immobilization for 4–6 weeks. Open reduction and interosseous wiring is usually undertaken within the first 7 days. The first step in LeFort repairs is to obtain proper occlusion with arch bars. Then the mobile fragments are attached to the maxilla, zygoma, and skull.

Occasionally, if there are multiple maxillary fractures that cannot be stabilized internally, external fixation to a halo frame or plaster head cap is undertaken. Often ophthalmologists and neurosurgeons will repair associated orbital and skull fractures. Associated CSF leaks usually resolve spontaneously; persistent leaks require exploration and repair of the cribriform plate.

Anesthetic Considerations

Special consideration should be given to the events leading up to the injury. Most serious accidents involve drug or alcohol intoxication. Also, a middle-aged or elderly person may have suffered a myocardial infarction or cerebrovascular injury leading to an automobile accident. A history of loss of consciousness might indicate a closed head injury.

Because of the patient's disfigurement and altered self-image (among other reasons), a preoperative visit is mandatory. This serves not only to help understand the patient's psychological state but also to minimize the patient's apprehension and to screen for associated injuries. Diazepam 10 mg orally provides good premedication without much danger of causing respiratory obstruction. Any disfigured patient should be kept well sedated and allowed privacy in the holding area.

For intraoral or mandibular surgery, a nasotracheal tube is desirable. For intermaxillary fixation, a nasotracheal tube affords free access to the upper and lower jaws for arch bar placement. Usually trismus from masseter spasm is present after mandibular and maxillary fractures. If repair of these fractures is performed within a week or 10 days, these muscles should relax after neuromuscular blocking agents are administered. However, after 2 weeks, fibrosis of these muscles may prevent adequate relaxation for laryngoscopy, and an alternative technique (awake nasal or nasal fiberoptic laryngoscopy) may be necessary. Another cause of inability to open the patient's mouth is fracture through the temporomandibular joint or joint dysfunction from posteroinferior displacement of a fractured zygoma.

For surgery elsewhere on the face, an orotracheal tube is preferred. Curved adaptors keep the endotracheal tube and airway tubing close to the lower chin and away from the surgical field. If the orotracheal tube is attached in the midline of the chin with a small amount of tape, there will be minimal distortion of facial features. However, the surgeon must warn the anesthesiologist prior to any manipulation of the head, to prevent accidental extubation or disconnection.

Despite the administration of general anesthesia, the surgeon usually infiltrates local anesthetic combined with epinephrine for the latter's vasoconstrictive effects. The total dose of both agents must be monitored and limited to avoid toxicity.

If a skull fracture or CSF leak is present, the presence of a pneumocranium should be suspected and nitrous oxide avoided. In addition, cerebral edema or mass effect may be present, which may warrant hyperventilation and diuretic therapy to correct elevated intracranial pressure (ICP).

Several methods can be utilized to minimize operative bleeding, which may be both venous and arterial. Postural hypotension can be achieved with a head-up tilt of 15–30° to reduce arterial pressure at the operative site and to eliminate venous congestion. Alternatively, controlled hypotension minimizes operative blood loss and provides a cleaner operative field. Controlled hypotension can be safely achieved with high concentrations of inhalation agents, adrenergic and ganglionic blocking agents, or arterial vasodilators.

Contraindications to induced hypotension include the presence of neurologic injury (elevated ICP, cerebral contusion, or hemorrhage), vascular disease (carotid occlusive or coronary artery disease), or an intrapulmonary shunt. Certain anesthetic techniques can cause synergistic hypotension, such as cardiodepression from inhalation agents, as well as diminished venous return from reverse Trendelenburg position and positive pressure ventilation.

Sedation with a combination of fentanyl and droperidol allows better toleration of the endotracheal tube in the recovery room. If the jaw has been wired shut, the nasotracheal tube should be left in place until the patient is alert enough to protect his airway should vomiting occur. Insertion of a nasogastric tube allows drainage of stomach contents and reduces the risk of aspiration. If extensive surgery has been performed, the endotracheal tube should be left in place for 24 h until the soft-tissue edema subsides. Dexamethasone 4–8 mg intravenously may help diminish surgical edema. If the jaw has been wired shut, then wire cutters must be immediately available in the recovery room should emergency access to the mouth be needed.

In conclusion, there are a multitude of factors that must be considered for proper handling of the airway in patients with maxillofacial injuries.

Optimal outcome is assured by the coordinated effort of anesthesiologists and surgeons from the time of the patient's arrival in the emergency room through the postoperative period.

References

1. Schultz RC: Facial Injuries. Chicago, Year Book Publishers, 1970.
2. Dingman RO, Converse JM: The clinical management of facial injuries and fractures of the facial bones, in: Converse JM (ed): Reconstructive Plastic Surgery, 2nd ed. Philadelphia, WB Saunders, 1977; vol. 2, 688–719.
3. James RB, Fredrickson C, Kent J: Prospective study of mandibular fractures. J Oral Surg 1981;39:275–81.
4. LeFort R: Experimental study of fractures of the upper jaw. Rev Chir de Paris 1901;23:208–27, 360–79. (Reprinted in Plast Reconstr Surg 1972;50:497–506.)
5. Manson PN, Hoopes JE, Su CT: Structural pillars of the facial skeleton: an approach to the management of LeFort fractures. Plast Reconstr Surg 1980;66:54–61.
6. Gotta AW: Maxillofacial trauma anesthetic considerations. ASA Refresher Course Lectures 1986;No.246.
7. Bailey BJ, Gaskill JR: Fractures of the mandible. Laryngoscope 1967;77:1137–54.

CHAPTER 17

The Patient with Hydrocephalus

Ross A. Malley

Case History. *A 75-year-old woman with a history of a large subfrontal lobe meningioma and new-onset seizure disorder was admitted for surgical resection of the lesion. Past medical history was significant for obesity, questionable history of congestive heart failure (CHF) without known myocardial infarction, and hypertension. Medications on admission included phenytoin 300 mg b.i.d., propranolol 20 mg t.i.d., and hydrochlorothiazide 50 mg q.d.*

The patient underwent an uneventful bifrontal craniotomy with complete resection of the meningioma. Her postoperative course was complicated by evidence of worsening CHF with subjective dyspnea, bibasilar râles, increased vascular pattern on chest x-ray, and PaO_2 of 55 mmHg on room air. The patient had also developed a persistent cerebrospinal fluid rhinorrhea that did not respond to lumbar draining. A head CT scan demonstrated enlarged ventricles and edema in the area of tumor resection. A diagnosis of communicating hydrocephalus was made, and the patient was scheduled for insertion of ventriculoperitoneal shunt.

Introduction

Hydrocephalus is a common problem that anesthesiologists must deal with in patients presenting for neurosurgical procedures. It is defined as an imbalance between the production and reabsorption of cerebrospinal fluid (CSF) within the central nervous system, resulting in increased intracranial pressure. The abnormality may affect patients of all ages, from the neonate to the centenarian. Uncorrected, it can result in significant nervous system dysfunctions, ranging from mental retardation and gait disturbance to coma and death.

Estimates of the incidence of the disease vary. The best information is

---

Reviewed by Dr. Allen B. Kantrowitz, Assistant Professor of Neurosurgery, Albert Einstein College of Medicine, Montefiore Medical Center, Bronx, NY.

for patients with congenital hydrocephalus: 0.9–1.5/1000 live births when it occurs as a single entity; 1.3–2.9/1000 live births with myelomeningocele.[1]

Cerebrospinal Fluid Dynamics

Cerebrospinal fluid is contained within the central nervous system and serves a supportive function for the neural elements. It acts both as a mechanical protector by cushioning the brain and spinal cord within their bony coverings and as a means of transporting nutrients and metabolic wastes.

CSF circulates within the substance of the brain itself, contained in the ventricles located in the cerebral hemispheres, the diencephalon, and the hindbrain. The paired lateral ventricles are found in the cerebral hemispheres. Horn-shaped, they are placed anterior to posterior from the frontal to the occipital lobes and then inferior to the temporal lobes. Within these ventricles are the major portions of the choroid plexus, which is the primary site of CSF production. The CSF exits the lateral ventricles via the paired foramina of Monro and enters the single midline third ventricle, which is bounded by the thalamic nuclei. From here the circulation transports the CSF caudally to the fourth ventricle via the aqueduct of Sylvius.

Additional areas of choroid plexus are located in both the third and fourth ventricles. Communication between the fourth ventricle and the cisterna magna is provided by the single foramen of Magendie (midline) and the paired foramina of Luschka (lateral). Once the CSF enters the subarachnoid space, it is able to flow over the cerebellar hemispheres, through the tentorial hiatus into the basilar cisterns, over the cerebral hemispheres, and eventually into the area of the arachnoid granulations. These are the sites of CSF reabsorption into the venous circulation. As detailed in Figure 17.1., the CSF also circulates within the spinal subarachnoid space.

The total volume of CSF in the adult ranges from 140 to 200 ml, with 25–50 ml contained in the ventricles.[2] Normal pressures in the laterally recumbent adult, measured in the lumbar subarachnoid space, range from 100 to 180 mm H_2O (5-15 mmHg).[3] Circulation of the CSF through the ventricles and subarachnoid space is effected by bulk flow propelled by pulsations within the ventricular system that are produced by arterial pulsations and by venous pressure changes transmitted from the respiratory system.

As noted previously, the major site for the production of CSF is the choroid plexus, located in the ventricular system. The balance of the constituents of CSF are derived from the metabolic activity of the central nervous system. The production of CSF by the choroid plexus is not a passive filtration process but involves active transport of ions and larger molecules. Light and electron microscopy of the choroid plexus reveals fenestrated capillaries that are believed to be evidence of the absence of the normal blood-brain barrier that limits the movement of solutes from the general circulation into the parenchyma. The plasma ultrafiltrate in the interstitial space is modified as it passes into the ventricular system by the pumps located in the choroidal epithelial cells (Figure 17.2.). Comparison of the electrolyte content of CSF and plasma is outlined in Table 17.1.

The rate of production of CSF in the adult has been measured at approximately 0.35 ml/min.[4] Of the factors investigated, the perfusion pressure of the choroidal capillaries appears to be the most significant[5]; systemic hypertension increases CSF production. Pharmacologic manipulation has been attempted to decrease the volume of CSF. Carbonic

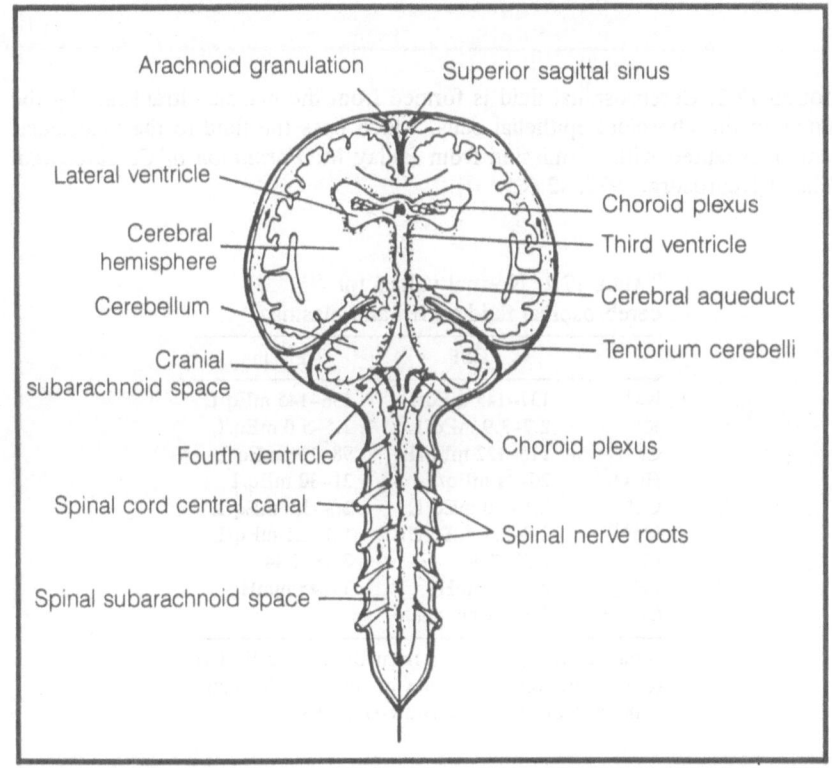

FIGURE 17.1. Sagittal section of the central nervous system, indicating the normal flow of cerebrospinal fluid. From Hockwald GM: *Cerebrospinal Fluid Mechanisms,* in Cottrell JE, Turndorf H (eds): *Anesthesia and Neurosurgery,* St. Louis, C.V. Mosby Co., 1986, p 37. Adapted with permission from Millen and Woollam: *The Anatomy of the Cerebrospinal Fluid,* London, Oxford University Press, 1962.

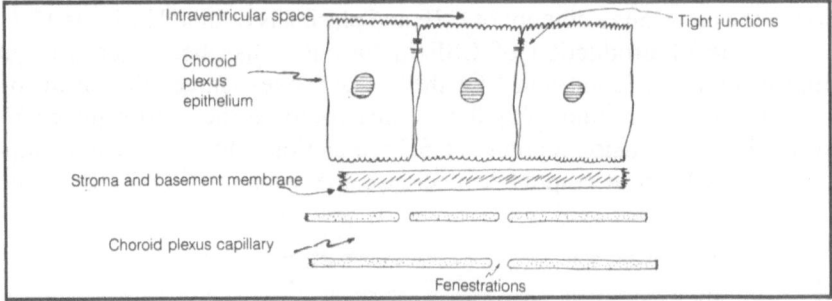

FIGURE 17.2. Cerebrospinal fluid is formed from the plasma ultrafiltrate by the pumps in the choroidal epithelial cells, which pass the fluid to the ventricular system. Adapted with permission from Pollay M: *Formation of Cerebrospinal Fluid,* J Neurosurg, 1975; 42:665.

TABLE 17.1. Normal values for cerebrospinal fluid (CSF) and plasma.

	CSF	Plasma
Na^+	137–145 mEq/L	136–145 mEq/L
K^+	2.7–3.9 mEq/L	3.5–5.0 mEq/L
Cl^-	116–122 mEq/L	98–106 mEq/L
HCO_3^-	20–24 mEq/L	21–30 mEq/L
Ca^{+2}	2.1–3.0 mEq/L	2.3–3.8 mEq/L
Mg^{+2}	2.0–2.5 mEq/L	1.3–2.1 mEq/L
pH	7.31–7.34	7.38–7.44
PCO_2	45–49 mmHg	35–45 mmHg
Glucose	2/3 plasma value	

Adapted with permission from Braunwald E et al (eds): Harrison's Principles of Internal Medicine, 11th ed; New York; McGraw-Hill, 1987.

anhydrase inhibitors have been used with limited success. Cardiac glycosides and steroids have been used experimentally and clinically to reduce CSF production, but with little reproducible success.

The sites of absorption of CSF are the arachnoid granulations in the sagittal sinus and other major venous sinuses in the cranium. The normal structure of the leptomeninges is modified with evagination of the arachnoid layer through the dura (Figure 17.3.). These evaginations balloon into the lumen of the sinus, and a thin layer of tissue separates the CSF from the venous circulation. On microscopic examination, numerous vacuoles are found in this cell layer. Current opinion holds that the CSF is carried through this layer in bulk form within these vacuoles.[6] Studies have shown that where there is increased CSF pressure, the number of vacuoles increases.

Etiology

The etiology of hydrocephalus is diverse, and the condition occurs in a broad spectrum of patients. Historically, it has three hypothetical etiologies. The first is an overproduction of CSF by the choroid plexus with an otherwise normal ventricular and absorption system. There are reports of relief of hydrocephalus in children by resection of choroid papillomas, although relief of concomitant ventricular obstruction is also suspected.[7] The second etiology is one of obstruction of venous drainage, increased pressure within venous sinuses, and resultant "back pressures," decreas-

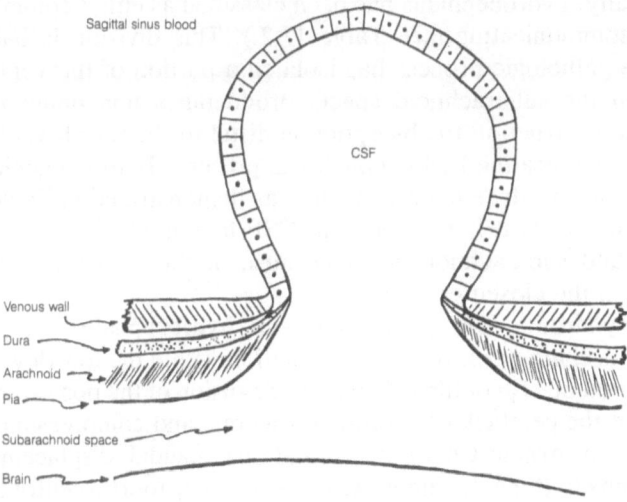

FIGURE 17.3. Evagination of the arachnoid layer through the dura forming granulations that absorb CSF.

TABLE 17.2. Classification of hydrocephalus.

Noncommunicating
  Congenital
    Aqueductal stenosis caused by septa, forking, scarring
    Obstruction of 4th ventricle (Dandy-Walker cyst)
    Obstruction by masses such as vascular malformations and benign and malignant
      tumors (neural-based and metastatic)
  Acquired
    Aqueductal stenosis caused by infection, reaction to intraventricular bleeds
    Ventriculitis
    Masses
Communicating
  Congenital
    Arnold-Chiari malformations
    Meningitis
    Congenital absence of arachnoid granulations
  Acquired
    Meningitis: infectious, hemorrhagic (esp. in newborns, trauma, postop, aneurysm
      bleeds)
    Masses

Adapted with permission from Wilkins RH, Rengachary SS (eds): Neurosurgery; New York, McGraw-Hill, 1985.

ing CSF absorption and producing hydrocephalus. Experimental data are lacking for this assertion.[8] Finally, obstruction of the CSF flow between sites of production and of absorption has the strongest experimental and clinical causative evidence and provides the basis for surgical treatment of this condition.

Traditionally, hydrocephalus has been classified as either communicating or noncommunicating (see Table 17.2.). This division is based on whether the pathologic process has isolated a portion of the ventricular system from the subarachnoid space, producing a noncommunicating lesion. If the obstruction to absorption is distal to the fourth ventricular outlet, a communicating hydrocephalus is present. Both congenital and acquired lesions produce hydrocephalus, as demonstrated in Table 17.2. Whatever the cause, it is possible that CSF flow is blocked at both the ventricular and subarachnoid level because of the pressure effects of masses within the closed cranium.

Specific syndromes are associated with hydrocephalus. A Dandy-Walker cyst is characterized by cyst formation within the fourth ventricle and obstruction of CSF outflow. There is expansion of the posterior fossa, separation of the cerebellar lateral hemispheres, and compression of the brain stem. In Arnold-Chiari malformations, caudal displacement of cerebellar tonsils (type 1), along with the vermis, fourth ventricle, and medulla (type 2), occurs with obstruction of CSF flow in the subarachnoid space. Approximately 90% of patients with meningomyelocele will have hydrocephalus with Arnold-Chiari type 2 malfunction. Of the acquired lesions, an extremely common cause in the pediatric patient, especially the preterm infant, is intracranial bleeds with resultant ventriculitis and inflammation of the meninges. This also occurs in adults as a result of aneurysm rupture or hemorrhagic infarcts, after head trauma, or, as in this case, as a consequence of iatrogenic subarachnoid blood and subsequent scarring.

Clinical Syndromes

The presentation of a patient with hydrocephalus is variable, both in the extent of dysfunction and the rapidity with which accumulation of CSF has increased intracranial pressure (ICP) and compensation by the central nervous system has occurred. In the pediatric age group with open fontanelles and sutures, the most obvious feature is an enlarged head relative to the body size. This may be grossly obvious at birth or become apparent with serial head-circumference measurements after birth. Associated signs include large "domed" forehead with low-set eyes and ears due to cranial-facial disproportion. The anterior fontanelle is full, even in the upright, relaxed position. Cranial nerve compromise occurs, with optic atrophy or abducens nerve palsy. In advanced cases, if the expansion of the ventricles is extensive and the cerebral cortex is extremely thin, transillumination of the skull is possible. If the obstruction occurs rapidly and the rise in ICP is faster than the open sutures can accommodate, there will be increased irritability, vomiting, seizures, lethargy, and brain stem compromise with respiratory failure and death.

Not uncommonly in children, pressure and traction around the brain stem may result in an inability to handle oropharyngeal secretions. The child appears to have a "runny nose," and there is a temptation to cancel the case pending resolution of the apparent upper respiratory tract infection. However, if the patient is afebrile, has no other constitutional symptoms, and has a normal white count, surgery should proceed to correct the elevated ICP.

In the child and adult with closed sutures, the presentation will depend on the rapidity at which the obstruction to CSF drainage and the rise in ICP occur.

In acute hydrocephalus, there is a sudden, rapid rise in ICP. The patient presents with nausea, vomiting, and headache. Further increases in ICP result in mental status changes with lethargy, confusion, and obtundation. On examination, papilledema is seen. Transtentorial herniation may occur, and decorticate or decerebrate posturing may appear. If untreated, brain stem function is further compromised, respiratory function deteriorates, and ECG abnormalities and hypertension may occur as preterminal events. This is a group of patients for whom rapid diagnosis and drainage of CSF can be lifesaving.

When the onset of obstruction and increased ICP is slower, presentation with "chronic" hydrocephalus is less dramatic; patients present with headache, nausea, and vomiting. Evidence of higher-function disturbances is present in the form of mental retardation, memory loss, decreased cognitive function, behavioral changes, and gait disturbances. On examination, papilledema is present in approximately 80% of patients, with varying degrees of optic atrophy due to longstanding pressure effects on the optic nerve. Abducens nerve palsy also is common. In children, endocrine abnormalities may occur, including obesity, giantism, precocious puberty, menstrual irregularity, and diabetes insipidus.[9]

Finally, note is made of a clinical entity termed normal-pressure hydrocephalus. In adults it is characterized by a triad of gait disturbances, dementia, and incontinence.[10] These signs are insidious in onset, and exclusion of other dementias, due to cerebrovascular disease, trauma, infections, and the like, must be made. In children the syndrome includes head enlargement, mental retardation, developmental delay, and mild spasticity. There is slowly progressive ventricular enlargement with minimal increase in intraventricular pressure. Diagnosis is established by neurologic examination, serial CT scans, and neuropsychologic testing.[11]

Treatment

Surgical shunting procedures, coupled with resection of obstructing lesions in appropriate cases, is the treatment of choice for patients with hydrocephalus.

Two nonsurgical approaches have been utilized with poor success. The first is wrapping a child's head to produce an increase in ICP, decreasing production and increasing absorption of CSF and thus encouraging compensation.[12] The other approach has been to reduce CSF formation by drugs such as the carbonic anhydrase inhibitor acetazolamide.[13] Neither technique has proved to be effective for longterm therapy.

Surgical placement of an artificial shunt is designed to divert the CSF from the area proximal to the block to an alternative resorption site. Currently, the indications for shunt placement include progressive hydrocephalus, either communicating or noncommunicating, with worsening or reversible defects.

Contraindications for shunting include active ventriculitis, extreme cortical atrophy with irreversible defects, systemic infection processes, and an obstruction amenable to complete surgical removal. Patients may require a simple ventricular drain to manage the acute phase of their disease. Currently, shunts are most frequently placed ventriculoperitoneally and ventriculoatrially. Other sites are listed in Table 17.3.

The system used consists of a ventriculostomy tube connected to a pressure-controlled valve and reservoir and a distal draining tube constructed of tissue-compatible materials. The valves include one-way slit,

TABLE 17.3. Sites for shunt placement.

Ventriculoperitoneal
Ventriculoatrial
Ventriculocholedochal
Ventriculovesicular
Ventriculopleural
Lumboperitoneal

ball-spring, and diaphragm, with low to high opening pressures depending on the type used. The patient is placed supine, and the head is manually rotated to the left to allow access to the right (nondominant) side of the cranium. Also, the patient's shoulder may be raised with a roll. After a scalp flap is turned, a small burr hole is drilled and the meninges are coagulated and nicked. The ventriculostomy tube is inserted with a stylet into the frontal horn of the lateral ventricle, and once CSF is obtained, the valve/reservoir assembly is attached. Alternative sites include parietal and occipital ventriculostomy sites.

In a ventriculoperitoneal (VP) shunt, a right-upper-quadrant incision is carried down to the peritoneum. A subcutaneous tunnel to the reservoir site is established with a blunt trocar, and the distal shunt tubing is passed through it. When the tubing is connected to the reservoir, the free end is passed into the peritoneum and the incision is closed. In adults and large children a supplemental incision at the level of the clavicle may be needed.

In ventriculoatrial (VA) shunts, an incision into the internal jugular vein is performed. The distal shunt is inserted through a venotomy, and the distal position is checked with either fluoroscopy or plain x-ray. The reservoir is connected proximally as for a VP shunt.

The advantage of the VP shunt versus the VA shunt is that a longer length of the tubing can be used in the abdomen, partially reducing the need for revision and avoiding invasion of the central circulation by a foreign body. VA shunting is useful in patients with intraabdominal processes such as extensive adhesions, which make the placement of the distal shunt difficult and reduce free flow of CSF over the peritoneum for absorption.

There are immediate and longterm complications associated with each type of shunt, as listed in Table 17.4.

Preanesthetic Assessment

The preanesthetic evaluation of patients for shunt placement or revision allows the anesthesiologist to gather the information needed for appropriate management. Concurrent or associated disease processes must be sought for and corrected, if possible, or stabilized before the patient is anesthetized.

TABLE 17.4. Complications of shunting procedures.

Most common for both VA and VP shunts
  Obstruction, both proximal and distal
  Disconnection of shunt tubing
  Infections in or around shunt (63% *Staphylococcus* sp.)
  Failure of valve system

Specific for VA shunts
  Air embolus during shunt insertion
  Perforations of great vessels and heart
  Pulmonary emboli, superior vena cava (SVC) thrombosis, pulmonary hypertension
  Renal insufficiency due to recurrent bacteremia/septic emboli
  Congestive heart failure
  Shunt nephritis

Specific for VP shunts
  Bowel obstruction or perforation
  Peritoneal cysts
  Erosion of catheter with extrusion through rectum, vagina

Adapted with permission from Keucher TR, Mealey J Jr: Longterm results after ventriculoatrial and ventriculoperitoneal shunting for infantile hydrocephalus. J Neurosurg 1979;50:179.

Nervous System

As the major system affected by hydrocephalus, the nervous system must be assessed by the anesthetist for degree and type of dysfunction present. Characterization of the symptoms—their onset, progression, and current status—will provide an index of compromise and compensation. The presence of old, fixed neurologic deficits should be documented for postoperative comparison. In the adult, concurrent atherosclerotic cerebrovascular disease must be identified, especially if the patient has symptoms that change with head position and may be exacerbated during positioning.

Respiratory System

The respiratory system also must be evaluated. Intercurrent respiratory illness, its degree of activity, and current therapy must be evaluated. Processes such as acute upper respiratory tract infections, bronchospastic pulmonary diseases, chronic obstructive pulmonary disease, and chronic bronchitis will impact on patient management. In patients in whom intracranial compliance is already reduced, even small increases in $PaCO_2$ may cause devastating increases in ICP. Quantifying smoking history is important to gauge the effect on lung function. Specific pulmonary problems associated with hydrocephalus and increased ICP may include the occurrence of recurrent aspiration and pneumonias caused by lower cranial nerve dysfunction and, as already mentioned, increased nasal secretions.

Cardiovascular System

In the pediatric age group a history of perinatal cardiac dysfunction, such as persistent cyanosis, history of CHF, or murmur, may be indicative of structural lesions in the heart and great vessels. These include problems such as intra- and extracardiac shunts and valvular anomalies, which may occur more frequently in patients with other developmental anomalies.

In the adult the presence of atherosclerotic cardiovascular disease, its functional significance, and the patient's compensation should be assessed. The use of daily activity to quantify this impairment is often difficult, as there may be limitations imposed by the primary neurologic dysfunction, and in such cases more intensive laboratory evaluation (echocardiography, angiography, etc) is indicated.

Cardiac changes due to elevated ICP in untreated hydrocephalus primarily manifest as ECG abnormalities such as U waves, ST-segment changes, notched T waves, and QT-interval abnormalities.[14] However, all cardiac dysrhythmias have been described in association with elevated ICP. There may be complications associated with patients with preexisting VA shunts, as previously noted (see Table 17.4).

Fluid and Electrolyte Balance

The frequent disruption of normal oral intake that can occur in both pediatric and adult patients with hydrocephalus requires an assessment of fluid and electrolyte status. Persistent nausea and vomiting may result in significant dehydration. The fact that the patient has been hospitalized is no guarantee that normal fluid balance has been reestablished. The obtunded or paretic patient may be unable to obtain or ingest fluids orally. A brisk osmotic diuresis also may have been established by contrast materials used in neuroradiologic procedures, together with a practice of keeping the neurosurgical patient "dry." As in any patient undergoing an anesthetic procedure, failure to correct or modify the anesthetic technique for dehydration will increase the degree of hemodynamic instability perioperatively.[15]

Electrolyte disturbances also can result from the effects of hydrocephalus on pituitary function and from the use of carbonic anhydrase inhibitors.

Past History

The balance of the usual preoperative evaluation should be completed, including (a) past neurosurgical and nonneurosurgical procedures; (b) anesthetic problems for either the patient or family; (c) allergies to medications, tape, or cleansing solutions; (d) current medications, including those administered in the hospital, that may affect level of consciousness or prolong emergence, especially sedation used for neuroradiologic procedures.

Physical Examination

The physical examination confirms previously identified problems and screens for unreported problems requiring attention during the anesthetic process. Examination of the head will reveal the extent of cranial expansion in the pediatric patient, and palpation of the fontanelle will provide an index of the degree of elevated ICP. Mouth and neck movement allows assessment of the ease of intubation. Range of motion of the neck in the elderly also indicates potential problems with positioning. In the presence of concurrent cerebrovascular disease, any changes in sensory or motor function or mentation should be noted. Chest auscultation identifies pulmonary and cardiac changes. Extremities should be examined for intravenous access, presence of contractions, or skeletal abnormalities that will hinder positioning of the patient.

Laboratory Evaluation

The laboratory evaluation consists of both routine and specific tests based on the extent and type of concurrent disease present.

Routine examination, including CBC, urinalysis, chest radiograph, ECG, and serum electrolytes, is essential. Additionally, ascertaining blood levels of antiseizure medications, blood gases, and the like may be indicated.

Currently, the "gold standard" for radiologic evaluation of hydrocephalus is the computed tomograph of the head. A CT scan allows for accurate characterization of the extent of ventricular dilation and the presence of obstructing masses, midline shifts, and, with the use of contrast agents, vascular abnormalities or tumors. Since it is a minimally invasive test, the serial CT scan can follow the progression of dilatation and confirm more chronic cases of hydrocephalus. This test has rapidly replaced the more traditional studies—pneumoencephalography and cistern dye/tracer—because of its minimal morbidity and essentially zero mortality.[16] Magnetic resonance imaging is becoming established as a sensitive and complementary method of imaging in hydrocephalus.

Anesthetic Plan

Premedication

The choice of premedication for the patient is based on the anesthetist's synthesis of the psychologic needs, the physiologic perturbations, and the surgical requirements for the patient's care.

At a minimum, patients should receive their current oral and transcutaneous medications, including antiseizure, antihypertensive, cardiac, and bronchodilatory agents, to maintain appropriate intraoperative levels.

The use of sedatives in patients with disturbed intracranial dynamics requires cautious utilization of reduced doses or titration of the drugs under observation. In patients with decreased levels of consciousness or other evidence of elevated ICP, all sedatives should be avoided to eliminate the risks of worsening ventilatory depression, hypercarbia, and increased cerebral blood flow.

Monitoring

Intraoperative monitoring needs include routine ECG, blood pressure, FIO_2, heart tones, temperature, pulse oximetry, and capnography. As recently reported,[17] the occurrence of clinically unrecognized episodes of hypoxia, especially in children, can be rapidly detected with modern pulse oximetry. Since the patient's airway is remote from the anesthesiologist and the positioning of the head can cause either unintentional extubation or endobronchial intubation, this technology is an important monitor.[18] The use of capnography provides a noninvasive means of assessing PCO_2 and can direct appropriate ventilatory modifications to modulate cerebral blood flow and ICP.

Other monitors, such as invasive arterial or venous pressure monitoring or precordial Doppler, are added as indicated by the patient's condition and planned procedure.

Induction

The induction of patients with hydrocephalus ideally should produce an anesthetic state with minimal changes in the ventilation, cerebral blood flow, and cardiovascular parameters. Since the condition of intracerebral dynamics is unknown, maintenance of the preanesthetic state in patients who are mentating, ventilating, and self-supporting of cerebral perfusion should not further compromise CNS function.

In the fasting patient with intravenous access established, induction with barbiturates, narcotics, or etomidate can be performed, the dose being titrated to achieve the necessary reduction in responsiveness. Because of its deleterious effect in increasing cerebral blood flow, ketamine is contraindicated.[19] Intubation of the patient should be facilitated by the addition of a neuromuscular blocking agent. Currently, the agents of choice appear to be the nondepolarizing agents, such as pancuronium, atracurium, and vecuronium, as they produce minimal changes in cerebral dynamics.[20] Succinylcholine should be avoided, as it may cause catastrophic hyperkalemia in paretic patients and produce increases in ICP not effectively blocked by defasciculating doses of a nondepolarizer.[21] Immediately prior to intubation, supplemental doses of barbiturate (1 mg/kg thiopental) or lidocaine (1 mg/kg) will help to blunt the stimulus of laryngoscopy and elevations in ICP.[22]

If the patient has a full stomach, the risks of aspiration must be weighed against the risks of elevating ICP with laryngoscopy and intubation in a patient who is not fully anesthetized. Intubation after administration of intravenous barbiturates, a priming and intubating dose of a nondepolarizer, and lidocaine, along with appropriate preoxygenation and cricoid pressure, appears to minimize or eliminate the risks of development of sudden intracranial hypertension.

Induction of pediatric patients with hydrocephalus adds another dimension to the risk/benefit decision. If intravenous access cannot be obtained without producing a crying, screaming, struggling, intracranially hypertensive child who may suddenly herniate, what is "Plan B"? The use of rectal barbiturates such as methohexital is one option that can produce an acceptable induction. The potential disadvantages include respiratory depression and prolonged emergence, both of which dictate careful observation for these complications.[23] The other option is an inhalational induction. The agents best accepted by the patient are nitrous oxide and halothane, yet both are associated with increased cerebral blood flow and elevated ICP.[24] Isoflurane has less effect on cerebral dynamics but is associated with more airway irritability. The best technique may be a slow, gentle induction using isoflurane and oxygen, with rapid establishment of I.V. access and reduction in the inspired concentration of isoflurane when narcotics, barbiturates, and muscle relaxants can be added.

Maintenance

With the airway now secure, the final positioning established, and breath sounds rechecked, surgery may begin. Maintenance of the anesthetic can be achieved with an appropriate combination of intravenous and inhalational agents that will allow for prompt awakening and extubation.

Of the available fixed agents, the narcotics—particularly small incremental doses or infusions of fentanyl, sufentanil, or alfentanil—provide acceptable analgesia/anesthesia. Barbiturates and benzodiazepines are less suited because of accumulation and long half-lives.

Nitrous oxide has the advantage of rapid onset and reversal, augmenting analgesia and amnesia, but it is associated with marked elevations in ICP in patients with intracranial pathology. Of the potent inhalational agents, isoflurane appears to have the most favorable profile, causing less increase in cerebral blood flow than either halothane or enflurane.[25] Enflurane is also associated with seizurelike ECG activity confounded by hypocarbia and with increased CSF production and decreased absorption.[26]

Marked ECG abnormalities may occur during the sudden decompression caused by CSF withdrawal during ventriculostomy. Although bradycardia may be partially corrected by atropine administration, replacement of some of the fluid and slower initial withdrawal are preferable.

Emergence

Given an uneventful procedure, the patient can be awakened and the trachea extubated promptly.

As the dressings are applied, the anesthetist must be aware of manipulation of the head and its effect on endotracheal tube position and stimulation. Coughing and bucking, hypertension, extubation, and endobronchial intubation are all possible.[27] The response to these maneuvers can be blunted by small doses of lidocaine. The potential for change in tube position is best managed by keeping a hand on the tube and a strong sense of suspicion.

If any question exists as to the patient's ability to sustain ventilation spontaneously, blockade by peripheral nerve stimulator should be evaluated. If the potential for narcotic-induced respiratory depression exists, incremental doses of naloxone can be administered. If neither condition exists, continued intubation and observation are indicated, along with mechanically assisted ventilation as needed to maintain adequate PaO_2 and $PaCO_2$ levels. Little analgesia is required postoperatively.

Conclusion

The patient with hydrocephalus presents a common problem that anesthesiologists are called on to manage intraoperatively, namely, that of disrupted cerebral dynamics. With an understanding of the underlying pathophysiology, the disease can be safely and effectively managed by means of techniques and agents currently available. As information concerning the effects of anesthetic agents on the brain continues to be refined, management will become more precise and the areas of current controversy settled.

References

1. Milhorat TH: Hydrocephalus and the Cerebrospinal Fluid. Baltimore, Williams and Wilkins Co, 1972; p 50.
2. Bull JWD: The volume of the cerebral ventricles. Neurology 1961;11:1–9.
3. Hakin S, Adams RD: The special clinical problem of symptomatic hydrocephalus with normal cerebrospinal fluid pressure. Observations on cerebrospinal fluid hydrodynamics. J Neurol Sci 1965;2:307–12.
4. Polley M: Formation of cerebrospinal fluid. J Neurosurg 1975;42:665–73.
5. Corey ME, Vela AR: Effects of systemic hypotension on the rate of cerebrospinal fluid formation in dogs. J Neurosurg 1974;41:350–55.
6. Tripathi R: Tracing the bulk outflow route of cerebrospinal fluid by transmission and scanning electron microscopy. Brain Res 1974;80:503–6.
7. Milhorat TH, Hammock MK, Davis DA, Fenstermacher JD: Choroid plexus papilloma: Part 1. Proof of cerebrospinal fluid overproduction. Childs Brain 1975;2:273–81.

8. Milhorat TH: Hydrocephalus and the cerebrospinal fluid. Baltimore, Williams and Wilkins Co, 1972; p 48.
9. Kim CS, Bennett DR, Roberts TS: Primary amenorrhea secondary to noncommunicating hydrocephalus. Neurology 1969;19:533–35.
10. Myer JS, Kitagawa Y, Tanahashi N, et al: Pathogenesis of normal pressure hydrocephalus. Preliminary observations. Surg Neurol 1985;23:121–33.
11. Milhorat TH: Hydrocephalus: Pathophysiology and clinical features, in Wilkins RH, Rengachary SS (eds): Neurosurgery. New York, McGraw-Hill, 1985; p 2138.
12. Epstein F, Hochwald GM, Ransoff J: Neonatal hydrocephalus treated by compressive head wrapping. Lancet 1973;1:634–36.
13. Rubin RC, Henderson ES, Ommaya LK, et al: The production of cerebrospinal fluid in man and its modification by acetazolamide. J Neurosurg 1966;25:430–36.
14. Arancibia CU, Shapiro K: Pediatric neurologic surgery in clinical anesthesia, in Frost E (ed) Neurosurgery. Boston, Butterworth, 1984; pp 235–64.
15. Campkin TV, Turner JM, Beasley J: Neurosurgical Anaesthesia and Intensive Care. London: Butterworths, 1980; p 56.
16. Naidich TP, Epstein F, Lin FP, et al: Evaluation of pediatric hydrocephalus by computed tomography. Radiology 1976;119:337–45.
17. Cote CJ, Goldstein EA, Cote MA, et al: A single-blind study of pulse oximetery in children. Anesthesiology 1988;68:184–88.
18. Conrady PA, Goodman LR, Lainge F: Alterations of endotracheal tube position. Flexion and extension of neck. Crit Care Med 1976;4:8–12.
19. Gardner AE, Olson BL, Lichtiger M: Cerebrospinal fluid pressure during dissociative anesthesia with ketamine. Anesthesiology 1971;35:226–28.
20. Rosa G, Sanfilippo M, Vilardi V, et al: Effects of vecuronium bromide on intracranial pressure and cerebral perfusion pressure. Br J Anaesth 1986;58:437–43.
21. Minton MM, Grosslight K, Stirt JA, Bedford RF: Increases in intracranial pressure from succinylcholine: Prevention by prior nondepolarizing blockade. Anesthesiology 1986;65:165–69.
22. Shapiro HM, Calindo M, Wyte SR, Harris AB: Rapid intraoperative reduction of intracranial pressure with thiopentone. Br J Anaesth 1973;45:1057–62.
23. Goresky GV, Steward DJ: Rectal methohexital for induction of anaesthesia in children. Can Anaesth Soc J 1979;26:213–15.
24. Hendrichsen H, Jorgensen PB: The effects of nitrous oxide on intracranial pressure in patients with intracranial disorders. Br J Anaesth 1973;45:486–92.
25. Frost EAM: Is isoflurane best for the cerebral circulation? Mt Sinai J Med (NY) 1987;54:283–89.
26. Artu AA, Nugent M, Michenfelder JD: Enflurane causes a prolonged and reversible increase in the rate of CSF production in the dog. Anesthesiology 1982;57:255–60.
27. Leech P, Barker J, Fitch W: Changes in intracranial pressure and systemic arterial pressure during the termination of anaesthesia. Br J Anaesth 1974;46:315–16.

CHAPTER 18

The Patient for Prostatic Surgery

William T. Gentry

Case History. *The patient, a 70-year-old man, was admitted to the hospital with progressive urinary hesitancy of 2 years' duration. Significant past medical history included hypertension and mild chronic obstructive pulmonary disease (COPD). The patient had been taking clonidine 0.1 mg po b.i.d. and theophylline 300 mg po b.i.d. On physical examination blood pressure was 140/80 mmHg; heart rate was 68/min and regular. On auscultation the heart sounds were normal, without murmurs, gallop, or friction rub. The ECG was reported as essentially normal with nonspecific ST-T wave changes. Auscultation of the lungs revealed decreased breath sounds on both sides but no wheezing.*

Laboratory values on admission showed serum sodium level 141 mEq/L, potassium 4.6 mEq/L, chloride 103 mEq/L, and total CO_2 content 26 mEq/L. Fasting blood glucose level was 100 mg/dl, and creatinine 0.9 mg/dl. The hematocrit was 42%, and urine specific gravity was 1.012.

The patient was scheduled for transurethral prostatectomy (TURP). It was anticipated that the procedure would last about 90 min, and spinal anesthesia was selected.

Introduction

Transurethral prostatectomy is one of the most common surgical procedures performed in men over 60 years of age. Overall mortality and morbidity after TURP may be higher than after other surgical procedures in the same age group.[1] These patients are particularly vulnerable to complications of anesthesia and surgery not only because of their advanced age but also because of a high incidence of systemic disorders (Table 18.1.). Cardiovascular disorders have been reported in 62% and

---

Reviewed by Dr. Irene Osborn, Assistant Professor of Anesthesiology, Department of Anesthesiology, Beth Israel Medical Center, New York, NY.

TABLE 18.1. Incidence of preoperative
problems in patients for TURP.

Medical Problem	% Patients
Cardiac disorder	50
Abnormal ECG	76
Chronic obstructive pulmonary disease	29
Hypertension	30
Obesity	9
Diabetes mellitus	8

50% of patients.[2,3] In another series, the preoperative ECG was abnormal in 23 of 30 patients. The incidence of chronic obstructive pulmonary disease (COPD) was 29%, hypertension 30%, obesity 9%, and diabetes mellitus 8%.[4]

Transurethral resection of the prostate is fraught with the risk of a particular complication—the excessive absorption of irrigation solution. This may cause circulatory overloading, severe hyponatremia, and toxicity due to the solute. The most common complication is congestive heart failure, which may deteriorate into frank pulmonary edema. Some patients may present with neurologic symptoms caused by hyponatremia and water intoxication. A few patients may develop toxic signs of glycine absorption such as transient blindness and high serum ammonium levels.

Surgical Procedure

The surgical procedure is performed by passing a resectoscope transurethrally. The resectoscope contains an electrically energized wire loop that resects the prostatic adenoma tissue. Bleeding is controlled by a coagulation current. Continuous irrigation is used to clear the surgical field of blood and particles of tissue. During surgery larger prostatic venous sinuses are opened, which may facilitate the absorption of significant amounts of irrigation solution. Also, particles of thromboplastins from prostatic tissue may be propelled into the circulation and initiate coagulopathy.

Normally, the prostatic capsule remains intact. Occasionally, however, the capsule is violated, promoting the absorption of irrigation solution into the retroperitoneal and periprostatic spaces. Perforation of the bladder wall may occur accidentally. Clinical signs of this complication are particularly insidious under general anesthesia and make early diagnosis difficult.

Preoperative Assessment

As for any elderly patient undergoing a surgical procedure, a detailed history and physical examination should be performed, with special emphasis on the cardiopulmonary and renal systems. Elderly patients usually receive multiple medications, including cardiac, antihypertensive, and diabetes preparations and aspirin. Laboratory data should include hemoglobin, hematocrit, electrolytes, and renal function tests (BUN/creatinine). Preoperative dehydration and depletion of sodium is common among TURP patients because of long-term diuretic therapy and restricted fluid intake, with consequent chronic hypovolemia. In addition, following bladder catheterization for relief of acute prostatic obstruction, patients often lose large amounts of water and sodium as a result of brisk diuresis. In one series 92% of patients were found to be dehydrated preoperatively.[5]

Cardiovascular System

Results of an ECG and chest x-ray should be available. Patients with a history of angina, previous myocardial infarction, or symptomatic coronary artery disease should be evaluated by an internist or cardiologist, especially if symptoms are not well controlled. It is important to be aware of the cardiovascular changes that occur with aging. The major change in cardiovascular function is loss of large-artery elasticity, resulting in stiffening of the arterial tree. Impedance to ejection of stroke volume is increased, systolic blood pressure rises, and there is generalized hypertrophy of the left ventricular wall.[6]

Congestive heart failure should be treated before surgery with appropriate and therapeutic doses of diuretics and/or digoxin. Bacteremia is often produced in surgical and manipulative procedures of the lower urinary tract. If valvular disease is present, infectious endocarditis can rapidly destroy the involved valve and result in chronic and debilitating bacteremia and intractable heart failure. Antibiotic prophylaxis is strongly reommended.

Operative Complications

As mentioned above, TURP may be complicated by several events. In assessing patients, the anesthesiologist should be aware of the difficulties that might occur intraoperatively, how they might impact on the patient's general medical condition, and what constitutes appropriate therapy.

Absorption of Irrigation Solution

The dangers of absorbing large quantities of irrigation fluid during surgery have been recognized for many years (Table 18.2.). Since the prostate contains large venous sinuses, it is inevitable that irrigating solution will be absorbed. The phenomenon is recognized by profuse dark-red venous bleeding and inadequate return of the irrigating solution. Both of these signs are perceived only by the surgeon and may or may not be indicated to the anesthesiologist.

The amount of absorption is governed by the height of the container of irrigating solution above the surgical table, which determines the hydrostatic pressure driving fluid into prostatic veins and sinuses, and the length of time of resection.[9] Several estimates and measurements suggest that as many as 8L of fluid may be absorbed during TURP, the average rate of absorption being approximately 20 ml/min. The average weight gain during surgery is about 2 kg.[10] Absorption of irrigating solution is greater during resection of a cancerous prostate gland than if the pathology is simple hypertrophy.

Oester and Madsen reported an average absorption of 889 ml in 34min during TURP.[11] Using a double-radioisotope technique, they concluded that only 29% of the irrigating solution was absorbed directly into the vessels. The remainder was absorbed extravascularly from the perivesical and retroperitoneal space through the defects in the prostatic capsule. Fluid that is absorbed interstitially has no immediate impact on the circulation and is gradually absorbed postoperatively. A simple method to determine the approximate amount of solution absorbed is to compare serum sodium levels before and after surgery.[12]

The following equation estimates intravascular absorption:

Volume absorbed = (preop serum Na^+/postop serum $Na^+ \times ECF$) − ECF where ECF (extracellular fluid) is estimated from body weight (20%–30% of body weight in kilograms).

Over the years many types of irrigating fluids have been used for TURP. The ideal solution should be optically satisfying (transparent), isosmolar, nonhemolytic, electrically inert, and nontoxic. No solution used at present has all of these qualities. For many years distilled water was used because it interfered least with visibility. However, it is

TABLE 18.2. Complications caused by absorption of irrigating fluids.

Circulatory overload
Hyponatremia
Solute toxicity

extremely hypotonic, and when absorbed by the circulation it often causes hemolysis and sometimes circulatory shock and renal failure. Because of this, distilled water was abandoned in favor of isosmotic or near isosmotic solutions. Normal saline or Ringer's lactate solution would be well tolerated intravascularly, but these electrolyte solutions are highly ionized and facilitate dispersion of high-frequency current from the resectoscope.

Some of the common irrigating solutions used for TURP are listed in Table 18.3. Modern solutions do not cause significant hemolysis but still can cause complications such as hyponatremia and circulatory overload. Some solutes can have adverse effects when absorbed, eg, glycine, mannitol, and glucose. The excessive absorption of irrigation solution is termed the TURP syndrome.

Hyponatremia

The use of nonelectrolyte isosmolar irrigating solutions has reduced the incidence of severe intracranial complications because extreme extracellular fluid hypoosmolality does not occur, and subsequent development of cerebral edema is avoided. Central nervous system (CNS) changes are due mainly to hyponatremia. Even moderate reductions of serum sodium levels may compromise brain function as well as myocardial contractility and conductivity. Minor degrees of hyponatremia may increase somnolence in the recovery room and the response to small doses of narcotics.

When extracellular Na^+ levels drop below 120 mEq/L, CNS symptoms, usually restlessness and confusion, may occur. Also, below 120 mEq/L, hypotension and reduced myocardial contractility develop.[13] Below 114 mEq/L bradycardia, widening of the QRS complex, ventricular ectopic beats, and T-wave inversions are evidenced. Generalized seizures, coma, respiratory arrest, and cardiac standstill are caused by levels below 100 mEq/L.[12]

TABLE 18.3. Commonly used irrigating solutions for TURP

Solution	Percent	Osmolality (mOsm)
Mannitol	5	275
Glycine	1.5	200
Cytal		
Sorbitol	2.7	
Mannitol	5.4	195
Sorbitol	3.3	165–180
Glucose	5	280

Respiratory System

Pulmonary changes that occur with aging affect the musculoskeletal supporting structure of the lung as well as the parenchyma of the lung. Maximal lung capacity, total lung capacity, and vital capacity all decline. Patients with pulmonary disease (asthma, COPD) are at increased risk when undergoing any surgical procedure. Deep breathing and coughing are important to clear secretions. Preoperatively, patients should be adequately medicated and if necessary should undergo respiratory therapy. Cessation of smoking, which decreases carboxyhemoglobin levels, is also helpful in preparing the patient for surgery.

The patient must be able to lie comfortably in the lithotomy position, whether regional or general anesthesia is selected. Coughing may disrupt the procedure or accidentally contribute to perforation of the bladder. Cautious sedation with narcotics may help, or tracheal intubation and control of respiration may be required. Preoperative arterial blood gases should be obtained in those with significant pulmonary disease. Intraoperative monitoring with a pulse oximeter is required.

Renal System

The patient with renal insufficiency can present serious management problems. Etiologic factors include obstruction of the urinary tract and intrinsic renal parenchymal diseases of the glomerular, tubular-interstitial, or vascular variety. Aging has a profound effect on the renal vasculature and hence on renal function. The linear fall in glomerular filtration rate (GFR) is more important than the modest loss of tissue mass, although the ability to concentrate urine and conserve free water is also progressively impaired.[7]

A decreased creatinine load associated with a declining skeletal muscle mass results in net serum creatinine concentrations nearly identical to those of young adults. There is sufficient residual function to avoid gross azotemia or uremia, but renal functional reserve to withstand gross water and electrolyte imbalance is minimal. The pharmacologic consequences are most significant in that the elimination half-time of virtually every anesthetic drug requiring renal clearance is prolonged.

Chronic renal parenchymal insufficiency leading to accumulation of nitrogenous wastes such as urea, creatinine, and uric acid may be present in the patient undergoing TURP. The main problems caused by chronic azotemia are easy bleeding due to qualitative platelet defect, anemia related to bone marrow suppression, hypernatremia, and, if far advanced, nausea, vomiting, and gastrointestinal bleeding.

Preoperative evaluation to determine the presence of any renal insufficiency is essential and includes measurement of serum creatinine, blood urea nitrogen, serum potassium, calcium, phosphorus, and hemoglobin. A serum creatinine level between 1.5 and 3 mg/dl indicates mild to moderate insufficiency. Renal failure is far advanced when levels exceed 7.5 or 8.0 mg/dl. Patients with renal failure should undergo hemodialysis or peritoneal dialysis prior to TURP. This is most important, as any large infusion of water and electrolyte solution may be excreted slowly or not at all.

Other diagnostic tests may be performed by urologists to distinguish benign prostatic hypertrophy from carcinoma. Serum acid phosphatase is elevated in patients with cancer, particularly in those with bony metastases.[8]

Choice of Anesthetic

In considering anesthesia for TURP, regional anesthesia (spinal, epidural) is preferred over general anesthesia because fluid overload, hyponatremia, and bladder perforation can be diagnosed earlier and treated more promptly. While under regional anesthesia the patient may complain of shortness of breath, tightness in the chest, and symptoms of hypoxia with fluid overload. Hyponatremia causes restlessness, confusion, and agitation. If severely hyponatremic, the patient may develop seizures and coma. If the bladder is perforated under regional anesthesia, the patient may complain of sudden onset of shoulder or abdominal pain and nausea, complaints that would not be recognized under general anesthesia. Thus, the diagnosis of such complications is often delayed when the patient is in this state.

Another advantage of regional anesthesia may be venodilation and reduced cardiac preload, which increases the margin of safety in absorption of irrigating solution.

Circulatory Overload

Excessive absorption of irrigating solution during TURP causes hypertension, pulmonary edema, and congestive heart failure. The degree and rate of development of symptoms of circulatory overload depend on the stability of the patient's cardiovascular system, the amount and rapidity of the absorption of the irrigating fluid, and the extent of the surgical field. Patients must be monitored carefully. Cardiac patients are particularly susceptible to circulatory overload caused by intraoperative absorption. Conservative administration of intravenous fluids during TURP is important. The use of a microdrip system for infusion is recommended.

Regional anesthesia (spinal, epidural) supplemented with only light sedation has the advantage of accessing awake patients. Another advantage of regional anesthesia is that sympathetic block increases venous capacitance and tends to work against fluid overload. Caution must be taken when the block dissipates because venous capacitance acutely decreases, and circulatory overload could occur.

Solute Toxicity

Glycine is a nonessential amino acid that is used commonly as a solute in irrigating solutions for TURP. It is toxic to the heart and the retina of the eye, causing transient blindness when absorbed intravenously. Glycine has a distribution similar to that of γ-aminobutyric acid (GABA), which is an inhibitory transmitter in the brain. It is postulated that glycine is also a major inhibitor transmitter, acting in the spinal cord and brain stem.[14] In animals, glycine has been shown to inhibit neuronal pathways of vision. In dogs, intravenously administered glycine suppressed visual evoked potentials.[15]

When glycine solution is used during TURP, glycine blood levels may become high. In some patients the concentration of glycine in the retina reaches a critical level that inhibits transmission of visual electrical signals and thus causes blindness. As soon as glycine blood levels start to decline, the glycine in the retina diffuses back into the blood, and vision is gradually restored.[16] If it is operating room practice to use glycine solutions, the patient and his family should be aware of this rare and reversible complication.

Ammonia is a major metabolic by-product of glycine; therefore, hyperammonemia is another potential complication of glycine irrigation. Although in most TURP patients ammonia blood levels remain within normal limits, glycine solutions should be avoided if encephalopathy preexists.

Absorption of other solutes in irrigating solutions also may cause problems. Diabetic patients may be particularly susceptible to side effects of absorption of sorbitol solution. This substance, although rapidly excreted by the kidneys, is metabolized to glucose, which may lead to hyperglycemia. Sorbitol solution is also metabolized to lactate from pyruvate and may compound lactic acidosis caused by sepsis, hypotension, or hypothermia.

When mannitol, in isosmolar solution, is used as irrigation, there is both volume expansion and an osmotic effect when the irrigation fluid is absorbed. Since the mannitol is not distributed evenly throughout the total body fluid space, hypervolemic changes may be compounded and further contribute to manifestations of the TURP syndrome.

Bladder Perforation

Another possible complication of TURP is perforation of the bladder. During difficult transurethral resection, perforation may be caused by the cutting loop or knife, the beak of the resectoscope, or overdistention of the bladder and prostatic fossa with irrigating medium. Most perforations are extraperitoneal, and in the conscious patient they result in pain in the periumbilical, inguinal, or suprapublic regions. The urologist may note the irregular return of irrigating fluid. Less often, the perforation is through the wall of the bladder and is intraperitoneal. A large extraperitoneal perforation may extend into the peritoneum. In such cases pain may be generalized in the upper abdomen or referred from the diaphragm to the shoulder. Other signs and symptoms include pallor, sweating, abdominal rigidity, nausea, vomiting, hypotension, and hypertension.[9]

Quick diagnosis of bladder perforation is important for survival. A urethrocystogram should be performed for definitive diagnosis. Bladder perforation is treated by performing suprapubic cystotomy. The most significant contributory factor in mortality after perforation is delay of more than 2h before placement of a suprapublic cystotomy.[1] Symptoms of perforation are realized much more quickly under regional than under general anesthesia. Again, the advantage of using regional anesthesia is underscored.

Sepsis

Bacteremia, a common complication following TURP and one of the more common causes of death, occurs because the prostate often harbors a variety of bacteria that may be the source of toxins and bacteremia. In addition, the patient with an indwelling bladder catheter often has significant bacterial growth in the urethral lining, with organisms that differ from prostatic bacteria. Therefore, urine cultures may not identify prostatic infection. The most common pathogens in bacteremia patients are *Aerobacter aerogenes* and *Escherichia coli.*[17]

Bacteremia can be devastating to geriatric patients who may have a lowered resistance to infection. It is therefore of paramount importance to control prostatic infection before surgery and to recognize and treat promptly any bacterial invasion of the bloodstream during TURP. Symptoms of bacteremia usually occur in the recovery room and include fever, chills, hypotension, and tachycardia or bradycardia. Blood should be drawn immediately for culture and sensitivity. Because of the high death rate, patients with septicemia should be treated with broad-spectrum antibiotics before culture and sensitivity results are available.[18]

Coagulopathy and Occult Blood Loss

Perioperative bleeding is a common complication of TURP. The exact mechanism is not clear, although several possibilities exist. Elderly patients may be confused because of either preexisting dementia or abnormal response to medications or drug interactions. When, in pain postoperatively, they become combative and tug on their bladder catheter, raw surfaces of the prostatic bed may be traumatized, causing bleeding. The provision of analgesia, sedation, replacement of blood loss, and observation may suffice in some cases. In other cases reoperation for fulguration of the bladder under anesthesia may be required.

Another possible cause of perioperative bleeding is dilution of thrombocytes. When a large volume of irrigation solution is absorbed, the platelet count may decrease, increasing bleeding time and causing hemorrhage. When perioperative bleeding occurs for no obvious reason, the coagulation profile should be determined, and if indicated, platelets should be administered.

Perioperative bleeding due to coagulopathy is far more ominous. The currently prevailing theory is that excessive bleeding after TURP is due to disseminated intravascular coagulation (DIC). The prostate gland and, particularly, malignant prostatic tumors are rich in tissue thromboplastins.[19] The tissue thromboplastins apparently enter the circulation during surgery and trigger DIC. Typically, TURP patients with a coagulopathy have a low platelet count, hypofibrinogenemia, prolonged partial thromboplastin and prothrombin times, and an increase in fibrin split products, all of which suggest a consumptive coagulopathy.

The symptoms, diagnosis, management, and outcome of 7 patients with coagulopathy related to TURP have been described.[20] In 4 of the 7 bleeding was excessive during or at the conclusion of surgery. Generalized oozing from the prostatic fossa accompanied by sudden bright-red bleeding without clots, concomitant bleeding from venous puncture sites, and submucosal hemorrhage were noted. All patients had heavy hematuria at 4h after surgery. Five of the 7 patients were treated with heparin, 2000 units loading dose and 750 units per hour by infusion, combined with fibrinogen 3–4 gm infused rapidly. Severe deficiencies in platelet and other clotting factors were corrected with platelet and fresh-frozen plasma administration. Bleeding from venipuncture sites stopped, and the extension of ecchymosis under the skin was arrested. In the 2 untreated patients surgical revision that included cystotomy and ligation of the hypogastric artery was required. Patients who survived the first postoperative day showed parallel rise in all clotting factors, although platelet count remained low for 3–5 days. Despite thorough hematologic workup and intense therapy, all 7 patients in this series eventually expired. Thus, the prognosis of TURP patients with coagulopathy is dismal.

It is very difficult to determine blood loss during TURP because visual estimates are grossly inaccurate as a result of dilution with irrigating fluid. Blood volume determination studies estimate blood loss to be from 200–2000 ml, with an average loss of 500 ml.[17] The geriatric patient who has compromised cardiovascular reserve may not tolerate this hidden loss without replacement.

Treatment of TURP Syndrome

Prompt recognition and treatment of TURP syndrome is absolutely necessary for survival (Table 18.4.). The following diagnostic and therapeutic steps are recommended:

1. Terminate the surgical procedure as soon as possible.

2. Administer furosemide 20 mg I.V.

3. Administer oxygen by nasal cannula or face mask. If the patient develops pulmonary edema, tracheal intubation and positive pressure ventilation with oxygen are indicated.

4. Draw arterial blood for blood gas analyses and sodium determination.

5. If the blood sodium level is below 120 mEq/L, hypertonic saline 3% should be administered at a rate no faster than 100 ml/h. Usually, infusion of no more than 300 ml is needed to correct the deficit. Often, spontaneous or induced diuresis corrects the hyponatremia within a few hours without therapy.[21] Certainly it is not necessary to replace the calculated deficit of sodium. Indeed, rapid correction of hyponatremia with hypertonic saline may lead to further complications. Pulmonary edema, pontine myelinolysis, and death have been reported. Hypertonic saline should be administered slowly after infusion of a diuretic.

6. If the patient develops seizures, barbiturate administration and tracheal intubation are indicated. Phenytoin (diphenylhydantoin) may be given slowly (50 mg/min) to a loading dose of about 10 mg/kg. The benzodiazepine derivatives (diazepam and midazolam), although effective anticonvulsant agents, have a very long half-life (24 h) in therapeutic doses in elderly patients and are best avoided. As a last resort, a paralyzing dose of an intermediate-acting muscle relaxant should be considered to protect the patient from seizure-induced trauma.

7. If pulmonary congestion, hypotension, bradycardia, or new-onset dysrhythmias are evident, the insertion of a pulmonary artery catheter

TABLE 18.4. Immediate prophylactic measures to decrease mortality and morbidity associated with TURP syndrome

Correct dehydration and electrolyte imbalance preop.
Treat congestive heart failure patients vigorously preop.
Preserve prostatic capsule.
Keep height of irrigation fluid pole no more than 60 cm.
Limit duration of surgery to less than 1 h.
Monitor serum Na$^+$ every 30 min.
Administer I.V. fluids conservatively during TURP.
Choose regional anesthesia over general anesthesia.
If patient is critically ill, use conservative surgical approach.

should be considered to guide the pharmacologic support with inotropes, vasodilators, and vasopressors.

8. If a significant loss of red blood cell mass is suspected, blood transfusion is indicated. Only red blood cells should be used, to avoid circulatory overload.

9. If a patient exhibits excessive bleeding, the coagulation profile should be studied and hematologic consultation urgently requested.

Preventive Measures

The incidence of complications from TURP depends to a great extent on the skill and technique of the operative team (Table 18.4.). Proper preparation and close monitoring during surgery are also important. Dehydration and electrolyte abnormalities should be corrected preoperatively, with special attention paid to serum sodium levels, particularly in patients receiving diuretics and low-sodium diets.

Cardiac patients are very susceptible to circulatory overload from irrigating solutions. In patients with congestive heart failure, conditions should be optimized before surgery. In patients who are very ill, a conservative surgical approach should be considered, such as staged prostatectomy, which would reduce the incidence of excessive absorption of irrigation solution.

A very important prophylactic measure during surgery is the preservation of the prostatic capsule, where the largest venous sinuses lie adjacent to the capsule. Other prophylactic measures include adjusting the height of the irrigation fluid pole to no more than 60 cm, limiting the duration of resection to no more than 1h, and avoiding over-distention of the bladder by frequent emptying.[22]

During surgery, serum sodium level determinations should be made every half hour. If there is a sudden fall, the surgeon should be notified. If levels below 130 mEq/L or obvious signs of TURP syndrome appear, surgery should be terminated as soon as possible. During TURP fluids should be infused slowly, by means of a microdrip technique.

Regional anesthesia is favored, since most of the complications cause mental signs or pain, and the diagnosis can be made promptly. The required level of anesthesia is up to T10. Levels higher than T10 should be avoided, because hypotension can develop. Should this complication occur, ephedrine (12.5–25 mg) is preferable to brisk intravenous fluid administration.

Summary

Anesthesia for TURP is often considered a simple procedure performed in sequestered parts of operating room suites. Yet the operation involves insidious and extensive alteration in circulatory volume and electrolyte imbalance. Other complications include occult blood loss, bladder perforation, coagulopathy, and sepsis. The patient is usually elderly with one or more medical problems. The anesthesiologist must evaluate such patients carefully and make sure they are in optimal condition before surgery, and also must understand the inherent problems, complications, and appropriate therapy in performing the surgery.

References

1. Malchior J, Valk WL, Foret JD, et al: Transurethral prostatectomy: Computerized analysis of 2,223 consecutive cases. J Urol 1974;112:634–42.
2. Desmond J: Serum osmolality and plasma electrolytes in patients who develop dilutional hyponatremia during transurethral resection. Can J Surg 1970; 13:116–121.
3. Mebust MK, Brody TW, Valk WL: Observations on cardiac output, blood volume, central venous pressure, fluid and electrolyte changes in patients undergoing transurethral prostatectomy. J Urol 1970;103:632–36.
4. Fox M, Hammonds JC, Copland RF: Prostatectomy in patients of 70 and over. Eur Urol 1981;7:27–30.
5. Harrison RH, Boren JS, Robinson JR: Dilutional hyponatremia: Another concept of the transurethral prostatic resection reaction. J Urol 1956;75:95–110.
6. Muravick S: The physiologic and pharmacologic implications of aging. ASA Annual Refresher Course Lectures, 1986, p 275.
7. McLesky CH: Anesthesia for the elderly patient. IARS Review Course Lectures, 1986, pp 136–38.
8. Sagalowsky AI: Hyperplasia and carcinoma of the prostate, in Harrison's Principles of Internal Medicine. New York: McGraw-Hill, 1987; p 1583.
9. Mazze RI: Anesthesia for patients with abnormal renal function and genitourinary operations, in Miller RD (ed): Anesthesia. New York: Churchill Livingstone, 1986; pp 1651–59.
10. Taylor RO, Maxson ES, Carter FH, et al: Volumetric gravimetric and radioisotopic determination of fluid transfer in transurethral prostatectomy. J Urol 1958;79:490–99.
11. Oester A, Madsen PO: Determination of absorption of irrigating fluid during transurethral resection of the prostate by means of radioisotopes. J Urol 1969;102:714–19.
12. Henderson DJ, Middleton RG: Coma from hyponatremia following transurethral resection of prostate. Urology 1980;15:267–71.
13. Logie JRC, Keenan RA, Whiting PH, et al: Fluid absorption during transurethral prostatectomy. Br J Urol 1980;52:526–28.
14. Aprison MH, Werman R: The distribution of glycine in cat spinal cord and roots. Life Sci 1955;4:2075.
15. Wang JM, Wong KC, Creel DJ, et al: Effects of glycine on hemodynamic responses and visual evoked potentials in the dog. Anesth Analg 1985;64:1071–77.
16. Ovassapian A, Joshi CW, Brumer EA: Visual disturbances: An unusual symptom of transurethral prostatic resection. Anesthesiology 1982;52:332–34.

17. Brechner T, Krechel S: Anesthesia for urologic procedures in the aged, in Krechel SW (ed): Anesthesia and the Geriatric Patient. New York: Grune & Stratton, 1984, pp 209–19.
18. Robinson MRG, Cross RJ, Shetty MB, et al: Bacteremia and bacteriogenic shock in district hospital urologic practice. Br J Urol 1980;52:10–14.
19. Marx GF, Orkin LR: Complications associated with transurethral surgery. Anesthesiology 1962;23:802–13.
20. Friedman NJ, Hoag MS, Robinson AF, et al: Hemorrhagic syndrome following transurethral prostatic resection for benign adenoma. Arch Intern Med 1969; 124:341–49.
21. Osborn DE, Rao PN, Green MJ, et al: Fluid absorption during transurethral resection. Br Med J 1980;281:1549–50.
22. Madsen PO, Naber KG: The importance of the pressure in the prostatic fossa and absorption of irrigating fluid during transurethral resection of the prostate. J Urol 1973;109:446–52.

CHAPTER 19

The Patient for Thyroidectomy

Svetlana Bonner

Case History. *A 67-year-old man was electively admitted to the hospital after needle aspiration of a nodule in his neck indicated the presence of follicular neoplasm. During routine physical examination two weeks earlier, a 2 cm nodule was palpated in the area of his thyroid gland. He had no history of palpitations, sweating, fatigue, dizziness, or recent weight loss.*

His past medical history was notable for adult-onset diabetes mellitus, controlled by oral hypoglycemic agents. He had a longstanding history of hypertension, treated with metoprolol. He had smoked heavily for years and had occasional mild asthma.

Physical examination revealed a healthy-appearing man in no acute distress. Blood pressure was 140/90 mmHg, pulse 66/min and regular. Electrocardiogram (ECG) showed left anterior hemiblock. All other laboratory values were within normal limits, except for blood glucose of 281 mg/dl. Routine thyroid function tests indicated a euthyroid state.

The patient was scheduled for partial thyroidectomy.

Introduction

In 1696 Wharton first introduced the term "thyroid glands" to describe the secreting structures adjacent to the part of the larynx named thyroid cartilage because of its shieldlike form (from Greek *thyreoides,* shield-shaped). The function of this "glandula thyroidea" remained an enigma for years and consequently became the subject of some very interesting speculations. Wharton himself suggested that the gland existed to round out the neck by filling otherwise vacant spaces about the larynx, "particularly in females to whom for this reason a larger gland has been assigned."[1] Other possible functions of the thyroid were related to the

Reviewed by Dr. Joseph Feldshuh, Assistant Professor of Medicine, Cornell University Medical College, New York, NY.

lymphatic, vascular, or digestive systems, with some very picturesque descriptions accompanying each theory. Werner[1] attributes the first description of endemic cretinism to Paracelsus, and that of hyperthyroidism to Parry (1825).

Many prominent scholars have contributed to our present understanding of thyroid anatomy, function, and pathophysiology, enabling us to promptly diagnose, treat, and frequently cure diseases of this organ. Patients are usually hyper- or euthyroid. Nowadays it is rather uncommon to see a hypothyroid patient presenting for thyroid surgery. Hyperthyroidism is 10 times more common in women than in men. Data from Whickham's study in England[2] indicated a prevalence of established hyperthyroidism of 2% in women and an estimated incidence of approximately 3 cases per 1000 women annually. A recent U.S. study demonstrated similar figures.[3]

According to the National Cancer Institute's SEER (Surveillance, Epidemiology and End Results) Program, the 1982 estimated incidence of new cases of thyroid carcinoma in the U.S. totaled 10,000 (2800 male, 7200 female). The estimated total deaths due to thyroid carcinoma approximated 1050 (350 male, 700 female). Furthermore, from 1973 to 1978 thyroid carcinoma ranked third among the five most frequent tumors in women aged 15–34 and was the fifth most common tumor in men aged 30–34.[4]

Physiology

The major thyroid hormones are thyroxine (T_4, a product of the thyroid gland) and the more potent 3,5,3-triiodothyronine (T_3, a product of both the thyroid and the extrathyroidal enzymatic deiodination of thyroxine). Whether all effects of thyroid hormones are mediated by T_3 or whether T_4 possesses its own biologic activity remains unclear.

Hormone Biosynthesis

The synthesis of the primary thyroglobulins monoiodotyrosine (MIT) and diiodotyrosine (DIT) takes place in the thyroid gland from amino acids, hexoses, and oxidized iodine (Figure 19.1.). The first step in the synthetic pathway is uptake (or trapping) of plasma iodide, which then becomes thyroid iodide and is further oxidized to iodine by the enzyme peroxidase. Formation of normal quantities of thyroid hormone depends on the availability of adequate exogenous iodine, for which dietary iodide is the major source.

Iodide is absorbed from the gastrointestinal tract and actively transported from the extracellular fluid into the thyroid gland. Transport occurs against both chemical and electrical gradients, achieving thyroid/plasma (T/P) iodide ratios of 30 to 40. Several ions act as competitive

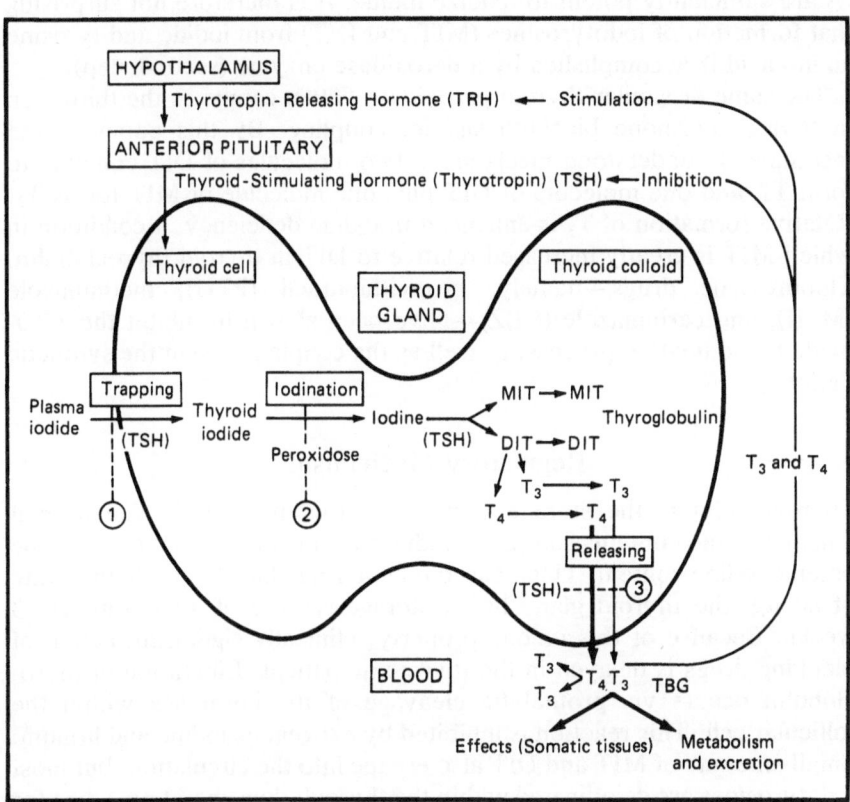

FIGURE 19.1. Summary of thyroid hormones pathway, TSH = thyrotropin-dependent process. 1-3 = main inhibition sites; inhibited by (1) perchlorate, thiocyanate, methimazole; (2) thiouracil; (3) iodide, lithium. MIT = 3-monoiodotyrosine. DIT = 3,5-diiodotyrosine. TBG = thyronine-binding globulin. T_4 = 3,5,3',5'-triiodothyronine (reverse T_3). Reprinted with permission from Halevy S: *Effects of Anesthesia and Surgery on Thyroid Function*, in Brown B (ed): *Anesthesia and the Patient with Endocrine Disease*, Philadelphia, F.A. Davis Co.

inhibitors of iodide transport by thyroid, including perchlorate, which has been used successfully in the treatment of hyperthyroidism. Thiocyanate also acts as a competitive inhibitor; hence, patients on prolonged sodium nitroprusside (SNP) therapy can develop signs of hypothyroidism.

Before iodide can act as an effective iodination agent within the thyroid gland, it has to be transformed to a higher oxidative state. Only H_2O_2 and O_2 are sufficiently potent to oxidize iodide. It is therefore not surprising that formation of iodotyrosines (MIT and DIT) from iodide and tyrosine amino acid is accomplished by a peroxidase enzyme (second step).

The same or similar thyroid peroxidase (TPO) catalyzes the third step in thyroid hormone biosynthesis, ie, coupling. By this complex and incompletely understood mechanism, two molecules of DIT combine to form T_4, and one molecule of DIT plus one molecule of MIT forms T_3. Relative formation of T_3 is enhanced in iodine deficiency, a condition in which MIT is greatly increased relative to DIT in thyroid thyroglobulin. Thioureylene drugs—namely, propylthiouracil (PTU), methimazole (MMI), and carbimazole (CBZ)—have been shown to inhibit the TPO-mediated iodination process, as well as the coupling step in the synthetic pathway.

Regulatory Mechanisms

Thyroglobulin is the storage form of thyroid hormones. The normal human thyroid contains 8000 μg of iodine; T_4 constitutes about 35% of the organic iodine content. Thus, based on a normal daily T_4 production rate of 80 μg, the thyroid gland has a storage reserve of approximately 3 weeks. Because of this unique property, clinically significant action of blocking drugs is delayed in the thyrotoxic patient. Liberation of thyro-globulin occurs via proteolytic cleavage of the hormones within the follicular cell. This reaction is inhibited by exogenous iodine and lithium. Small amounts of MIT and DIT also escape into the circulation, but most iodotyrosines are deiodinated within the thyroid, thus liberating iodine for the intrathyroidal pool.

A complex feedback relationship exists between thyroid hormone production and the hypothalamic-pituitary system (Figure 19.2). Thyro-tropin-releasing hormone (TRH) is synthesized in the supraoptic and paraventricular nuclei of the hypothalamus. It then travels to the anterior pituitary via the hypophyseal portal venous system, where it activates thyroid-stimulating hormone (TSH) synthesis through a cAMP-mediated process. Thyroid hormones have a negative feedback effect on TSH synthesis and secretion. This effect appears to be mediated by an inhibitory protein.[5]

The thyroid gland also possesses an autoregulatory mechanism that helps maintain a constant store of thyroid hormone, independent of serum

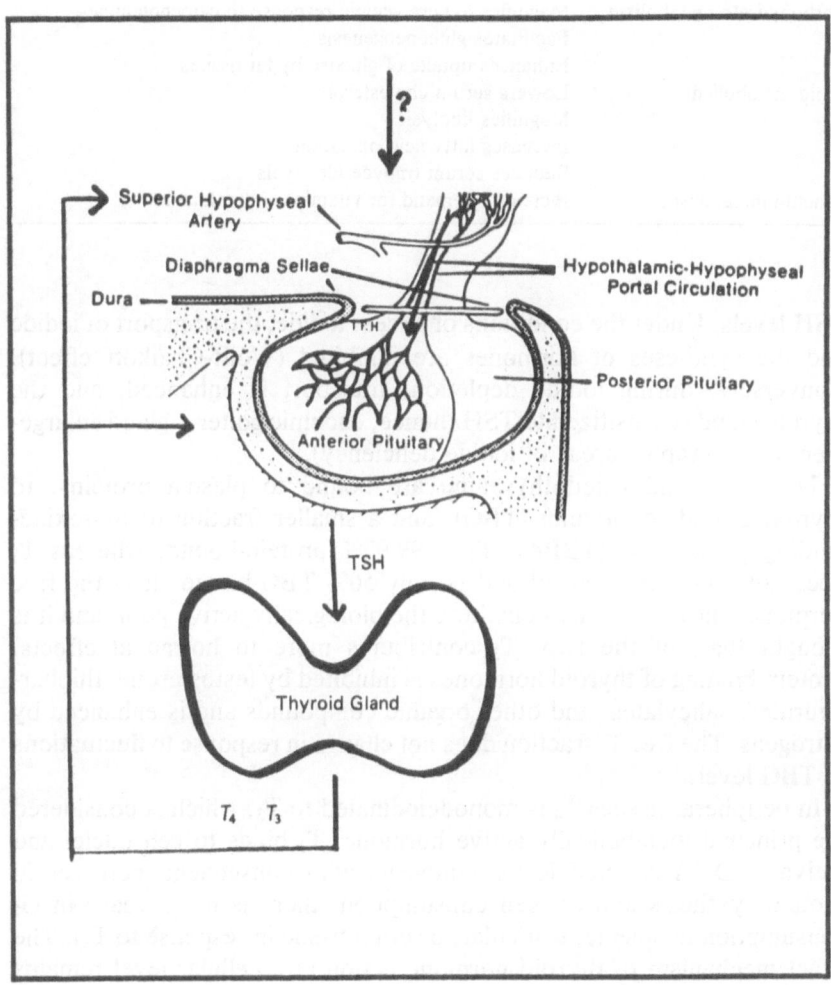

FIGURE 19.2. Hypothalamic-pituitary-thyroid axis. Thyroid hormones (T_4 and T_3) inhibit secretion of thyroid-stimulating hormone (TSH) in pituitary. Modulation may also occur at hypothalamic level by inhibition of thyrotropin-releasing hormone (TRH). TRH secretion is probably also controlled by neurotransmitters from higher brain centers.

TABLE 19.1. Thyroid hormone effects on metabolic processes.

Process	Thyroid Hormone Action
Basal metabolic rate	Increases
Protein metabolism	Enhances synthesis; needed for growth and maturation
Carbohydrate metabolism	Magnifies hyperglycemic response to catecholamines
	Facilitates gluconeogenesis
	Enhances uptake of glucose by fat tissues
Lipid metabolism	Lowers serum cholesterol
	Magnifies lipolysis
	Increases fatty acid oxidation
	Reduces serum triglyceride levels
Vitamin metabolism	Increases demand for vitamins and cofactors

TSH levels. Under the conditions of excess iodide, the transport of iodide and the syntheses of hormones are inhibited (Wolff-Chaikoff effect). Conversely, during iodide depletion, transport is enhanced, and the thyroid gland is sensitized to TSH (hence, endemic goiter—gland enlargement in geographic areas of iodide deficiency).

Thyroxine and triiodothyronine are bound to plasma proteins, to thyroxine-binding globulin (TBG), and a smaller fraction to thyroxine-binding prealbumin (TBPA). T_4 is 99.97% protein-bound, whereas T_3 does not bind TBPA at all and is only 50% TBG-bound. It is the free hormones, however, that constitute the biologically active pool, and it is thought that, of the two, T_3 contributes more to hormonal effects. Protein-binding of thyroid hormones is inhibited by testosterone, thiobarbiturates, salicylates, and other organic compounds and is enhanced by estrogens. The free T_4 fraction does not change in response to fluctuations of TBG level.

In peripheral tissues T_4 is monodeiodinated to T_3, which is considered the principal metabolically active hormone. T_3 binds to cell nuclei and activates DNA-directed RNA synthesis, with consequent increases in protein synthesis and oxygen consumption (there is no increase in O_2 consumption in splenic, testicular, or brain tissue in response to T_3). The exact mechanism of thyroid hormone action at a cellular level remains unclear. One of the proposed mechanisms is that of stimulation of Na^+/K^+ ATPase, but this theory is not universally accepted. Enhancement of basal metabolic rate as evidenced by increased O_2 consumption is one of the classic actions of thyroid hormones.

A more comprehensive summary of thyroid hormone effects is listed in Table 19.1.

One feature of thyroid hormones deserves special mention: Hyperthyroidism mimics sympathetic overactivity without altering catecholamine kinetics. It seems probable that excess thyroid hormone magnifies catecholamine effects by mechanisms that are poorly elucidated.

Diagnostic Tests

Tests are designed to determine the level of thyroid function. Routine laboratory screening of patients with suspected thyroid disease usually involves determinations of T_4 and TSH levels. TSH level is a measure of pituitary response. The hormone is involved in a reciprocal feedback loop. In primary hyperthyroidism, TSH is secondarily suppressed. Elevated TSH levels associated with hyperthyroidism indicate pituitary disease.

There is no test currently available to determine directly the free T_4 fraction. An indirect method of determination is provided by the T_3 resin uptake, a test that measures unoccupied hormone-binding sites on an ion-exchange resin and is thus inversely proportional to the free hormone concentration. Free T_4 index (the product of the in vitro uptake value and the serum total T_4 concentration) provides some correlation with free T_4 concentration.

Thyroid imaging studies are especially useful in assessing the presence of thyroid pathology, both anatomic and functional. Routine diagnostic scanning is usually performed with ^{123}I or ^{99m}Tc. Both isotopes have short half-lives, and both expose patients minimally to radiation. Most thyroid scans are performed to determine the degree of hyperfunction in suspected cases of thyrotoxicosis or to localize and determine the function of palpable thyroid nodules. Nodules may be hot (functioning) or cold (nonfunctioning) with respect to the surrounding normal thyroid image. Lack of function in a single nodule increases the likelihood of malignancy; however, 80% of cold nodules are benign.[5]

Ultrasonography is also employed for evaluation of thyroid nodules. The sonogram differentiates between solid, cystic, and mixed lesions. Pure cystic lesions have a low incidence of malignancy. Mixed and solid lesions suggest a 20% possibility of neoplasm. Needle biopsy (fine-needle aspiration [FNA]), coupled with cytologic examination of the specimen (aspiration biopsy cytology [ABC]), has become an integral part of diagnosing the nature of thyroid nodules (Figure 19.3.).

In addition, a battery of tests is available to evaluate the function of the hypothalamic-pituitary axis, including tests of pharmacologic stimulation or suppression that determine the precise hormonal defects in conditions manifested by altered thyroid function. A detailed discussion of these assays is available elsewhere.[6]

Preoperative Evaluation and Preparation

Patients presenting for thyroid surgery are likely to be hyper- or euthyroid. Conditions involving decreased activity of the thyroid gland rarely require surgical correction except in the presence of massive goiter.

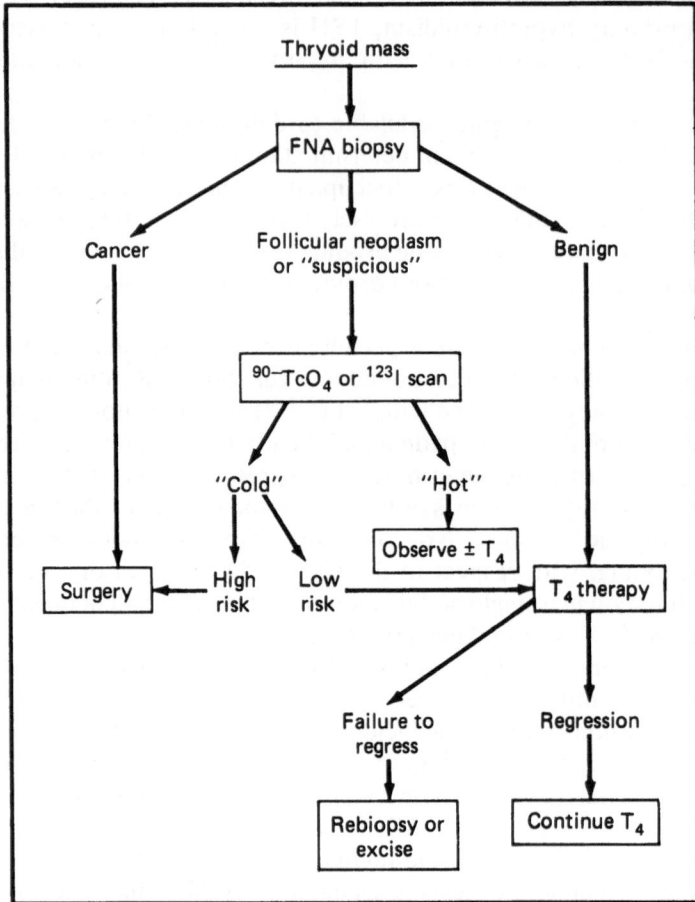

FIGURE 19.3. Decision matrix for diagnosis and management of thyroid nodule. Reprinted with permission from Greenspan FS and Forsham PH (eds): *Basic ana Clinical Endocrinology,* 2nd ed. Los Altos, Calif, Lange Medical Publications, 1985.

TABLE 19.2. Indications for thyroidectomy (partial and total).

Group I	Unusually large goiters or multinodular toxic goiter
	Continuous goiter growth while patient is undergoing maximal tolerated therapy
	Failure of antithyroid therapy secondary to its side effects, ie, bone marrow suppression by thionamides (PTU and MMI)
	Toxic goiter with symptoms of progressive CHF
	Symptoms of thyrotoxicosis in pregnant patients or women who wish to become pregnant
	Patient noncompliance
Group II	Goiter compressing the airway
	Thyroid mass causing dysphagia or pain
	Cosmetic correction
Group III	Fine-needle aspiration (FNA) cytology indicative of malignancy
	Recurrent cysts
	Palpable "cold" nodules in a patient with exposure to ionizing radiation

Patients with unsuspected thyroid pathology presenting for unrelated surgery are not uncommonly hypothyroid, especially those in the elderly population (up to 0.8% of the total adult population may be hypothyroid).[7]

A separate subpopulation of patients deserves special mention: patients who had chemical or surgical thyroid ablation for cancer and now present with recurrence of the tumor. As a rule, thyroid hormone replacement therapy is discontinued once the diagnosis of recurrent carcinoma is made. Patients present for surgery in a hypothyroid state, thus constituting a challenge for the anesthesiologist since no easy management decisions are available. Major complications of untreated hypothyroidism during general anesthesia have been reported. These include severe hypotension or cardiac arrest following induction of anesthesia, extreme sensitivity to narcotics and inhaled anesthetics with prolonged unconsciousness, and hypothyroid coma following anesthesia and surgery.[8,9]

Patients may be candidates for a partial or complete thyroidectomy (Table 19.2.). Patients with symptoms of thyrotoxicosis in whom medical suppressive therapy is either contraindicated or has failed, constitute one group (pregnant women, patients with a history of congestive heart failure, and patients who have developed bone marrow suppression on antithyroid medication). A second group comprises those with thyroid gland enlargement, causing local symptoms such as pain, dysphagia, or respiratory embarrassment. Yet another group are patients in whom thyroid malignancy is suspected or diagnosed during evaluation of a thyroid mass (Figure 19.3.).

This classification of patients for thyroidectomy into three main groups simplifies the approach to a rather complex and diversified pathologic problem. Thus, the issues that constitute major concern to the anesthesiologist during the preanesthetic visit are addressed systematically.

Level of Thyroid Function

The first concern is the level of thyroid function. In patients presenting for partial or total thyroidectomy it is unusual to find hypothyroidism because those patients are frequently controlled by thyroid hormone replacement therapy. Therefore, the assessment should be made as to the presence of a hyperthyroid state. Besides the indexes of thyroid function (eg, T_4, T_3, TSH) and imaging studies, clinical features should alert the physician to poor control and the existence of a hyperactive thyroid gland. The most common symptoms are increased nervousness, heat intolerance, increased perspiration, palpitations, fatigue, and weight loss. Common physical findings include goiter, tachycardia, skin changes, and tremor.

Cardiovascular manifestations of hyperthyroidism are palpitations, tachycardia, and dyspnea. Atrial fibrillation occurs in approximately 10%–20% of patients and is more common after age 45.[10] Some patients develop congestive heart failure and angina pectoris. There are no specific ECG findings, although varying degrees of heart block may occur in 3%–30% of patients. Hyperthyroid patients have increased blood volume, cardiac output, and systolic blood pressure and decreased peripheral resistance, resulting in a wide pulse pressure.

Antiadrenergic drugs should be used with caution in such patients because of the dependence of the failing heart on catecholamines. No attempt should be made to revert supraventricular dysrhythmias in hyperthyroid patients because 30%–70% of the patients will spontaneously convert to normal sinus rhythm following return to the euthyroid state.[10] Refractoriness to cardiac glycosides is the rule, and cardiac failure is more properly termed a "hyperkinetic circulatory state." Cardiac output is raised in excess of requirements imposed by the hypermetabolic state. Also, ventricular contractility is enhanced.

Hematocrit, hemoglobin, and total red blood cell count are usually normal, although Graves' disease is associated with pernicious anemia in 1% of patients.[7] White blood cell count is usually normal, but antithyroid medications can cause granulocytopenia. Rarely, thrombocytopenia or prolongation of the coagulation time may be manifest. Muscular weakness, especially in the proximal muscle groups, and, rarely, muscular atrophy can occur. About 1% of patients with hyperthyroidism also have myasthenia gravis.[5] Another associated neuromuscular condition is periodic paralysis, frequently accompanied by hypokalemia. Episodes of periodic paralysis and myasthenia improve once hyperthyroidism is treated successfully.

Common gastrointestinal symptoms associated with hyperthyroidism are weight loss despite hyperphagia, and increased bowel frequency. It is therefore particularly important to assess hydration status and electrolyte balance prior to anesthesia and to make appropriate correction.

Control of Hyperthyroidism

Even though clinical manifestations of hyperthyroidism have been well studied and active research has focused on thyroid hormone action, the exact mechanism of the latter remains speculative. Research in thyroid hormone production and release have led to the development of antithyroid medications.

The mainstays of endocrinologists' therapy have been iodine, which blocks the output of thyroid hormone temporarily; thioureylenes (PTU, MMI), which block organification of iodine within the gland; and propranolol, which controls tremor, nervousness, and thyroid, and thus the traditional "steal" of the hyperthyroid patient to the operating room after heavy premedication is unnecessary.[13]

Anesthetic Management

Local and regional anesthesia have been used for surgery on the thyroid gland but have not become popular for a variety of reasons, including patient discomfort and the need for excessive draping and covering of the head. Moreover, the innervation of the upper poles of the thyroid does not arise from the cervical somatic segments but rather is part of the vagus innervation, and thus an adequate block is difficult to achieve. Local anesthesia occasionally has a place in the biopsy and removal of obvious thyroid nodules, but the stress placed on the precariously euthyroid patient may tip the delicate balance toward the thyrotoxic state.[14]

High spinal anesthesia has been used for thyroid surgery. Currently, however, there is very little disagreement on the issue—general endotracheal anesthesia is considered the anesthetic method of choice.

No specific additional intraoperative monitoring is required for patients undergoing thyroid surgery; blood pressure cuff, ECG, temperature probe, esophageal stethoscope, pulse oximetry, and capnography are used routinely. A cooling blanket, refrigerated solutions, and ice should be readily available to deal with possible complications. Immediate access to corticosteroids, propranolol, and nitroprusside is also recommended. Patients frequently become hypothermic in the cool operating room; therefore, even slight elevations in temperature (0.5–1°C) should be regarded with suspicion. Some authors advocate that Lugol's solution (K^+ or Na^+ iodide) be available for intravenous administration.[15]

Protection during positioning of the patient is often the responsibility of the anesthesiologist. A soft roll under the shoulders or an inflatable "thyroid pillow" allows the head to fall backward so that the neck arches and the thyroid gland is presented at approximately the position preferred by most surgeons. Hyperextension should be avoided since it can cause both neurologic complications from cervical nerve compression and obstruction to the cerebral circulation to the head. The head should not be allowed to hang free but should be supported by a "doughnut" made of soft material. Slightly raising the torso (ie, Fowler's position) is helpful to reduce venous bleeding and improve operative conditions. The arms and hands must be protected against nerve injuries. The arms placed at the sides may be subject to considerable pressure by the surgeons. Proper padding at the elbows and hands and avoidance of excessive downward traction at the shoulders will prevent nerve damage. If exophthalmos is pronounced, tarsorrhaphy may be indicated.

Lidocaine administered endotracheally prior to intubation helps decrease bucking caused by neck movement.

Controlled studies have not demonstrated clinical advantages of any one anesthetic drug. A review of cases since 1968 from the University of California, San Francisco, reported that virtually all techniques and agents have been employed without any adverse effects.[5] The thiobarbiturates are considered by many to be the induction agents of choice.[15] Their antithyroid activity may be related to the thiocarbamate structure. Inhalation anesthetics have been used widely, as have intravenous narcotics in combination with an oxygen/nitrous oxide mixture.

Whatever the technique, the patient must be adequately anesthetized prior to laryngoscopy and intubation. The key to a safe anesthetic is assuring a depth of anesthesia adequate to eliminate stimulation of the same sites of activity that are related to thyrotoxicity. Hypercarbia should be avoided because it stimulates the sympathoadrenal axis. Therefore, capnography and appropriate manipulation of ventilation are essential during thyroidectomy procedures. Prior to extubation, direct laryngoscopy should be performed to assess the movement of the vocal cords. Even when there seems to be no impairment of vocal cord motion, airway management may be a problem during emergence.

Following thyroidectomy, patients should be extubated under optimum conditions so that reintubation, if necessary, will be facilitated.

Complications

Several complications have been described perioperatively (Table 19.3.). By far the most feared is the *"thyroid storm."* It is best described as an extreme case of thyrotoxicosis and can occur intraoperatively and up to 6–18 h postoperatively. Thyroid storm was uniformly fatal prior to the introduction of antithyroid therapy at the beginning of this century. The highest quoted mortality now is 10%, and the crisis itself is extremely rare, since most patients present to surgery in a euthyroid state.

TABLE 19.3. Complications associated with thyroidectomy.

Intraoperative	Postoperative
Thyroid storm	Thyroid storm
Venous air embolism	Nerve injury (recurrent laryngeal, phrenic, or cervical sympathetic)
Carotid sinus reflex	
Pneumothorax	Hematoma formation
Pneumomediastinum	Hypoparathyroidism
	Tracheal malacia
	Tracheoesophageal fistula

The thyroid storm has an abrupt onset, the clinical picture being dominated by the effects of excessive tissue concentration of thyroid hormone. Sinus tachycardia or atrial fibrillation with rapid ventricular response, marked increase in systolic and pulse pressure, hyperpyrexia rising rapidly to 106°F or higher, profuse sweating, tremulousness, flushing, and obvious high oxygen usage and carbon dioxide production are among the symptoms. In a patient with heart disease, pulmonary edema and other signs of congestive heart failure develop. If the condition arises postoperatively, delirium and frank psychosis may occur. As the disorder progresses, apathy, stupor, and coma with hypotension supervene.

The aims of therapy are to (1) control the heart rate and prevent heart failure by rapid digitalization and the administration of β-blockers; (2) control the temperature by external cooling, including gastric and colonic lavage, administration of cold intravenous solutions, and application of cooling blankets; (3) block further release of thyroid hormone by administering intravenous iodide (1–2 gm), intravenous corticosteroids, and large doses of thionamides via nasogastric instillation; and (4) achieve general sympathetic blockade with guanethidine or reserpine.

Adequate oxygen delivery to the patient is of paramount importance during the thyroid storm, which must be differentiated from *malignant hyperthermia*.[16] The distinction is frequently difficult, and several clinical parameters should be considered: presence or absence of muscle rigidity, high serum levels of CPK, family history. Both conditions are extremely serious and must be recognized promptly and treated appropriately. Treatment of thyroid storm generally requires 5–7 days before the manifestations of hyperthyroidism can be brought under control. The high mortality underscores the importance of achieving the euthyroid state prior to surgery.

Two other possible problems can confront the anesthesiologist during a thyroidectomy procedure: *carotid sinus reflex* and *venous air embolism*. The latter, although uncommon, may occur if a large vein is opened. As much as 200 ml of air can be aspirated during a deep negative-pressure breath. Flooding the surgical field with saline is the primary emergency measure.

Manipulation of the carotid sinus can cause severe hypotension with marked bradycardia. Treatment consists of cessation of the stimulus and infiltration of the area around the bifurcation of the common carotid artery with local anesthetic solution. Intravenous administration of atropine (0.4 mg) is beneficial.

A complication of concern to the anesthesiologist postoperatively is unilateral or bilateral *recurrent laryngeal nerve injury*. In about half of the population the recurrent laryngeal nerve lies within the body of the thyroid gland. Since currently it is rare for total thyroidectomy to be performed, unilateral damage is more likely. There has been considerable controversy about the end result when one or both nerves are cut or injured. The recurrent nerve supplies both the abductor and adductor muscles of the vocal cords and larnyx, and varying degrees of injury may result in partial paralysis in one set of muscles versus the other.

Of importance to the anesthesiologist is the fact that in the acute phase immediately after extubation, unopposed adductors, either uni- or bilaterally, may produce stridor or even total airway obstruction. The anesthesiologist can make a tentative diagnosis based on observation of the cords, provided the patient is breathing. Partial movement of the cords in a back-and-forth direction is suggestive of temporary weakness.

If there is a degree of airway obstruction, the endotracheal tube should be left in place until the patient is fully awake and a careful assessment can be made. If both recurrent nerves are cut, accommodation may take place over time, and both cords may be in midposition. Tracheostomy is required immediately postoperatively in most instances. If one nerve is cut, stridor may be present but will decrease with slow and measured breathing. Injury to the superior laryngeal nerve results in loss of sensation in the larynx and piriform sinus. Aspiration occurs easily.

References

1. Werner SC: Historical resume, in Ingbar SH, Braverman LE (eds): Werner's the Thyroid: A Fundamental and Clinical Text, Philadelphia, JB Lippincott Co. 1986; pp 3–6.
2. Turnbridge WMG, Evered DC, Hall R, et al: The spectrum of thyroid disease in a community: The Whickham Survey. Clin Endocrinol 1977;7:481–93.
3. Dos Remedios LV, Weber PM, Feldman R, et al: Detecting unsuspected thyroid dysfunction by the free thyroxine index. Arch Intern Med 1980; 140:1045–49.
4. Silverberg E: Cancer statistics 1982. CA 1982;32:15–31.
5. Clark OH: Endocrine Surgery of the Thyroid and Parathyroid Glands. St. Louis, CV Mosby Co., 1985.
6. Hellman DE: The thyroid gland, in Brown BR (ed): Anesthesia and the Patient with Endocrine Disease. Philadelphia, FA Davis Co, 1980; pp 109–46.

7. Murkin JM: Anesthesia and hypothyroidism: A review of thyroxine physiology, pharmacology and anesthetic implications. Anesth Analg 1982;61: 371–83.
8. Kim JM, Hackman L: Anesthesia for untreated hypothyroidism: Report of three cases. Anesth Analg 1977;56:299–302.
9. Senior RM, Birge SJ, Wessler S, et al: The recognition and management of myxedema coma. JAMA 1971;217:61–5.
10. Leonard JJ, Degroot WJ: The thyroid state and cardiovascular system. Mod Concepts Cardiovasc Dis 1969;38:23–7.
11. Stehling LC: Anesthetic management of the patient with hyperthyroidism. Anesthesiology 1974;41:585–95.
12. Shires GT: Questions and answers on anesthesia for thyroid surgery. Clin Anesth 1963;1:(3)206.
13. Roizen MF: Endocrine abnormalities and anesthesia: Implications for the anesthesiologist. ASA Refresher Courses in Anesthesiology, 1984;12(14): 161–77.
14. Benson DW: Anesthesia for thyroid surgery. Seminars in Anesthesia 1984; 111:168–73.
15. Stehling LC: Anesthetic implications of hyperthyroidism, in Brown BR (ed): Anesthesia and the Patient with Endocrine Disease, Philadelphia, FA Davis Co, 1980; pp 147–58.
16. Nance P, Wingard DW: Malignant hyperthermia. Anesth Analg 1981;60: 613–15.

CHAPTER 20

The Patient with Chickenpox

Anil de Silva

Case History. *A 20-year-old, 60-kg Asian man was brought to the emergency room with a complaint of abdominal pain. He stated that he had been in good health until 5 days previously, when he developed fever and muscle pain. The following day he noticed multiple fluid-filled lesions distributed mostly on his trunk. He was treated at home with fluids, bed rest, and acetaminophen. Two days prior to hospitalization he developed a cough, followed by abdominal pain.*

Physical exam revealed a fever of 102°F. Blood pressure was 130/60 mmHg, with a pulse of 84/min. Skin examination showed erythematous papules and vesicles in singlets and in clusters in a truncal distribution. Some lesions were beginning to crust. Auscultation of the chest was significant for fine crackles throughout the lung fields. Cardiac examination was unremarkable. Abdominal examination revealed absent bowel sounds, with rebound tenderness and guarding at McBurney's point.

Laboratory data included a white cell count of 13,000 and a BUN and creatinine of 24 and 2.0, respectively; SGOT, 140; ECG, occasional premature ventricular complexes; chest x-ray, an interstitial infiltrate in both lung fields. Blood gas analyses revealed a pH of 7.45; PCO_2, 35: PO_2, 87. All other laboratory values were within normal limits.

The patient was scheduled for emergency appendectomy.

Introduction

Varicella, or chickenpox, is a generally benign childhood disease caused by the varicella-zoster (VZ) virus. The name *varicella* is thought to be a French appellation given to the less malignant form of the dangerous variola, or smallpox, virus. The term chickenpox is thought by some to

---

Reviewed by Dr. Miguel Rosa, Assistant Professor, Department of Anesthesia, Albert Einstein College of Medicine, Bronx, NY.

describe the shape of the skin lesion, akin to that of a chick-pea. VZ is a species of herpesvirus. The name *herpes* is derived from ancient Greek, meaning "to creep," signifying the capacity of the disease for local spread. *Zoster* is a Greek term for "belt," denoting a common site for the skin lesions, around the waist.[1]

Morphology of the Virus

VZ is a herpesvirus primarily because of its structure. Other herpesviruses that affect humans are the simplex virus (a close cousin of VZ virus), cytomegalovirus, and Epstein–Barr virus. The virion is composed of a capsid (an outer envelope) and a core. The capsid comprises 162 protein subunits called capsomers. The core is composed of double-stranded DNA, as are those of all herpesviruses. The virion weighs approximately 80 million daltons and is about 200 nm in diameter.[2]

Epidemiology

Varicella is highly contagious. Ninety-six percent of adults in the United States are seropositive to VZ virus.[3] The highest incidence of disease occurs between the ages of 5 and 9 years, although it is possible to acquire the infection at any age. Chickenpox is generally a benign disease and is only rarely fatal. Between 1972 and 1978 approximately 2,800,000 cases were recorded in the United States, with 735 deaths. Seventy percent of the deaths involved those 10 years old or younger. Mortality was much higher in patients over the age of 20. The reported mortality risk for patients less than 1 year of age was 1 : 13,000. Patients aged 1 to 4 years had a risk ratio of 1 : 50,000; those 20 years or older, 1 : 1500.[1]

Clinical Course

The clinical course of chickenpox may be divided into several distinct stages, as outlined in Table 20.1. The primary varicella infection after exposure is acquired by absorption through the mucous membranes of the

TABLE 20.1. Clinical course of chickenpox.

Stage	Day	Systemic Event
1	1	Viral absorption via mucous membranes
2	5	Primary viremia and secondary replicative sites
3	12	Secondary viremia, eruption of exanthem
4	12–19	Spreading of rash
5	20	Secondary infection of papules

oropharynx and conjunctivae of droplets containing viral particles. The lymphatic system transports the virus to local tissues, where incubation begins.

About 5 days later a primary viremia occurs, and virions in large quantity are released into the bloodstream. The virus is spread throughout the body to secondary sites for replication. These sites include epithelial derivatives of liver, lung, kidney, intestines, adrenals, and blood vessels. As occurred in our case, replication may also take place in the appendiceal lymphatic tissue, with presentation as acute appendicitis.

Seven days later a secondary viremia occurs that heralds the appearance of the characteristic exanthem. The lesions appear rapidly and begin as clusters of small erythematous papules on scalp and trunk. Over a 1-week period these lesions spread centrifugally. The skin lesions are in varied stages of development. The papules turn vesicular, and the contents become cloudy within 24 hours, after which the vesicles begin to crust. The patient is infectious from 24 to 48 hours prior to the appearance of the exanthem and until all lesions are crusted.[1,4,5]

Systemic Complications

Although varicella has a normally benign course, it exerts multisystem changes, and the complications that ensue may be severe. Some of the major complications that affect anesthetic management are listed in Table 20.2. The most frequent complication of varicella is secondary infection of the skin lesions, with *Staphylococcus aureus* and *Streptococcus pyogenes* as the most common pathogens. Fifty-seven percent of all complications in children appear to involve bacterial superinfection.[4] Other, less common complications include pneumonitis, encephalitis, cerebritis, myelitis, myocarditis, nephritis, vasculitis, hepatitis, arthritis, and thrombocytopenia. Involvement of some of these systems carries particular concern for the anesthesiologist. Careful review during the preanesthetic assessment is essential.

TABLE 20.2. Multisystem complications of chickenpox.

System	Complication
Respiratory	Pneumonia, embolism
CNS	Encephalitis, transverse myelitis
Cardiovascular	Myocarditis
Hepatobiliary	Hepatitis
Renal	Glomerulonephritis
Hematopoietic	Thrombocytopenia

Pulmonary Involvement

Although varicella pneumonia has an incidence of only 0.8% in the pediatric age group, the adult population exhibits a significantly increased incidence of this complication. Most of the increased morbidity associated with chickenpox in the adult population is secondary to pneumonia. The pneumonitis generally begins 1 to 6 days after the appearance of the exanthem and is typified by cough and dyspnea. Pleuritic chest pain may be present. The pneumonitis in most cases is short-lived, resolving within 2 to 3 days. A severe case, however, can result in worsening tachypnea, dyspnea, cyanosis, hypoxia, and death.

Chest x-ray in most cases of varicella pneumonitis demonstrates bilateral infiltrates with perihilar nodular densities.[1] Pulmonary biopsy shows areas of focal necrosis and consolidation, with mononuclear infiltration. In rare cases pulmonary embolism has been reported associated with varicella pneumonitis. In such cases diagnostic lung scan or angiography may be crucial for appropriate therapy.

The treatment of varicella pneumonitis is primarily directed toward maintaining oxygenation. To that end, clearance of secretions, careful monitoring of blood gases, and provision of sufficient oxygen are all-important. Worsening pulmonary status may result from the increase in ventilation-perfusion inequalities found in patients with interstitial pneumonitis. Tracheal intubation and ventilation with a slow inflation rate and end-inspiratory pause will allow redistribution of inspired gas to better-perfused alveoli. The application of positive end-expiratory pressure (PEEP) may reduce shunt fraction by increasing functional residual capacity above closing volume, thus opening otherwise collapsed alveoli.[6]

Neurologic Complications

Meningoencephalitis and cerebellar ataxia are the primary neurologic manifestations of chickenpox. Approximately 0.2% of people with chickenpox develop encephalitic findings. Encephalitis generally occurs about 3 to 7 days after the appearance of the exanthem. Symptoms include nuchal rigidity, headache, vomiting, and fluctuations in consciousness. Seizures and psychoses may develop.

Pathologic examination reveals areas of demyelination, mononuclear infiltration, and microglial proliferation. Cerebritis commonly manifests as ataxia and nystagmus. Lumbar puncture reveals mildly increased lymphocytes, polymorphonuclear leukocytes, and granulocytes (fewer than 100 cells/ml). There may be a slight elevation in protein. Intracranial pressure is usually elevated.

Symptoms generally resolve within 24 to 48 hours, although ataxia may last longer. There have been reports of transverse myelitis associated with varicella. Sensory deficit and loss of sphincter control may be problematic. In most cases symptoms of spinal involvement tend to resolve without lasting deficit.[1] Intracranial pressure (ICP) monitoring may be helpful in the management of these patients. Hyperventilation to a PaCO$_2$ of 25–30 mmHg is recommended to reduce cerebral blood flow and thus decrease ICP.[7] Mannitol (0.5 gm/kg) and/or furosemide (0.5 mg/kg) may be indicated.

Cardiac Assessment

Although rare, varicella myocarditis does occur, sometimes with accompanying pericarditis. The cardiac symptomatology generally develops about 3 days after the appearance of the skin manifestations of chickenpox. Pathologic examination shows focal necrotic areas of myocardium with perivascular inflammatory infiltrates. Inflammation of the myocardial conduction system sometimes presents as atrial and ventricular dysrythymias. Occasionally, they have been fatal.[8] ECG changes may include ST or Q-wave abnormalities. Therapy for myocarditis is primarily supportive, with adjunctive use of digitalis and antidysrhythmic agents.[3]

Hepatic Lesions

Some patients with varicella exhibit evidence of abnormal liver function. A study of otherwise healthy children with varicella showed that 49% of them had mild SGOT elevation. Twenty-eight percent had elevation to greater than 50 IU/L, and some had SGOT levels in the 200–800 IU/L range.[1] Jaundice may be apparent. Pathologic examination of hepatic tissue reveals isolated foci of necrosis throughout the hepatic parenchyma.[9,10]

The implication for the anesthesiologist is that halothane should probably be avoided because it is metabolized in significant quantities by the liver. In addition, there are reports of greater reduction in splanchnic blood flow and concomitant hepatocyte hypoxia with halothane as compared to isoflurane or enflurane. The use of muscle relaxants may help reduce the dosage of inhalational agent required, but care should be taken to use an agent that is primarily nonhepatically metabolized, such as isoflurane.

Renal Function

The patient with varicella may develop glomerulonephritis. It generally occurs within the first 3 days after the appearance of skin lesions, with characteristic urinary findings of hematuria and proteinuria. Plasma values show an elevated BUN and creatinine. Renal parenchyma, on histologic examination, exhibits areas of focal necrosis and interstitial infiltration, with accompanying glomerular hypercellularity. The formation of crescents within the glomerulus is caused by anti-basement-membrane antibody–antigen complexes that may cause oliguria or complete anuria. Dialysis is necessary until renal function returns. The complication is self-limiting, and complete reversal is possible with supportive care. Anesthetic and neuromuscular agents requiring good kidney function for excretion should be avoided.

Hematologic Changes

Diffuse bleeding as a severe complication of chickenpox is generally the result of thrombocytopenia. The clinical picture is characterized by fever, mucosal bleeding, petechiae, and hemorrhagic vesicles. Should the complication develop into purpura fulminans, ecchymotic areas of the trunk and extremities may coalesce. Intracerebral hemorrhage has occurred; hemorrhagic shock is possible.[11]

The pathologic basis for the disease is the degeneration and vacuolization found in the megakaryocytes. Platelet counts may fall below 50,000. Blood and platelet transfusions may be required if emergency surgery is contemplated. If the platelet count is below 100,000, general anesthesia, rather than a regional technique, is probably preferable. The choice should be weighed against the risk of aspiration in an emergency situation or the possibility of airway bleeding should the intubation be traumatic. Nasotracheal or nasoesophageal instrumentation should be avoided.

Specific Therapy

Some protection against the complications of chickenpox is afforded by the administration of varicella immune globulin, a commercial preparation made from plasma. Optimally, the globulin should be given within the first 3 days of exposure to VZ virus, although it may have efficacy up to 5 days later. Despite the VZ globulin, up to 66% of exposed people will develop the disease, but the course is much attenuated.[12] Studies have shown that VZ immune globulin given to high-risk children exposed to chickenpox is protective and safe. The high-risk group comprises those who are immunosuppressed because of chemotherapy, leukemia, or other immunosuppressive disease processes. Immune globulin has not been found useful for the amelioration of symptoms in adults.

Other antiviral therapeutic regimens are currently under investigation. Vidarabine, a nucleoside analog, acts competitively to inhibit VZ-viral and host-cellular DNA polymerase. Intravenous administration of 10 mg/kg significantly reduces the incidence of life-threatening complications from varicella.[1]

Acyclovir is a synthetic purine nucleotide that also inhibits DNA polymerase. The incorporation of acyclovir into a newly forming DNA chain causes its termination. The drug is used in doses of 15 mg/kg/day. Both drugs are without significant toxicity in the immunosuppressed population studied so far. They are not routinely used in a varicella-infected population that is otherwise healthy.

Isolation Techniques

Operative preparation for a patient with chickenpox must include attention to the timing of the operation as well as careful selection of appropriate personnel. If patient safety allows, the scheduling of an elective operation should occur after the period of contagion. If it is possible to operate on an urgent rather than emergent basis, the operation may be performed at the end of the day. Such an approach will minimize the risks of varicella infection to susceptible patients and operating room personnel. In most cases previous infection with chickenpox confers immunity; therefore, if at all possible, anesthetic, surgical, and nursing personnel who are immune to the disease should be selected to perform the operation.

The bacterial and viral contamination of the anesthetic breathing system should be considered. The concentrations of oxygen, temperature, and humidity found in an anesthetic circuit are bactericidal although not necessarily viricidal. Studies have not shown any certain benefit from using filters and disposable breathing circuits. Nevertheless, it is prudent to use disposable equipment to safeguard the health of other patients.

Anesthetic Plan

Standard monitoring in this case should include assessment of a 5-lead ECG, pulse oximetry, temperature, blood pressure, and blood gas analyses. An inhalation technique is probably preferable; isoflurane, which is metabolized to the extent of approximately 0.7%, is the agent of choice. Prior to intubation, preoxygenation and application of cricoid pressure are indicated. Adequate muscle relaxation is best achieved with atracurium if the duration of the procedure is expected to be less than 1 hour, or pancuronium if a longer period of neuromuscular relaxation is required.

Fluid replacement should be with a non-glucose-containing solution if there is any indication of cerebral involvement by the VZ virus. Should dysrhythmias occur intraoperatively, bolus or continuous infusion of lidocaine is indicated.

Temperature should be controlled as close to normal levels as possible by surface-regulating techniques and adjustment of the temperature of infused and irrigating solutions.

References

1. Hyman R: Natural history of varicella-zoster virus. Boca Raton, Fla, CRC Press, 1987; pp 2, 5, 73, 76, 77, 167.
2. Brunell P: Varicella-zoster infections, in Feigin R, Cherry J (eds): Textbook of Pediatric Infectious Diseases. Philadelphia, WB Saunders, 1987; p 1602.
3. Schauf V, Tolpin M: Varicella-zoster virus, in Belske RB (ed): Textbook of Human Virology. Littleton, Mass, PSG Publishing Co, 1984; p 831.
4. Preblud S, Orenstein W, Bart K: Varicella: Clinical manifestations, epidemiology, and health impact in children. Pediatr Infect Dis 1984;6:505–9.
5. Betts R: Varicella zoster, in Stein J (ed): Internal Medicine. Boston, Little Brown & Co, 1983; p 1293.
6. Cimons IM, Lacher MJ, LaMonte CS, et al: Treatment of varicella pneumonia. JAMA 1968;206:372–74.
7. Andreasson S,: Severe acute encephalitis: Improved outcome after barbiturate therapy. Scand J Infect Dis 1984;16:25–30.
8. Coppack SW, Doshi R, Ghose AR: Fatal varicella in healthy young adults. Postgrad Med J 1985;61:529–31.
9. Harris R: The newer hyperbilirubinemias. Disease-a-Month. Chicago: Year Book Medical Publishers, March 1968.
10. Hook EB, Orandi M, Bensel RW, et al: Familial fatal varicella. JAMA 1968;206:305.
11. Benoit P, Raymond R, Glorieux FH: Purpura fulminans. Can Med Assoc J 1969;101:42–6.
12. Gershon A: Prevention and treatment of varicella-zoster virus infection. Pediatr Infect Dis 1984;3(suppl):534–37.

CHAPTER 21

The Patient with Rheumatoid Arthritis

Werner Pfisterer

Case History. *A 56-year-old woman who had suffered from severe progressive rheumatoid arthritis for ten years was scheduled for elective replacement of a severely degenerated right hip. Medical history was positive for hypertension, dysphagia, and occasional tingling of the hands on excessive neck movement. Medications included prazosin 2mg q.d., hydrochlorothiazide 50mg q.d., prednisone 10mg q.d., and a six-month course of gold.*

Laboratory results indicated the following: hemoglobin 11gm/dl; hematocrit 31%; electrolyte levels within normal limits; BUN/CR, 17/1.1; urinalysis, normal; chest x-ray: diffuse haziness but no acute infiltrate, no cardiomegaly; cervical spine x-ray: atlantoaxial subluxation, subaxial subluxation C4-5; ECG: no acute changes, normal sinus rhythm, left ventricular hypertrophy; arterial blood gas analysis on room air: pH, 7.42; CO$_2$, 38mmHg; O$_2$, 72mmHg; saturation, 93%. On physical examination vital signs were BP 160/96mmHg, pulse 86/min, respiration 22/min, temperature 36.8°C; weight was 74kg, height 5'4".

Airway assessment revealed mouth opening 3cm, reduced neck mobility in all directions, leftward laryngeal deviation, flexion deformity of neck. Chest: breath sounds clear but diminished in all fields, heart tones regular and without murmurs. Extremities: hands with marked bilateral deformities and ulnar drift, rheumatoid nodules over both elbows, swelling and tenderness of wrists, elbows, and knees. Hips showed reduced mobility, right greater than left.

Epidemiology

Using the American Rheumatism Association criteria for diagnosis, the prevalence of rheumatoid arthritis (RA) is about 0.5% in the adult population. Women are afflicted three times more often than are men, the

Reviewed by Dr. H. Keisar, Director, Department of Rheumatology, Albert Einstein College of Medicine, Bronx, NY.

prevalence increasing with age into the seventh decade. Race is not a factor, and familial spread is not clear. Insidious onset is common, but variability in presentation occurs. Prognosis is best when onset is acute, involving few joints, in a male patient. Poor prognosis exists when a female patient exhibits polyarticular arthritis, positive rheumatoid factor, eosinophilia, thrombocytosis, elevated sedimentation rate, elevated C-reactive protein levels, vasculitis, or Sjogren's syndrome. Juvenile arthritis (Still's disease) has bimodal onset at age 2 and age 12. A salmon-colored rash with fever, iridocyclitis and blindness, and hypoplasia of the mandible, contributing to an extremely difficult intubation, are some characteristic features of the juvenile form.[1]

Pathophysiology

Immunoglobulin M and immunoglobulin G antiglobulins (rheumatoid factors) are complexed with complement in the synovial lining layer, liberating chemotactic factor. Phagocytosis of the immune complexes by responding macrophages and polymorphonuclear cells releases lysosomal proteases, resulting in local inflammation and necrosis. Macrophage migration inhibitory factor and mitogenic factor propagate the inflammatory response and, together with the antigenic reservoir of joints and synovial membrane, produce chronic granulation tissue. Erosion and destruction of bone and cartilage cause fibrous tissue scarring, leading to ankylosis, subluxation, and distortion of the affected joints.[2]

Clinical Presentation

The stages in the clinical presentation of RA are listed in Table 21.1. Myalgia, malaise, and early fatigue may precede arthritic changes. Joint involvement is nonmigratory and symmetrical in distribution, with the metacarpophalangeal, proximal interphalangeal, and metatarsophalangeal joints affected early, although all diarthrodial joints are at risk. Ligament

TABLE 21.1. Clinical stages of rheumatoid arthritis.

Stage	Signs
Early	Myalgia, malaise, fatigability
Middle	Symmetrical joint swelling (hands first)
	Subcutaneous nodules
	Ligamentous involvement
Advanced	Joint deformity
Middle	Subluxation
Late	Atrophy of bone, muscles, skin

TABLE 21.2 Clinical findings in rheumatoid
arthritis (seven must be present to establish
the diagnosis).

Morning stiffness
Pain on motion, with joint tenderness
Swelling over at least one joint
Symmetrical nonmigratory joint involvement
Nodules on bony or extensor surfaces
X-ray changes of periarticular demineralization
Positive rheumatoid factor test
Decreased mucin clotting of synovial fluid
Histologic change in synovial biopsy
Histologic changes in nodules

---

involvement results in joint instability, with extensor/flexor muscle group
imbalance, and the joint becomes deformed. Subluxation occurs when
deformity is coupled with articular surface erosion. Atrophy occurs in
bone, muscles, and skin adjacent to the affected joints. Subcutaneous
nodules, which occur in 20%–30% of patients, are considered the most
characteristic lesion of rheumatoid arthritis.[1]

Diagnosis and Classification

The diagnosis of classical RA requires 7 of the 10 criteria listed in Table
21.2. The presence of 5 or more criteria is considered definitely indicative
of RA; 3 indicate probability, and 2 may be considered a possible
diagnosis. Functional classification is made into one of four categories:
class 1—able to carry on all usual duties without handicaps; class 2—able
to conduct normal activities despite limited mobility; class 3—able to
perform few occupational or self-care activities; class 4—wholly incapac-
itated.[1] Our patient qualifies as class 3.

Preoperative Assessment

Virtually all organs can be affected by rheumatoid changes. Those of
lesser clinical importance for the anesthesiologist include the eyes
(scleromalacia perforans when rheumatoid nodules develop in the sclera)
and the skin (subcutaneous nodules on bony prominences). Of greater
concern for anesthesiologists are the changes that occur in the following
systems: cardiovascular, pulmonary, hematologic, immunologic, and
renal. Perhaps of greatest import are those alterations involving the
airway and the cervical spine.

Airway Assessment

Securing and maintaining the airway in the patient with RA is often a challenge. Taking a careful history for the presence of dysphagia, dysarthria, fullness in the throat, hoarseness, or stridor (especially when asleep) is a critical first step in the proper management of such patients. Examination of the oropharynx becomes more important if any of these findings is present, as cricoarytenoid arthritis should be suspected. Commonly arthritic, the cricoarytenoid is considered a true diarthrodial joint because two cartilages, complete with synovial membrane lining both the joint capsule and the joint cavity, move freely in opposition. Indirect laryngoscopy reveals tense, edematous, reddened arytenoid mucosa, swollen aryepiglottic folds, false cords, and a marked decrease in true cord mobility.[3] This finding should alert the anesthesiologist that a smaller endotracheal tube may be required. Necessity for fiberoptic intubation or elective tracheostomy should be anticipated and discussed with the patient and surgeon. Induction and/or emergence may result in airway obstruction as the laryngeal muscles lose tone.[4]

Evaluation of the temporomandibular joint includes assessment of the upper-to-lower incisor distance with the mouth maximally opened (at least 5 cm, or three fingers, is required normally) and ability to visualize the uvula. Lateral profile inspection is considered part of the airway assessment of the mandible. Intubation difficulty is encountered especially in patients in whom the combination of cricoarytenoid arthritis, temporomandibular joint ankylosis, and a receding chin (often seen in the juvenile RA patient) exists. Inspection and palpation should ascertain the presence of laryngeal deviation. RA of the cervical spine produces consistent conformational changes in laryngeal and tracheal alignment, as may be noted fiberoptically.[5] Shortening of the cervical neck caused by the rheumatoid process, together with a tethering effect from the aortic arch, produces a rightward rotation, left anterior/lateral displacement, and a forward tilt on the larynx and trachea.[5]

Smooth induction and intubation does not ensure an uneventful postoperative course, as trauma from intubation to the arthritic cricoarytenoid apparatus can require emergency tracheotomy. Patients can develop airway difficulty even after a benign postoperative six-day course.[4]

Cervical Spine Assessment

The incidence of cervical spine involvement in RA patients has been variably reported (6.4%–90%).[5] History of decreased neck mobility, neck pain with radiation to the occiput, and upper extremity radiculopathy should raise suspicion of cervical spine arthritis and additional airway management difficulty. Patients must be evaluated for active flexion, extension, and lateral rotation on physical exam. The results of a careful neurologic examination ruling out long tract signs, posterior column dysfunction, and urinary sphincter abnormality should be documented.

The process of synovial destruction, ligament involvement, and vertebral erosion produces cervical spine instability. The most common cervical spine instability in the RA patient is atlantoaxial subluxation. Cervical neck films in flexion and extension may signal impending neuropathology if the atlas/odontoid interval is greater than 3 mm in flexion. The normal relationship within the first cervical ring has been described by Steel's rule of thirds: the first cervical ring area is normally divided into equal thirds occupied by the odontoid, free space, and the spinal cord. The free space allows for some degree of movement without immediate cord compression.[6]

Normally, the odontoid process of the axis is fixed against the anterior arch of the atlas by the transverse ligament. When RA affects this transverse ligament, the atlas is free to shift anteriorly over the axis. Preventing cord compression is then dependent on the other two members of the axial cruciform ligament: alar ligaments (connecting the odontoid to the anterior edge of the foramen magnum) and the superior and inferior longitudinal bands (attaching the atlas to the occiput above and the axis below). Anterior displacement of the atlas greater than 3 cm in the adult or 4 cm in the child implies that all three ligaments are affected and cord compression is likely. Values less than these imply that only the transverse ligament is involved and lessens the chance of cord compression.

Lateral cervical neck x-rays are also important for the detection and assessment of vertebral subluxation, the second most common cervical spine pathology. Subaxial subluxation (when two or more cervical vertebrae below the level of C2 are involved) is considered significant when a superior vertebra is displaced more than 15% on an inferior vertebra. The incidence of subluxation is greatest at C1–2 and lessens progressively to C6–7, where the incidence is lowest.[5] Normally, the odontoid process is just inferior to the foramen magnum. With cervical spine rheumatoid changes, the odontoid process migrates superiorly into the foramen magnum. Odontoid migration, associated with severe bone erosion, is the least common cervical rheumatic change reported (incidence 3.8%–15%).[5,6] Measurement of the perpendicular distance between the arch of C1 and the pedicle of C2 on lateral cervical x-ray indicates impending cord compression when it is less than 13 mm.[8] Computerized axial tomography and magnetic resonance imaging have replaced cervical tomograms for detection of odontoid migration.

Evidence of any of the three classical spine deformities necessitates neck stabilization during laryngoscopy and intubation. In addition to bony involvement, occlusion of the vertebral arteries causes dizziness on head movement, especially in patients with cervical abnormalities.

Cardiovascular Assessment

Granulomatous changes are known to affect both the myocardium and heart valves, resulting in conduction defects and regurgitance. Restriction of cardiac output may result from congestive failure, amyloidosis, pericarditis, and pericardial effusion. Focal vasculitis causing myocardial damage and diffuse arteritis have been reported. Although clinically evident RA-related heart disease may be rare, inquiry about signs and symptoms of pump dysfunction, dysrythmia, or chest pain is appropriate in the elderly. The incidence of heart disease is 35% in RA patients and only 15% in control patients.[9] Physical exam and ECG with rhythm strip are basic. Myocardial depressants should be deleted, and invasive monitoring with cardiac profiling may be considered in selected patients.

Pulmonary Assessment

Three types of lung pathology are encountered: diffuse interstitial fibrosis (most common); multiple or coalescent granulomatoid nodules seen as honeycombing cysts on x-ray; and diffuse, large silicotic nodules often associated with coal mining. These changes can restrict lung function, diminish diffusing capacity, and lower oxygen saturation.[10] Costochondral arthritis and thoracic flexion deformity result in marked decrease in chest wall compliance. History of dyspnea, restrictive breathing pattern, and inability to inspire deeply is not unusual. Chest x-ray, arterial blood gas analyses, and pulmonary function testing are important in selected patients. Steroid therapy may incite active tuberculosis in those with prior exposure to the bacillus.

Hematologic Assessment

Hypochromic microcytic anemia is seen in patients with ulceration and bleeding secondary to chronic acetylsalicylic acid treatment. Irreversible platelet dysfunction is also a common side effect. A history of weakness, dizziness, and tachycardia may indicate the presence of anemia. Complete blood count, bleeding time, and testing for occult blood in the stool to evaluate the side effects of medical treatment are indicated. Anemia in RA patients is often resistant to oral iron, making transfusion necessary preoperatively.[11] A hyperviscosity syndrome, secondary to changes in immune globulins, may result in neuropathy and retinopathy. Epistaxis, petechiae, and purpura are also associated with this syndrome.

Immunology Assessment

Humoral and cellular defenses can be altered, increasing the frequency of infection and neoplasms. Virtually all components of the immune system may undergo changes in production and function. Felty's syndrome, a combination of splenomegaly, leukopenia, and RA, puts these patients at risk for serious opportunistic infections.[12] A history of infection, knowledge of the present drug treatment, and results of a white cell count with differential should identify patients at great risk.

Kidney Assessment

Renal dysfunction in RA is most often related to drug therapy, resulting in proteinuria and a nephrotic syndrome. Amyloidosis of the kidney is common and is found in 20% of patients at autopsy.[13]

Drug Therapy Assessment

Preoperative assessment of the patient's medical regimen should generate questions about drug efficacy and potential side effects and should guide the anesthetic management. Initial therapy for RA is usually with salicylates (optimal serum levels 25 mg/dl) unless sensitivity or a bleeding diathesis exists. Platelet function is of concern if major surgery is planned, and discontinuation of salicylates 10 days prior to surgery should be considered. Other adverse effects of chronic salicylate use, such as gastric erosion and renal toxicity, are well known.

Nonsteroidal anti-inflammatory drugs (NSAID) are no more effective than aspirin for pain relief. Besides blood dyscrasias, bleeding, and peptic ulcerogenesis, drug interaction because of high protein binding by NSAIDs may displace drugs given concomitantly, leading to relative overdose. Current recommendations to discontinue NSAIDs preoperatively should be considered.

Remittive therapy for progressive disease includes gold salts, D-penicillamine, hydroxychloroquine, and immunosuppressant agents. Thirty-three percent of patients treated with gold fail to respond or develop toxic manifestations, including mucocutaneous reaction, proteinuria with serious renal disease, and hematologic complications (leukopenia, thrombocytopenia, agranulocytosis). Toxicity from D-penicillamine is primarily hematologic and renal. Retinal damage, although rare, may be progressive despite the discontinuation of hydroxychloroquine. Immunosuppressive drugs (cyclophosphamide, chlorambucil, azathioprine, and methotrexate) in low doses are regarded as second-line therapy. If remittive therapy fails, or to help boost this phase, prednisone is given in a low dose (<10 mg/day), or in a high dose (>60 mg/day) in cases with severe rheumatoid vasculitis.

Patients receiving steroids are at risk for adrenal suppression and should be given a stress dose pre-, intra-, and postoperatively until newer recommendations are founded.[13] Anesthesiologists should be aware that patients at risk for adrenal suppression are difficult to identify preoperatively and that the stress of minor surgery is sufficient to incite an adrenal crisis. Current evidence suggests that plasmapheresis is not effective in cases of refractory RA. Total lymphoid irradiation is currently under investigation for use in patients with refractory illness.

Anesthetic Plan

In addition to the usual types of surgery performed in nonarthritics, RA patients are scheduled for numerous reconstructive and palliative ortho-pedic procedures. Upper and lower extremity surgery, total hip repair, and cervical spine stabilization constitute the majority of these. Each RA patient must be managed according to the following: severity of arthritis; degree of airway, neck, and organ involvement; medical therapy; type and extent of planned surgery. Preanesthetic assessment, properly com-pleted, will alert the anesthesiologist to discuss special needs with the patient and surgeon and to prepare additional equipment. These patients require special care in positioning because of deformities, osteoporosis, and delicate skin and mucous membranes. Intravenous placement may be difficult, especially in those receiving steroid therapy. Monitoring re-quirements are essentially similar to those for other patients, except when deformities demand ingenuity. Finger deformity may make recording from a pulse oximeter difficult, prompting probe application to the earlobe or nasal septum. In patients with an existing neurologic deficit of a hand, it may be wise to avoid cannulation of the ipsilateral artery.

Intubation for general anesthesia requires impeccable airway assess-ment, knowledge of characteristics of laryngeal deviation, assistance with cervical spine stabilization, and dexterity with the fiberoptic bron-choscope. Elective tracheostomy and retrograde intubation are effective techniques in selected patients. Attempts at nasal intubation may result in bloody trauma because of mucous membrane fragility and drug side effects, making it the least desirable choice. Regional anesthesia has been used effectively in severe arthritis.[14] Interscalene block for operations on the upper extremity and shoulder can be useful. Axillary block is used if deformities do not prevent abduction. Intravenous regional block, be-cause of deformed extremities and fragile skin, is less desirable. Spinal or epidural block is often performed without difficulty, as the lumbar spine is not usually affected. Ankle block can be utilized in forefoot procedures. Sedation during regional anesthesia is risky in RA patients; judicious use is recommended because obstruction from cricoarytenoid arthritis can be sudden and difficult to manage.

References

1. Committee of the American Rheumatism Association: Primer in rheumatic diseases. Special contribution, Part 1. JAMA 1964;190:127–28.
2. Mowat AG, Baum J: Chemotaxis of polymorphonuclear leucocytes from patients with rheumatic arthritis. J Clin Invest 1979;50:2451–59.

3. Funk D, Raymon F: Rheumatoid arthritis of the cricoarytenoid joints: An airway hazard. Anesth Analg 1975;54:742–44.
4. Gardner DL, Holmes F: Anaesthetic and postoperative hazards in rheumatoid arthritis. Br J Anaesth 1961;33:258–59.
5. Keenan MA, Siles CM, Kaufman RL: Acquired laryngeal deviation associated with cervical spine disease in erosive polyarticular arthritis. Anesthesiology 1983;58:441–49.
6. Steel HH: anatomical and mechanical considerations of the atlanto-axial articulations. J Bone Joint Surg [Am] 1968;50-A:1481–82.
7. Pellicci PM, Ranawat CS, Tsairis P, et al: A prospective study of the progression of rheumatoid arthritis of the cervical spine. J Bone Joint Surg [Am] 1981;63-A:342–50.
8. Ranawat CS, O'Leary P, Tsairis P, et al: Cervical spine fusion in rheumatoid arthritis. J Bone Joint Surg [Am] 1979;61-A:1003–10.
9. Cathcart ES, Spodick DH: Rheumatoid heart disease: A study of the incidence and nature of cardiac lesions in rheumatoid arthritis. N Engl J Med 1962;266:959–61.
10. Lee FI, Bain AT: Chronic diffuse interstitial pulmonary fibrosis and rheumatoid arthritis. Lancet 1962;2:693–94.
11. Syndas DA: The anemia of rheumatoid arthritis and its treatment with blood transfusions. Acta Rheum Scand 1961;7:95–6.
12. Felty AR: Chronic arthritis in the adult, associated with splenomegaly and leucopenia: A report of five cases of an unusual clinical syndrome. Bull Johns Hopkins Hosp 1924;35:6–20.
13. Eisele JH: Connective tissue diseases, in Anesthesia and Uncommon Diseases (2nd ed). Philadelphia: WB Saunders Co, 1981; pp 506–16.
14. Bernstein RL, Rosenberg AD: Anesthesia for orthopedic surgery. Seminars in Anesthesia: Anesthesia for Special Situations 1987;6(1):36–43.

CHAPTER 22

The Patient for Outpatient Cataract Surgery

C.J. Eagle and Jan M. Davies

Case History. *A 73-year-old retired farmer with hypertension and diabetes mellitus was admitted to the outpatient department for surgical treatment of cataract disease. His medications on admission included chlorpropamide 250 mg daily and hydrochlorothiazide 50 mg b.i.d. Before admission his ophthalmologic assessment showed a visual acuity of 20/80 in his right eye.*

Admission blood work included hematocrit 45% and fasting blood sugar 145 mg/dl. Other chemical analyses (serum electrolytes) were normal. This patient had been seen by an internist in the preoperative assessment clinic one week before admission, at which time his ECG and chest x-ray were normal. There were no other significant abnormalities. The patient was scheduled for elective right cataract extraction and intraocular lens implantation. Regional anesthesia was requested by the ophthalmologist.

Introduction

Cataract removal and intraocular lens implantation is an increasingly common surgical procedure. This trend has resulted from the confluence of several factors, including a growing population of elderly people and widespread availability of surgical techniques involving use of the operating microscope and phacoemulsification devices. Escalating health care costs have not diminished the development of cataract surgery but have led to the far greater use of outpatient facilities. The ability to perform complex surgery on elderly patients without overnight hospital admission has been a major challenge for anesthesiologists, resulting in a refinement of the preoperative assessment facilities so that the patient's medical, surgical, and psychological preparation may be attended to before the day

Reviewed by Dr. L. Strunin, Professor and Chairman, Department of Anesthesia, University of Calgary, Calgary, Alberta, Canada.

of surgery. Concurrently, regional anesthesia for the eye has been improved by the development of the peribulbar block, which allows surgery to be performed with minimal, if any, sedation. In fact, patients frequently request videotape recordings of the operative procedures.

A cataract is an opacity of the crystalline lens of the eye resulting from changes in the lens fibers. The word *cataract* is derived from the Greek *katarrhegnynai,* to break down.[1]

TABLE 22.1. Importance of cataract disease

No. People	Region	Problem
50,000,000	Worldwide	Vision-disrupting cataract
17,000,000	Worldwide	Disabled or blind
4,000,000	U.S.A.	Vision-disrupting cataract
40,000	U.S.A.	Blind

Adapted with permission of from Kahn HA, et al: The Framingham Eye Study, *Am J Epidemiol* 1977; 106:17–32.

Incidence

Cataract disease is a widespread problem (Table 22.1.), although that is not necessarily evident from surgical booking lists. For example, between 1973 and 1975, 2675 of the 3977 still-living members of the Framingham, Massachusetts, study population were examined for eye disease. In subjects aged 52 to 85 years, 15.5% had a cataract-induced reduction in visual acuity of 20/30 or less.[2] Furthermore, the incidence of cataract disease increases with age (Table 22.2.), and this will become more evident with the "graying of America." In 1980, those aged 65 years or more represented 11% of the population of the United States; by 2020 this group will constitute approximately 16% of the population.[3]

TABLE 22.2. Incidence of cataract disease in the United States[a]

Age (years)	Incidence
52–64	5%
65–74	18%
75–85	46%

[a] Decrease in visual acuity to 20/30 or less. Adapted with permission from Kahn HA, et al: The Framingham Eye Study, *Am J Epidemiol* 1977; 106:17–32.

Pathophysiology

Progressively, aging produces physiologic changes in the lens, namely, increases in size, weight, and density. However, these must be distinguished from the pathophysiologic changes that occur with cataract disease, each of which defines a specific type of cataract (Table 22.3.). For example, an exaggeration of the normal hardening of fibers in the lens nucleus produces a nuclear cataract, a type that accounts for about 25% of senile cataracts.[4] Once present, cataracts may be defined by their degree of maturity, depending on the biochemical state of the lens protein. An incipient cataract shows increased fluid between the lens fibers. An immature cataract still has some transparent protein, whereas in a mature cataract, all protein is opaque. Finally, in a hypermature cataract, some cortical protein becomes soluble.

TABLE 22.3. Pathophysiologic changes in the lens

Change	Type of Cataract
Fibrous metaplasia of lens epithelium	Anterior subcapsular
Liquefaction of lens fibers and formation of Morgagnian globules anteriorly in cortex	Anterior cortical
Exaggeration of normal sclerosis of fibers in lens nucleus	Nuclear
Liquefaction and globular degeneration of posterior lens cortex	Posterior cortical
Posterior migration of epithelial cells under the capsule, forming large, irregular nucleated or bladder cells	Posterior subcapsular

Adapted with permission from Kahn HA, et al: The Framingham Eye Study, *Am J Epidemiol* 1977; 106:17–32.

Causes of Cataracts

As with many diseases, cataracts may be either congenital or acquired (Table 22.4.). Most frequently, cataract disease is idiopathic. However,

TABLE 22.4. Causes of cataracts

Congential
  Chromosomal
  Heredofamilial
  Infectious
  Inflammatory
  Nutritional
Acquired
  Idiopathic
  Systemic disease
    Diabetes, hypocalcemia
  Drugs and toxins
    Corticosteroids, metals
  Radiation, including ultraviolet light
  Trauma

there are conditions associated with cataracts that have anesthetic implications—for example, myotonic dystrophy. Furthermore, cataract progression may be accelerated by other conditions, such as poorly controlled diabetes mellitus with hyperglycemia and resultant osmotic changes in the lens. The vogue for winter tanning may produce a generation of patients with cataracts, as well as ultraviolet-induced skin cancers, although the relationship between sunlight and cataract disease is still controversial.[5]

Assessment of Cataract Disease

Once cataract disease is suspected, a general ophthalmologic consultation should be undertaken. The presence, nature, and severity of lens opacity are determined and the degree of visual disability established. Visual disability is related to the location and character of the cataract. The impact of the visual impairment depends on the activity of the patient and may be determined objectively (eg, inability to read) and/or subjectively (eg, depression). The time course of visual loss is also important. Sudden loss is unusual with cataracts, more common with primary retinal, vascular, or optic nerve disease. Cataracts cause a progressive loss of vision, but other diseases also may be present.

More-specific ophthalmologic investigations are then carried out—for example, tests of retinal/macular function and measurement of intraocular pressure. Finally, specific additional tests should be done if the patient's condition warrants them (Table 22.5.).

Treatment of Cataract Disease

Once the condition is diagnosed, treatment may be medical, surgical, or both. Medical management is directed at limiting progression of the cataract disease, for example, by controlling hyperglycemia, hypercalcemia, steroid intake, and exposure to ultraviolet light. Also important is provision of the best possible vision with eyeglasses or contact lenses,

TABLE 22.5. Additional
ophthalmologic investigations

Microbiologic studies of conjunctiva
Corneal endothelial cell counts
Diagnostic ocular ultrasound
Visual field testing
Angiography of retinal vessels
Lens photography
General medical evaluation: metabolic,
   genetic, or nutritional contribution to
   lens opacity

TABLE 22.6. Surgical Considerations

Visual need vs functional disability
Severity and maturity of cataract
Prognosis for visual improvement
Ocular and general medical health
Special ophthalmologic indications
    Lens maturity or hypermaturity
    Lens-induced glaucoma or uveitis
    Inability to visualize or treat disease in
        the posterior ocular segment

low-vision aids (magnifying glasses), dilation of the pupil, and regular observation and education of the patient.

Surgical treatment of cataract disease has been used for at least 3000 years, and should be contemplated in a variety of conditions (Table 22.6.). There are two surgical techniques, depending on the approach to extraction of the cataract: intracapsular (removal of entire lens with enveloping transparent capsule) and extracapsular (transparent posterior capsule left in place). Extracapsular extraction is the more popular technique (66% of more than 490,000 cases in 1983).[2] Surgery involves two major steps. A 3-mm incision is made in the cornea, through which an ultrasonically activated titanium cannula is inserted. With this instrument the nucleus and cortex of the lens are emulsified (phacoemulsification) and the debris is aspirated from the eye. The incision is then enlarged to 7 mm to allow placement of the intraocular lens. The three types of intraocular lens are listed in Table 22.7. Of these, the posterior chamber lens is currently the most popular.

Preoperative Evaluation

General Assessment

Once the ophthalmologist has made the diagnosis of surgically correctable cataract disease, the next question to be decided is the suitability of the patient for outpatient care versus preoperative admission to the hospital. This decision is made initially by the ophthalmologist, who, by his or her

TABLE 22.7. Types of intraocular lens

Anterior chamber	—in front of iris
Iris-plane	—at level of iris
Posterior chamber	—behind iris

interaction with the patient, will have made a general assessment. Factors to be considered include patient refusal of regional anesthesia, patient cooperation, and postoperative care.

Patient refusal may stem from a combination of anxiety and ignorance, the latter contributing to the former. Anxiety is very susceptible to environmental factors. For example, our experience shows that patients scheduled later in the day are less anxious than those scheduled first thing in the morning. As the first patients of the day return to the outpatient unit, those who follow are reassured by the street-ready condition of the patients after operation.

Preoperative teaching is obviously extremely important. This is started by the ophthalmologist, continued in the anesthetic preoperative assessment clinic, and reinforced in the outpatient clinic by the nursing staff. While the goal of preoperative teaching to inform patients of the risks inherent in any medical or surgical procedure, so that he or she can give informed consent, a significant benefit is reduction of anxiety by repetition of material from numerous sources. The elderly patient may have difficulty understanding unfamiliar technical details, and instruction should be given slowly and clearly but without condescension.

Patient cooperation may be limited by communication difficulties due to the effects of aging on vision, hearing, and comprehension. Language difficulties are common in communities with large immigrant populations. Often a close family member may accompany the patient during the perioperative period, providing a supportive atmosphere plus invaluable interpretive skills.

Physical problems also may affect patient cooperation. Motor skills may be diminished by a number of age-related factors, such as Parkinson's disease, osteoarthritis, and cerebrovascular disease. Sufficient time must be taken to allow for patient preparation in a calm, unhurried environment, for positioning as comfortably as possible, and for safe provision of the anesthetic care. Continuous verbal reassurance aids at every stage of the procedure. Anesthesiologists need good communication skills, particularly for this patient group.

After surgery, patients are released to the care of a responsible adult. Without this person, outpatient anesthesia and surgery is not possible.

Medical Assessment

Once assured of the general acceptability of the patient for outpatient surgery, the ophthalmologist makes an assessment of the patient's medical condition. Frequently, this is done by referring the patient back to his or her primary care physician for preoperative assessment and reevaluation of any preexisting diseases. In addition to the physiologic alterations of aging (Table 22.8.), elderly patients have a greater risk of

TABLE 22.8. Anesthetic implications of age

Nervous system
   Selective attrition of cerebral and cerebellar cortical
     neurons
   Depletion of brain neurotransmitters
   Loss of peripheral nerve fibers
   Disseminated neurogenic atrophy of muscle
   Increased threshold for all forms of reception
Cardiovascular system
   Loss of large-artery elasticity
   Possible impaired adrenergic receptor quality
Respiratory system
   Generalized reduction of elasticity
   Impaired ventilation perfusion matching
   Reduced chest wall compliances
Renal system
   Reduced glomerular filtration rate
   Reduced renal plasma flow
   Reduced ability to concentrate urine and conserve
     free water
   Reduced renal drug clearance
Hepatic system
   Reduction in liver size
   Maintenance of hepatocellular function
   Reduced hepatic drug clearance
Sympathoadrenal axis
   Elevated plasma epinephrine and norepinephrine
   Reduced autonomic end-organ responsiveness
Body composition
   Cellular dehydration
   Loss of skeletal muscle
   Increased proportion of adipose tissue

Adapted with permission from Muravchicks: The Physiologic and Pharmacologic Implications of Aging, ASA
Annual Refresher Course Lectures, No. 275, Las Vegas,
1986.

acquired illness affecting any body system. The most frequent problems
are hypertension, coronary artery disease, diabetes, chronic obstructive
pulmonary disease, and obesity. Patients with extensive or unusual
disease may require additional investigation and treatment. In our institution, a preoperative assessment clinic allows patients with complications
to be seen by general internists, medical subspecialists, or anesthesiologists. The ophthalmologist makes the initial referral to this clinic—to a
general internist or anesthesiologist—for development of a preoperative
treatment plan. Where necessary, multidisciplinary consultations can be
obtained. This enables patients with extensive medical problems to be
assessed and treated and to undergo surgery as outpatients.

Disposition

Following review of the patient, the ophthalmologist decides whether or not to proceed with surgery. Surgery may be undertaken using general or regional anesthesia. Historically, the use of general anesthesia was predominant in many institutions. Since the late 1960s, however, regional anesthesia has been the technique of choice for reasons of cost, length of stay in hospital, decreasing duration of procedure, and resultant patient acceptance. Until recently, regional anesthesia was the domain of the ophthalmic surgeon, with the anesthesiologist providing patient monitoring and intravenous sedation. Currently, in many institutions anesthesiologists perform regional eye blocks (in most instances without sedation[6]) and monitor the patients. Intraoperatively, no sedation is required by patients. Furthermore, it is essential that the patient remain still. This requires an alert, cooperative patient, and it is our impression that some anxiety is not detrimental. Commonly, the anxious patient will become calm and relaxed during the procedure. The majority are amazed that the procedure can be accomplished so rapidly and with so little duress. In our institution, general anesthesia is required only for patients with severe behavioral, motor, or psychiatric disorders.

Management Plan

Regional anesthesia can provide analgesia, akinesia of the globe and orbicularis oculi, and an acceptable level of intraocular pressure. Until recently, regional anesthesia was produced by retrobulbar injection of

TABLE 22.9. Complications of regional anesthesia for cataract surgery

Complication	Incidence
Brainstem anesthesia	0.06%
Retrobulbar hemorrhage	0.04%
Scleral perforation	0.008%
Optic atrophy	0.008%
Contralateral orbital block	0.008%
Vasovagal reaction	0.7%
Minor local problems	3%
Ecchymosis	
Extraocular muscle paresis	

Adapted with permission of from Hamilton RC, et al: Regional anesthesia for 12,000 cataract extraction and intraocular lens implantation surgical procedures, *Can J Anaesth* 1988; 35:615–23.

local anesthetic drugs. Despite the long history of retrobulbar anesthesia, a significant number of complications have been documented (Table 22.9.). Recently, considerable experience has been achieved with peribulbar injection of local anesthetic agents.[6] In distinction to retrobulbar anesthesia, no attempt is made to penetrate the conus formed by the extraocular muscles and fascia (Figure 22.1.). The technique of peribulbar anesthesia, as performed in our institution, is described below.

When the patient is received in the operating room, the pupil of the affected eye is checked for adequate mydriasis, and 3 drops of Ophthaine (proparacaine) 2% solution (or another topical anesthetic agent) are placed on the conjunctiva. Before the block is performed, a heparin lock or cannula is inserted into a peripheral vein, and electrocardiographic, oximetric, and blood pressure monitoring is started.

Additionally, 4 ml bupivacaine 0.75%, 4 ml lidocaine 2% with 1 : 200,000 epinephrine, and 1 ml hyaluronidase solution are mixed in a 10 ml syringe. A 27-gauge, 1¼-inch needle is attached to the syringe. Once prepared, the lower lid of the affected eye is retracted, and the infero-lateral area of the conjunctive is exposed. The needle is then inserted through the anesthetized conjunctiva. It is advanced approximately 1 inch, taking care to avoid the glove, and then 5 ml of the local anesthetic mixture is injected slowly (Figure 22.2.). Before injection, attempts are made to aspirate through the needle. Gentle pressure is then placed on the eye with a folded 4 × 4 swab. After 2 minutes, a further 3 ml of the mixture is injected transcutaneously, again following aspiration, into the now-anesthetized superior medial quadrant of the orbit, avoiding the globe (Figure 22.3.). Gentle pressure is again applied to the globe for approximately 1 minute; then a Honan cuff is placed over the eye. The eye is left undisturbed for about 10 minutes. Approximately 75% of patients will have excellent paresis of the extraocular muscles and orbicularis oculi at this time. Twenty minutes after injection, 90% of patients will show excellent surgical conditions. In some patients specific muscle activity will be observed, and this can be blocked by additional 2–3 ml injections of the local anesthetic mixture into either the superomedial or inferolateral quadrant depending on the location of the unaffected muscle. Rarely, an additional retrobulbar block will be required.

During the course of the surgical procedure, special consideration must be paid to the awake patient. Unfortunate exclamations ("Oops"), inappropriate conversation among staff ("There's an arrest in room four"), and unnecessary noise in the operating room (dropping of instrument trays) may provoke undue anxiety in the patient. As mentioned above, use of a heparin lock may eliminate administration of excessive volumes of intravenous fluid and resultant patient discomfort and disquiet from a full bladder. Furthermore, patient position and comfort is ensured by covering the hard surface of the operating room

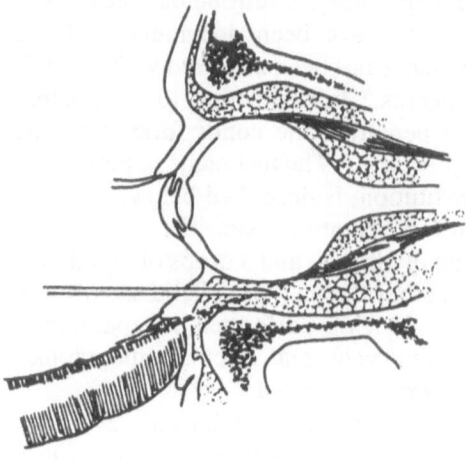

FIGURE 22.1. Peribulbar anesthesia—no attempt is made to penetrate the conus formed by the extraocular muscles and fascia.

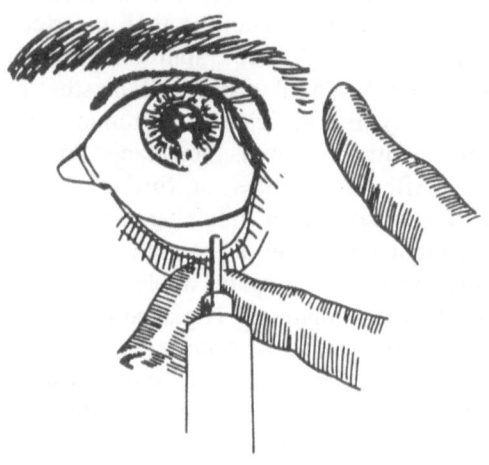

FIGURE 22.2. Peribulbar anesthesia—inferior injection through the inferolateral area of the conjunctiva.

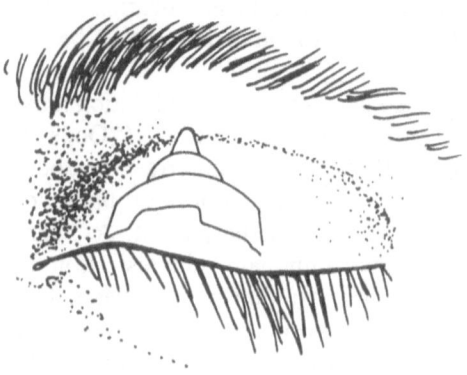

FIGURE 22.3. Peribulbar anesthesia—superior injection transcutaneously into the superior medial quadrant of the orbit, avoiding the globe.

table with a foam mattress and by adjusting the table (eg, hip/knee flexion) to accommodate the patient. Optimal head position can still be achieved.

Preoperative monitoring is continued because of the rare occurrence of delayed drug reactions and oculocardiac-reflex-induced bradycardia (seen rarely during the performance of the block and occasionally intraoperatively). Some patients may become claustrophobic because of the closely confining drapes. Verbal reassurance and flow of cool fresh air or oxygen around the patient's face can diminish this sensation. Once the procedure is finished, the patient is transferred to a reclining chair with wheels and is transported directly back to the outpatient area. There the patient is quickly assessed (vital signs) and given fluids by mouth (tea, coffee, juice). After 45 minutes, the patient is helped to dress and then assessed for street-readiness. Once fit, the patient is discharged to the care of a responsible adult.

Morbidity and Mortality

Anesthesia for cataract surgery is very safe. Several large series have not reported any mortality.[6-8] In more than 6 years of experience, encompassing 4000 procedures, we have had only one death: a patient who, at autopsy, was found to have had a silent, recent preoperative myocardial infarction.

Serious morbidity may occur after retrobulbar anesthesia. In a series of 910 patients, Petty et al[8] found 12 cases of major morbidity, including globe perforation (2), cardiovascular collapse (2), respiratory arrest associated with probable intradural injection (2), and central nervous system symptoms (3). However, no patient suffered lasting morbidity as a result of these complications, and surgery was successfully completed in all instances. Recently, Hamilton et al[6] have reported a series of 12,000 consecutive cataract extractions and intraocular lens implantation procedures under a variety of regional anesthetic techniques. Although a number of different regional anesthetic techniques were used, the overall safety is apparent (Table 22.9.). The incidence of brain stem anesthesia and retrobulbar hemorrhage seems to be greater with retrobulbar blocks, but the incidence of all complications is very low. Hamilton's experience with the dual peribulbar block (described above) shows more than 2000 cases performed without brain stem anesthesia or scleral perforation.[6] In our institution, more than 2000 peribulbar blocks have been performed, again with no brain stem anesthesia or known perforation. Similar results have been obtained by others.

Although proponents of peribulbar anesthesia feel that intravascular injection, scleral perforation, and intraneural (optic nerve) injection are less likely than with retrobulbar anesthesia, it must be remembered that the incidence of all complications is low and that large numbers of patients must be compared in order to assess relative risks.

References

1. Dorland's Illustrated Medical Dictionary, 25th ed. Philadelphia: WB Saunders, 1974.
2. Kahn HA, Leibowitz HM, Ganley JP, et al: The Framingham Eye Study. I. Outline and major prevalence findings. Am J Epidemiol 1977;106:17–32.
3. Kline D, Sekuler R, Dismukes K: Social issues, human needs, and opportunities for research on the effects of age on vision: an overview, in Sekuler R, Kline D, Dismukes K (eds): Aging and Human Visual Function. New York: Alan R. Liss, 1982; pp. 3–6.
4. Straatsma BR, Foos RY, Horwit J, et al: Aging-related cataract: laboratory investigation and clinical management. Ann Intern Med 1985;102:82–92.
5. Cotlier E: The lens, in Moses RA, Hart W Jr (eds): Adler's Physiology of the Eye. Clinical Application, St. Louis: C. V. Mosby, 1987; pp. 268–90.
6. Hamilton RC, Gimbel HV, Strunin L: Regional anesthesia for 12,000 cataract extraction and intraocular lens implantation surgical procedures. Can J Anaesth 1988;35:615–23.
7. Davis DB, Mandel MR: Posterior peribulbar anesthesia: an alternative to retrobulbar anesthesia. J Cataract Refract Surg 1986;12:182–84.
8. Petty JM, Davies JM, Strunin L: Retrobulbar block for cataract surgery: retrospective review of 910 patients. Anaesth Intens Care 1984;13:95.
9. Muravchick S: the Physiologic and Pharmacologic Implications of Aging. 1986 ASA Annual Refresher Course Lectures, Las Vegas: no 275.

CHAPTER 23

The Patient with Peripheral Vascular Disease

Raghubar P. Badola

Case History. *A 71-year-old woman with a history of insulin dependent diabetes mellitus and severe peripheral vascular disease was admitted with gangrene of the left big toe. The patient had undergone surgery one month previously for debridement of the toe and adjoining area. There was no history of trauma to the toe but the patient reported multiple infections at the site and had been treated with parenteral antibiotics. For the past year, the patient had experienced pain in her left calf on walking. She had expressive aphasia secondary to a cerebral vascular accident 6 months ago. There was no specific history of cardiac disease; she had never been told of hypertension. She had smoked heavily in the past but had stopped about 2 years ago. She enjoyed an occasional drink. Except for occasional hydrodiuril and "heart tablets," she did not regularly take any prescribed drugs apart from regular insulin (dosage range 12–40 units, adjusted according to the blood sugar level) and a 2–week course of oxacillin.*

Physical examination was significant for lack of all distal pulses, blood pressure, 175/100 mmHg, temperature: 99.5°F. The patient was acutely distressed and complained of considerable pain in her foot.

Laboratory findings were as follows: hematocrit 27.7, hemoglobin 9.5 gm, white blood count 10,200/mm³, serum electrolytes-potassium 4.7 mEq/L sodium 139 mEq/l, chloride 101 mEq/L, blood glucose 316 mg/dl, BUN 48 mq/dl, creatinine 2.1 mg/dl. Urine: negative for acetone; 2+ glucose. Angiogram revealed occlusion of the left tibioperoneal trunk and the posterior tibial artery. Electrocardiogram showed normal sinus rhythm with evidence of an old subendocardial infarction. Chest x-ray showed bilateral basal congestion.

Peripheral vascular disease with occlusion of the major vessels below the knee was diagnosed and the patient was scheduled for left femoral popliteal bypass graft.

Reviewed by Patricia Underwood, M.D., Associate Professor, Department of Anesthesiology, Albert Einstein College of Medicine/Montefiore Medical Center.

Introduction

Vascular surgery as we know today has developed only in the last thirty years, although its evolution is much longer.[1] Ambrose Paré, in 1552, used ligatures to control bleeding from vessels severed during amputations (he is also credited with obtaining regional anesthesia by compression of nerves. The first successful clinical arterial repair was done in 1759 by Hallowell, who repaired the opening in the brachial artery by a figure of eight suture after excising an aneurysm. In 1896, Murphy successfully performed the first clinical end-to-end arterial suture using an invagination technique. In the first decade of this century, Carrel and Guthrie experimentally resolved many problems of vascular reconstruction by refining suturing methods that allowed resection, transplantation and replacement of autogenic and allogenic arterial segments.

Rudolph Matas may well deserve to be called "The Father of Vascular Surgery." His work principally during 1888 to 1900 marks the turning point in aneurysm surgery. He introduced the concept of endoaneurysmorrhaphy both restorative and constructive. The latter is the forerunner of the widely used method of intravascular insertion of the graft popularized by Stanley Crawford some seventy years later.

The absence of an effective method of autoregulation limited wide application of these pioneer effects. Heparin, although discovered in 1916 by a second year medical student, Jay McLean at the Johns Hopkins University, was not clinically available until 1933 and not used in vascular surgery until 1937.[2] The advent of antibiotics and the ability to limit infection by the 1940's was another spur to the development of vascular surgery. Also, with the introduction of water soluble organic iodides in 1929, contrast angiography made in vivo exploration of the arterial system possible and opened new vistas for diagnosis and therapy of vascular disease.

The first direct attack on arterial obliterative disease is credited to J. Cid dos Santos, who in 1946 extracted a thrombus from an acutely occluded femoral artery, and noted that he had inadvertently removed intima and part of the media. The vessel remained patent and the idea of thromboendarterectomy was conceived. Kunlin in 1948 employed a venous bypass technique and successfully dealt with obliterative arterial disease. These two important contributions opened an entirely new era of vascular surgery.

Advances came rapidly in the fifties with successes in infrarenal graft substitution for aortic aneurysm, the advent of prosthetic grafts and availability of cardiopulmonary bypass. Contributors to surgical techniques were numerous, prominent among them were Debakey, Crawford and Cooley. Advances in anesthesiology had a direct bearing on the success of vascular surgery, including the introduction of safe and potent inhalation agents, ventilatory control, and precise, continuous monitoring. Careful preanesthetic assessment and optimization of cardiovascular dynamics are now two of the most important factors in ensuring success of the operation and good outcome for the patient.

Pathophysiology

Arteriosclerosis is a genetic term for three patterns of vascular disease all of which cause thickening and inelasticity of the arteries (Table 23.1.). Atherosclerosis is the dominant form of arteriosclerosis and is often loosely referred to as arteriosclerosis. It is characterized by the formation of intimal fibrofatty lesions (atherosclerotic plaques) that narrow the vascular lumen and are associated with degenerative changes in the media and adventitia. The center of these plaques contain a grumus lipid rich debris containing cholesterol and chlolesteryl esters. The Greek term "athera" means gruel or porridge and "atheroma" is a cyst full of gruel like pus. Atherosclerosis is a generalized degenerative disease process progressing erratically throughout the arterial tree. Lesions are irregularly distributed: different vessels are involved at different ages and to varying degrees. Atherosclerosis has a predilection for the coronary arteries, carotid arteries, intracranial cerebral vessels, the aorta and the arterial supply of the kidneys and lower legs. In the coronary arteries atherosclerosis causes ischemic heart disease or myocardial infarction; in cerebral arteries, strokes, cerebral ischemia, infarction or hemorrhage may result. The aorta may develop aneurysmal dilation and rupture. Vascular insufficiency or gangrene of the lower leg are caused by disease in the iliac, femoral or popliteal vessels.

Hypertension is an important accelerator of the atherosclerotic process. Dibetes mellitus and heavy cigarette smoking contribute to the degenerative process of atherosclerosis. Changes of aging and atherosclerosis though commonly found together, appear to be separate and distinct processes. Age related change in the arterial wall is a continuous symmetrical increase in the thickness of the intima due to accumulation of smooth muscle cells and connective tissue, coupled with progressive accumulation of sphingomyelin and cholesterol linoleate. Diffuse age related intimal thickening is distinguished from the focal discrete raised fibromuscular plaques, characteristic of atherosclerosis.

The second morphologic form of arteriosclerosis is Monckeberg's

TABLE 23.1. Arteriosclerosis may be divded into three groups.

Type	Characteristics
Atherosclerosis	Plaque formation; media and adventitia
Monckeberg's calcific sclerosis	Calcium deposits medial of muscular arteries
Arteriolosclerosis: hyaline	Small vessel narrowing
hyperplastic	

medial calcific sclerosis, characterized by calcification in the media of
muscular arteries. Medium sized arteries are mostly affected usually, in
patients over the age of fifty years. Occasionally the calcific deposits
undergo ossification. These medial lesions do not encroach on the vessel
lumen. However, arteries so affected may also develop atherosclerosis.

The third vascular disease, a disease of small arteries and arterioles is
known as arteriolosclerosis. Small vessel sclerosis is often associated
with hypertension and diabetes mellitus. There are two variants, hyaline
and hyperplastic that are related to the cause and rate of progression of
the disease. Both cause thickening of vessel walls with luminal narrowing
and may induce ischemic injury to tissues or organs (e.g. kidneys).

Risk Factors

The presence of distal disease is a poor prognostic sign. The mean
survival of patients with aorto-ilial disease is 10.7 years compared to 7.2
years in patients with femoro-popliteal disease.[3] Several risk factors have
been identified in patients with peripheral vascular disease (Table 23.2.).

Age

Patients about to undergo vascular surgery are generally in the sixth to
ninth decade of life or older.[4] Physiologic functions decline with age and
there is a decrease in reserve that manifests often at times of stress.
Cardiac output has been said to decrease linearly after the middle of the
fifth decade at the rate of about one percent per year in individuals
otherwise free of cardiac disease. Even though recent data refute these

TABLE 23.2 Several risk factors of significance to the
anesthesiologist have been identified in patients with
peripheral vascular disease.

Risk Factor	Effects
Increasing age	Decreased systems reserve
	Reduced drug
	Multisystem disease
	Multiple drug ingestion
Atherosclerotic	Myocardial ischemia
vascular disease	Cerebral hemmorage
	Stroke
	Aortic aneurysm
	Visceral Ischemia
Diabetes	Metabolic acidosis
Smoking	Hypoxia
	Chronic obstructive pulmonary disease
	Hypercarbia

earlier beliefs, older hearts have less reserve than their younger counterparts.[4] Blood pressure increases with age, probably due to an increase in the afterload imposed by an age related thickness of intima in the larger arteries. The aging heart is a less compliant biological pump that may demonstrate marked changes in atrial and ventricular wall tension with even minor fluctuations of venous return or peripheral resistance. Response to catecholamines is altered and the elderly heart requires a tenfold increase in isoproterenol to demonstrate a 25 beat per minute increase in heart rate. There is also a five fold increase in resistance to beta-adrenergic blockade suggesting altered receptor configuration. Tachycardic response to atropine is markedly reduced.[4]

Respiratory functions are compromised by age. Forced expiratory volume in one second (FEV_1) and forced vital capacity (FVC) have been said to diminish progressively about 20–30 ml/year. There is increasing reduction in gas exchange efficiency. Alveolar-arterial PO2 difference increases and by seventy years, arterial PO2 averages 75 mmHg when room air is inspired. Thus, intraoperatively the inspired concentration of oxygen should be increased in the elderly. Careful monitoring of O_2 saturation and frequent blood gas analyses are indicated.

Renal cortical mass, number of glomeruli, tubular function and glomerular filtration rate are all decreased in the elderly. Creatinine clearance declines linearly after age 45. Ability to concentrate urine after water deprivation is reduced. Thus, fluid and electrolyte balance require close monitoring and the half lives of drugs that depend on kidney function for elimination are prolonged. Digoxin level in the blood can be 2–3 times larger at any given dose because of decreased renal excretion. Cardiotoxicity can easily result.

Hepatic function is reduced either by decreased circulation or decreased enzyme levels. Drug metabolism may be significantly altered. Higher blood levels of free (active) drugs occur due to decreased plasma binding. The total blood pool is also reduced. Circulating blood volume averages 2.9 $1/m^2$ in young men which decreases to 2.1 $1/m^2$ by age 70. Although overall body weight decreases, total body water and lean body mass are reduced more and the percentage of fat is increased. These changes alter the distribution half life and plasma clearance of drugs and cause unexpected response.[4] For example, diazepam and midazolam have a long elimination half life that are markedly increased in the elderly. In addition, the number of drug receptor sites declines, delaying the response to drug action. Anesthetic requirements of inhalational anesthetics are reduced as MAC is decreased. Thus all drugs should be given in reduced doses and titrated slowly.

Perioperative morbidity and mortality increase with age. One analysis showed that death within seven days of surgery occurred in 1.5% of all surgical patients from 21 to 50 years of age, in 4.4% of those patients 61–70 years of age and in 8.2% in those patients over the age of 80.[5] The

National Institutes of Health in 1977 estimated that after 70 years of age there is approximately a three fold increase in mortality, related to surgical procedures.

Concomitant systemic disease is common in the elderly. A study of patients admitted to geriatric units revealed that the average number of diseases per patients is 6.[6] There is a high prevalence of coronary artery disease, hypertension, renal disease, diabetes and chronic obstructive pulmonary disease, especially associated with acquired vascular disease.

The preanesthetic assessment must focus on evaluation of an ill patient with serious multisystem disease, reduced systems reserves and one who is receiving multiple drugs.

Coronary Artery Disease

The presence of coronary artery disease in patients with peripheral vascular disease is common. At least 50–70% of patients undergoing vascular surgery have evidence of coronary artery disease; angina occurs in 10–20%; a history of previous myocardial infarction is obtained in 40–50% and significant heart disease may be found in 30–60% of asymptomatic patients. Hertzer and coworker, using routine preoperative coronary angiography detected coronary artery disease in 90% of patients.[7] In another series of 82 patients with vascular disease, 43 were without clinical evidence of coronoary artery disease.[8] However, on routine coronary angiography 67% of the asymptomatic group had stenosis of one or more coronary arteries. Postoperative myocardial ischemia occurred in 15% of patients, all with clinical evidence of coronary artery disease.

In an earlier study by Hertzer, in patients with an unremarkable clinical history, and a normal ECG, the 10 year survival was not significantly different from the general population and the five year survival rates were almost identical.[9] Based on these results, the need for more sensitive tests other than history and a resting ECG to detect significant coronary artery disease has been questioned.[10] In patients with associated coronary artery disease, the five year mortality is three times that of patients with healthy hearts.[11,12] In a Finnish study, the increased mortality in male claudicants appeared to correlate completely with concomittant heart disease.[13]

Several studies have focused on the mortality of patients with chronic leg ischemia.[14] After 5, 10 and 15 years of follow up, the mean mortality rate was approximately 30, 50, and 70 percent respectively. When compared to general population groups matched for age and sex, the mortality rate for claudicants was 3 times higher after 10 years and two times higher after 15 years. About 75% of deaths are due to atherosclerosis, 50% in the coronary circulation, 15% in the cerebral vessels and 10%

in the abdominal vasculature (aortic aneurysm). Large studies indicate that the life expectancy of patients with peripheral vascular disease is reduced by about 10 years.[14]

Diabetes

The presence of diabetes is of grave prognostic significance. In Hertzer's study about half the nondiabetic patients survived ten years as compared to one third of diabetic patients.[15] Another series indicated that the ten year mortality rate in nondiabetics was abut 50% compared to 100% in diabetics.[16]

Smoking

Continued smoking has been shown to triple mortality in 11 years in patients with vascular disease. The patient with chronic obstructive pulmonary disease is also at increased risk of respiratory complications in the postoperative period.[17]

Surgical Approach

Several therapies are used for patients with peripheral vascular disease. Synthetic materials have been developed to produce artificial vessels that may be used to replace occluded arteries. Free veins may be anastomosed to arteries to bypass obstructed areas. More recently LASER beams and mechanical devices have been developed to ablate intravascular lesions. Some of the LASER types with application to vascular surgery are listed in Table 23.3. LASER instrumentation has been used to open occluded arteries, in conjunction with percutaneous angioplasty and in welding of vascular tissue. Currently, hot tipped LASER beams (e.g. argon or YAG-neodynium) are used to recreate a lumen in an occluded vessel in conjunction with balloon angioplasty. Success rates vary from 40 to 75% and vessel perforation occurs in 10–20%.[18] In the developmental stage is

TABLE 23.3 Several LASERS are currently being used or are in the development stages for the treatment of patients with peripheral vascular diseases.

Carbon dioxide

Yttrium-aluminum garnet (YAG) ⟨ Neodynium
                                  Erbium

Holmium
Argon
Ultraviolet eximer dye

---

the dual bundle LASER that has one bundle for tissue recognition (angioscopy) and a second bundle for tissue ablation. An extension of this concept is the dual system with one bundle to recognize abnormal tissue and the second bundle to emit short pulsed LASER beams to destroy tissue. Though a feedback system, the LASER stops firing when normal tissue is detected by the spectroscopic bundle. Two types of intraarterial atherectomy devices are available. The Kensey device is designed to create a hole through an atheroma. The Simpson instrument incorporates a catheter mounted blade that pares the atheroma and collects the debris in a nosecone.[18]

Preanesthetic Assessment

As may be predicted by the identified risks, assessment must focus on several specific areas (Table 23.4.):

Cardiac Assessment

In patients who have sustained myocardial infarction, the risk of reinfarction in the perioperative period ranges from 5.8% to 37%; 2.3% to 16% and 1.7% to 6% if the previous myocardial infarction occurred less than 3 months prior to surgery, 3 to 6 months prior to surgery or more than 6 months previously.[19,20] Symptoms of coronary artery disease should be sought such as a history of angina, dyspnea, palpitations, orthopnea, paroxysmal nocturnal dyspnea, transient syncope or dizziness. Relevant hospitalizations for treatment and diagnostic studies should be documented. Previous myocardial infarction may have affected the heart by reducing the functioning myocardium and thus reducing the ejection fraction. It may predispose the patient to dysrrhythmias, and papillary muscle dysfunction producing mitral regurgitation. Infarction may also predispose to the formation of a ventricular aneurysm.

If a cardiac pacemaker has been placed, the indications should be known. Any previous episodes of conjestive heart failure must be noted and the treatment regimen elicited.

TABLE 23.4 Cardiac Assessment Laboratory testing.

Exercise electrocardiography	Localize ischemic areas quantitive exercise limits proke dysrhythmias
Thallium scan	Identify underperfused areas
Dipyridamole	Causes coronary vasodilation and steal (mimics exercise effects)
Gated blood pool scan	Identify chambers, shunts, regurgitation
2-Dimensional echocardiography	Identifies scarring from infarction

Both exercise and radionucleide studies have been developed to identify patients at risk of myocardial damage.

In the perioperative period, the electrocardiogram forms the basis for detection of ischemia. By employing leads V5/2, 96% of ischemic events detectable by ECG can be diagnosed. An ST segment depression of 1 mm or more indicates ischemia. Other signs of ischemia include alteration of T wave and onset of new dysrrythmias or conduction abnormalities, e.g., left bundle branch block. ECG changes from ischemia should be differentiated from other causes of ECG changes including left ventricular hypertrophy, effect of digitalis, hypokalemia and hyperventilation. ST elevation is always significant and denotes transmural ischemia. However, ECG changes due to ischemia are late signs. In many instances, the patient's history, ECG and Goldman Risk Index may not accurately reflect the amount of cardiac damage and additional evaluation may be necessary. Stress test ECG, although useful in assessing cardiac disease, is not feasible in most patients with peripheral vascular disease because claudication prevents treadmill stressing. Also if there are changes due to bundle branch block, or left ventricular hypertrophy on the resting ECG, a stress test ECG may not offer further information. Regional wall motion abnormalities and changes in ventricular compliance as seen on the echocardiogram are earlier signs of ischemia.

Thallium-dipyridamole non-stress tests have been recently introduced. Injected thallium 201 acts as a marker of coronary blood flow distribution. Reduced uptake of thallium in the left ventricular wall indicates reduced blood flow to that segment. Abnormalities are examined after exercise and if the defects disappear after some hours of rest, then it indicates that myocadial ischemia rather than infarction has occurred. If the patient is unable to exercise, dipyridamole (Persentine), a potent coronary vasodilator, produces coronary steal in the stenotic arterial leasions. (Patients with a positive Persentine-thallium scan have a 50% chance of developing significant cardiac complications following major surgery or a greater than 20-fold increase in risk of postoperative myocardial infarction).[21] Dipyridamole induced coronary vasodilation may reveal myocardial perfusion defects.[22] There is a correlation between perioperative thallium redistribution after dipyridamole-induced coronary vasodilation with the occurrence of a postoperative myocardial ischemic event. Thus a preoperative scan which shows thallium redistribution after dipyridamole would indicate the necessity for coronary angiography and possible coronary artery bypass surgery before proceeding with peripheral vascular surgery. An intraoperative ischemic event is more likely in a patient with a positive thallium redistribution.[22]

Other diagnostic tests include two dimensional echocardiography which uses multiple beams of sound to construct larger, spatially correct images of the heart and enable the measurement of end diastolic and end systolic dimensions. From these values the ventricular volume, cardiac output, ejection fraction, mean circumferential fiber shortening rate and systolic time intervals can be determined. Correlation between echocardiographic data and angiographic determinations of these variables is good.

Transesophageal two dimensional echocardiography (2D-TEE); provides a non-invasive method for continuous study of regional left ventricular wall motion during anesthesia. The incorporation of miniature phased array transducers into a flexible gastroscope, from which fiberoptics have been removed, permit the operator to direct the ultrasound beam in multiple planes from any position within the esophagus. The TEE is an immediate and sensitive indicator of myocardial ischemia. It detects any change in regional wall motion which reflects developing myocardial ischemia. Experimentally, in 80% of models of coronary occlusion, the ECG does not show motion abnormality for two minutes, but TEE changes in 15 seconds.[23] Hypokinesia indicates a 50% reduction in blood flow and dyskinesia means 95% reduction. In addition, TEE's high resolution, obtainable in 98% of cases, may also help to identify acute hypovolemia, acute left ventricular failure, and intravascular air. Because of the noninvasiveness of TEE there are fewer complications than occur following pulmonary artery catheterization. Insertion of the latter monitor is associated with 15% minor complications and 3-5% major complications including death.[24]

In yet another test, cardiac contractions may be gated by the ECG following injection of autologous red cells labelled with technetium (99mTc). About 400 cardiac contractions are examined and the left ventricular volume, and ejection fraction (EF) estimated. Normal ejection fraction is greater than 50% and after exercise it should increase by 5%. Patients with significant coronary artery disease often have a decrease in EF. This method can detect over 90% of cases with significant coronary artery disease.[24]

Should some of these more recent tests not be available, important information may be obtained by monitoring information from a pulmonary artery catheter. Among the earliest consequences of myocardial ischemia are changes in ventricular compliance which reflect changes in the pulmonary capillary wedge pressure (PCWP). A fixed cardiac output with increased PCWP suggests decreased left ventricular compliance. The presence of prominent AC waves in the PCWP tracing is consistant with myocardial ischemia.[25] The appearance of ''V'' waves in the tracing suggests ischemia of the papillary muscle causing dilation of the left ventricle and/or mitral valve apparatus.

Respiratory System

Especially in patients with a smoking history, baseline arterial blood gas analyses and bedside respiratory function tests should be performed. Preoperative respiratory therapy may be valuable to acquaint the patient with the aids that are available to promote better postoperative ventilatory function.

Other Systems

Diabetes is frequent in patients with peripheral vascular disease and causes multiorgan dysfunction. In addition to the association of myocardial infarction and hypertension, cardiac autonomic neuropathy is found in about 50% of insulin dependent diabetic patients. Degeneration of afferent and efferent components of the sympathetic and parasympathetic innervation of the heart and peripheral vasculature allow the development of painless myocardial ischemia and infarction and an impaired cardiovascular response to exercise and stress. Orthostatic hypotension is a reliable indicator of cardiac autonomic neuropathy. Cardiorespiratory dependence causing unexpected sudden death has been reported in the perioperative period in patients with severe diabetes and known autonomic neuropathy. It is suggested that an abnormal hypoxic drive in these patients increase the risks of hypoxia.[26]

While "tight" control of the diabetic situation may not be possible, especially if infection is recent, attempts should be made to control the blood sugar level between 100–200 mg/dl. These levels although somewhat arbitrary reflect overall control of the catabolic response to major surgery or stress. An insulin, dextrose and K^+ infusion is a reliable method of controlling metabolism. Coordination and agreement between the anesthesiologist, surgeon and internist and frequent blood sugar monitoring are essential to any protocol. Fluid replacement should be with saline or isolyte solutions. Lactated Ringer's solution contains 28 mEq/L of lactate and is a gluconeogenic substrate. Administration to the diabetic is inappropriate perioperatively as hepatic conversion to glucose and aggravation of stress induced hyperglycemia may increase blood sugar levels in excess of 400 mg/dl.[26]

Hepatic renal function should be assessed by laboratory analysis of liver enzymes, blood urea nitrogen and creatinine levels. The anesthesiologist must be able to assess the probable feasibility of appropriate drug clearance and modify the anesthetic technique to include agents metabolized by other pathways if necessary.

Neurologic function should be evaluated. Discussion with relatives and friends often reveals subtle and even not so subtle (e.g. involuntary seizure type movements) changes in mental or neurologic status that may indicate transient ischemic attacks or strokes. Succinylcholine should be avoided in patients with even mild hemiparesis because of the risk of ventricular dysrhythmias caused by hyperkalemia. Also, even moderate hyperventilation may prove catastrophic in some patients by causing cerebral vasoconstriction and infarcting a marginally ischemic area.

During the preanesthetic visit, radial pulses should be checked for volume, rate and rhythm, and Allen's test should be performed on both hands as there may be discrepancy in blood pressure between the two arms due to atheromatous changes or previous surgical interventions. Scars may be noted on the arms from prior cardiac catheterization and measuring blood pressure distally may give falsely lower values.

Anesthetic Plan

The goal of anesthetic management is summarized in Table 23.5. Several other factors must be considered.

Fluid Management

Maintenance of normovolemia or institution of moderate hemodilution is the basic principle of fluid management. During hypovolemia, blood flow to the lower extremities is dramatically decreased. Early graft thrombosis correlates closely with intraoperative graft blood flow. Little et al found that the incidence of early graft thrombosis was 80% when the graft blood flow was less than 60 ml/min but only 20% when flow was more than 60 ml/min.[27] Yates et al showed that a reduction of hematocrit from a mean of 45.2% to 35% was associated with a 56% increase in calf blood flow at rest and three fold increase in peak blood flow.[28] Mean hemoglobin delivery increased by 20% at rest and 111% at peak flow.

The physiological changes following moderate hemodilution include a decrease in blood viscosity and a fall in peripheral resistance. Blood

TABLE 23.5. Goal of Anesthetic Management in Patients with Vascular Disease.

Minimize O_2 Consumption	Maximize O_2 Delivery

Reduce ventricular wall Tension,
    Treat hypertension
    Decrease chamber size (LVEDV) with
    venous and arterial vasodilation
	Decrease heart rate
	    Maximize cardiac filling during diastole

Reduce contractility
    Ca^{2+} channel blockers
    Beta blockers
    Inhalational anesthetics
	Increase perfusion pressure
	    Increase aortic diastolic pressure
	    Reduce LVEDP with small doses of
	    neosynephrine and nitroglycerin

Reduce heart rate
    Narcotic
    Beta blockers
	Maximize O_2 carrying capacity
	    Supplemental oxygen
	    Red blood cell transfusion

Reduce response to stimulation
    Adequate anesthesia
    Short acting beta blockers
    Vasodilators	

pressure may decrease but is compensated by an increase in the venous return and increase in cardiac output. Stroke volume increases and blood pressure is maintained without an increase in pulse rate or sympathetic stimulation. Blood is a non-newtonian fluid and is most viscid at low flow rates. As flow increases, less pressure is required to move the blood. At high flow, blood behaves in a newtonian fashion and flow increases in direct proportion to the force applied. At low flows, red cells tend to aggregate proximal to an arterial stenosis where flow is turbulent and viscosity increases. In the major arteries where flow is fast, red cells migrate toward the center of the stream and orient themselves longitudinally such that their flat surfaces are parallel to the direction of the flow. In these fast flow situations, cell free plasma is in contact with the vessel wall and the flow is laminar. Minute oxygen delivery does not fall because the lowered hematocrit is balanced by an increase in cardiac output. Optimum hematocrit for tissue oxygenation approximates 30%. All these factors tend to suggest that a hematocrit in the region of 30–35% is adequate in patients for lower limb surgery.

Crystalloids are given at the rate of 5–10 ml/kg/hr. Hematocrit estimations are done frequently and if the hematocrit falls below 30%, blood loss is replaced by cross-matched packed red cells or, preferably, whole blood. If the hemocrit is above 30%, the blood loss is replaced by a plasma expander such as 5% albumin or other synthetic products (e.g., hydroxyethyl starch).

Colloid osmotic pressure of plasma (COPp) may correlate with the total amount of fluid retained during the day of operation.[29] A positive fluid balance of 3 L on the day of operation corresponds with a COPp of 25 mmHg. At a COPp of 20 mm or below the positive fluid balance is 5 L or more. When COPp is reduced below 20 mmHg, interstitial edema occurs. Edema includes cardiac muscle edema and pulmonary interstitial edema with consequent impairment of oxygen transport and wound healing, increased susceptibility to infection and difficulty in ambulating. Earlier reports that measurement of COPp would be of value have not been substantiated.

Monitoring

In patients undergoing major peripheral vascular surgery the extent of monitoring is dictated to a large extent by the cardiovascular status, other concomitant diseases, location of the arterial defect, and the surgical procedure planned.

In general, the following are appropriate in all cases: Blood pressure cuff, ECG (both lead II and V5), pulse oximetry, capnography, mass spectrometry, indwelling arterial pressure catheter, temperature probe, Foley catheter and esophageal stethoscope. Pulmonary artery catheter insertion is indicated in patients undergoing major peripheral vascular surgery, with clinical evidence of coronary artery disease and poor left ventricular function, i.e. patients with a history of a recent or multiple infarctions with signs and symptoms of conjestive heart failure, ejection fraction less than 0.4, LVEDP greater than 18 mmHg, low cardiac output and many areas of left ventricular dyskinesia. Its use is warranted in all procedures where the aorta is to be crossclamped. This maneuver is associated with a decrease in cardiac output of 15–35%, an increase in systemic vascular resistance of approximately 40%, an increase in pulmonary capillary wedge pressure, increase in mean arterial blood pressure and increase in myocardial work. The appearance of "V" waves on the pulmonary artery tracing may represent myocardial ischemia, and may be apparent before ECG signs of ischemia appear. Monitoring via a pulmonary artery catheter is invaluable in managing the rapid shifts in preload and afterload and estimating cardiovascular parameters and determining appropriate therapy with vasodilators and/or inotropes.

No consistant relationship between pulmonary capillary wedge pressures and central venous pressures (CVP) have been found in patients with both good and poor left ventricular function. Also, MUGA (multiple uptake gated acquisition) scans may not be reliable in predicting patients for whom monitoring with a CVP catheter would be adequate.[24]

Changes in the wave form of the pulse oximeter is a reliable indicator of decreased volume status.[30]

Somatosensory evoked potential (SSEP) monitoring is indicated where crossclamping of the aorta could compromise blood supply to the spinal cord. SSEP monitoring only tracts the integrity of the sensory pathways and a motor lesion may go undetected.

Choice of Anesthetic Techniques

Choice of anesthetic depends on the severity of the systemic disease, the skill of the surgeon and the patient's choice. Patients with angina may not tolerate several hours of surgery under regional anesthesia. Continuous epidural anesthetic may be relatively contraindicated in patients who are anticoagulated. However, in a large series, the safe use of epidural or subarachnoid catheters in heparinized patients undergoing vascular surgery has been documented provided low levels of anticoagulants (ACT 130–150 sec) were used and the catheter was placed prior to heparinization.[31] Continuous epidural anesthesia reduces peripheral vascular resistance and lessens the effects of aortic cross clamping on afterload.[32] Epidural anesthesia may also attenuate renocortical reflex vasoconstriction by blocking the sympathetic supply to the kidneys and may allow a higher graft flow to the extremities. Also, postoperative pain is more easily controlled if an epidural catheter is left in place. Postoperative pulmonary complications are fewer. An effective plan is therefore to combine light general anesthesia to control stress with a continuous epidural technique.

References

1. Szilagyi DE: Vascular Surgery: A propaedeutic of its past, present and future, in Wilson, ES, Veith, FJ, Hobson, RW, Williams RA (eds): Vascular Surgery—Principles and Practice, New York: McGraw-Hill, pp 3–10, 1987.
2. Murray DWG, Best CH: The use of heparin in thrombosis. Ann Surg 1938; 108:163–77.
3. Reid DD, Brett GJ, Hamilton PJS, et al: Cardiorespiratory disease and diabetes among middle aged male civil servants. Lancet 1974; i:469–73.
4. Miller RD: Anesthesia for the elderly, in Miller RD (ed): Anesthesia, 2nd ed, New York: Churchill Livingston, pp 1801–18, 1986.
5. Marx GF, Mateo CV, Orkin L: Computer analysis of postanesthetic deaths. Anesthesiology 1973;39:54–8.
6. Wilson LA, Lawson R, Porass W: Multiple disorders in the elderly. Lancet 1962; 2:841–43.
7. Hertzer NR, Beven EG, Young JR, et al: Coronary artery disease in peripheral vascular patients—a classification of 1000 coronary angiograms and results of surgical management. Ann Surg 1984; 199:223–33.
8. Bloombery PA, Ferguson A, Rosengarten DS, et al: Role of coronary artery disease in complications of abdominal aortic surgery. Surgery 1987; 101: 250–55.
9. Hertzer NR: Fatal myocardial infarction following lower extremity revascularization—Two hundred and seventy three patients followed six to eleven postoperative years. Ann Surg 1981; 193:492–98.
10. Dormandy JA, Mahir MS: The natural history of peripheral atheromatous disease of legs, in Greenhalgh, RM, Jamieson Crawford, W, Nicolaids, AN (eds): Orlando: Grune & Stratton, Vascular Surgery issues in Current Practice, ed, 1986; pp 3–17.
11. Crawford ES, Bomberger RA, Glasser DH, et al: Aorto iliac occlusive disease: Factors influencing survival and function following reconstructive operation over a twenty five year period. Surgery 1981; 90:1055–67.
12. Vecht RJ, Nicolaides AN, Brandao E, et al: Resting and treadmill electrocardiographic findings in patients with intermittent claudication. Int Angio 1982; 1:119–21.
13. Reunanen A, Takkunen H, Aromma A: Prevalence of intermittent claudication and its effect on mortality. Acta Med Scand 1982; 211:249–56.
14. Biland L, DaSilva A, Zemp E, et al: Occlusive peripheral artery disease (OPAD). Mortality and risk profile, in Proceedings of the 13th International Congress of Angiology, Athens, 9–14 June 1985.
15. Hertzer NR, Young JR, Kramer JR, et al: Routine coronary angiography prior to aortic reconstruction. Arch Surg 1978; 14:1336–44.
16. Malone JM, Moore WS, Goldstone J: Life expectancy following aorto-femoral arterial grafting. Surgery 1977; 81:551–55.
17. Gaensler EA, Weisel AD: The risk in abdominal and thoracic surgery. Postgrad Med 1973; 53:183.
18. White RA, Grundfest WS: LASERS in cardiovascular disease. Chicago: Year Book, Med Pub 1987.
19. Rao TLK, Jacobs KH, Adel AL: Reinfarction following anesthesia in patients with myocardial infarction. Anesthesiology 1983; 59:499–505.

20. Steen PA, Tinker JH, Tarhan S: Myocardial reinfarction after anesthesia and surgery. JAMA 1978; 239:2566–70.
21. Leppo J, Paja J, Gionet M, et al: Noninvasive evaluation of cardiac risk before elective vascular surgery. J Am Coll Cardiol 1987; 9:269–76.
22. Baucher CA, Brewster DC, Darling RC, et al: Determination of cardiac risk by dipyridamole-thalium imaging before peripheral vascular surgery. N Engl J Med 1985; 321(7):389–94.
23. Clements FM, deBruijn NP: Preoperative evaluation of regional wall motion by transesophageal two-dimensional echocardiography. Anesth Analg 1987;ii:66:249–61.
24. Barash PG: Non-invasive cardiovascular monitoring. Ann Refresher Course Lectures, American Society of Anesthesiology, San Francisco, 1988, No. 411.
25. Kaplan JA, Wells PH: Early diagnosis of myocardial ischemia using the pulmonary artery catheter. Anesth Analg 1981; 60:789–93.
26. Ammon JR: Perioperative management of the diabetic patient. Annual Refresher Course Lectures, San Francisco, No. 215, 1988.
27. Little JM, Sheil AGR, Lowenthal J, et al: Prognostic value of intraoperative blood flow measurements in femoropopliteal bypass vein grafts. Lancet 1968; 648–51.
28. Yates CJP, Berent A, Andrews, et al: Increase in blood flow by normovolemic hemodilation in intermittent claudication. Lancet 1979; 2:166–68.
29. Nielsen OM, Engell HC: The importance of colloid osmotic pressure for interstitial fluid volume and fluid balance after elective abdominal vascular surgery. Ann Surg 1986; 203:25–29.
30. Partridge BL: Use of pulse oximetry as a non-invasive indicator of intravascular volume status. J Clin Monit 1987; 3:263–68.
31. Rao TLK, El-Etr AA: Antiocoagulation following placement of epidural and subarachnoid catheters: an evaluation of neurologic sequelae. Anesthesiology 1981; 55:618–20.
32. Baron HC, LaRaja RD: Continous epidural analgesia in the Heparinized Vascular Surgical Patient: A Retrospective Review of 912 patients. J Vasc Surg 1987; 6:144–46.

CHAPTER 24

The Patient with Parkinson's Disease

Michael S. Ackerman

Case Report. *A 62-year-old man with a 6-year history of Parkinson's disease, treated with Sinemet 25/250 mg b.i.d. and Amantadine 100 mg. b.i.d., was brought to the ER by Emergency Services personnel. The patient's family had become alarmed when he did not answer the telephone that morning. They came to his home and found him on the floor, confused and unable to rise. It was estimated that the patient had been disabled for a period of 18–24 hours. On physical exam, the patient was a thin cachetic man, somewhat disoriented, displaying diffuse tremor, pinrolling movements, and stiff facial expresion. Blood pressure, supine, was recorded at 140/80, heart rate 90/min. Upon sitting, blood pressure was 90/60 and heart rate 116/min. The patient was also noted to have a marked deformity of the right hip which was extremely painful on attempted rotation. X-ray of the right hip revealed a fracture of the femur.*

Laboratory data was remarkable for a hematocrit of 47%, and BUN/ creat. of 41/1.3. Chest x-ray within normal limits.

He was scheduled for open reduction and internal fixation of the right hip as soon as possible.

Introduction

In 1817, James Parkinson described the disease which bears his name.[1] Parkinson's apt description of the symptomatology was as follows "involuntary tremulous motion, with lessened muscular powers, in parts not in action and even when supported; with a propensity to bend the trunk forward and to pass from a walking to a running pace, the senses and intellects being uninjured."

Parkinson's disease, known also as paralysis agitans, is characterized

---

Reviewed by Dr. Alan Hirshfeld, Assistant Professor of Neurosurgery, Albert Einstein College of Medicine/Montefiore Medical Center.

by a stooped posture, slowness of movement (bradykinesia), "masklike" facies, tremor of the limbs, involuntary pronation-supination of the upper extremities, "pinrolling" movements of the hands, a monotonous voice, hypokinesia, and stiffness. Most striking is the shuffling gait movement which, typically, accelerates with continued motion.

Pathophysiology

The etiology of Parkinson's disease is not completely understood. It is thought to arise from a deficiency of dopamine in the substantia nigra, an area concerned with regulation of movement. Dopamine exerts an inhibitory efect on the basal ganglia, thus controlling extrapyramidal movement.[2] Pathologically, changes are seen in the melanin-containing nerve cells in the brainstem (substantia nigra, locus ceruleus), with loss of nerve cells and reactive gliosis. In 1913,[1] F.H. Lewy described the eosinophilic, cytoplasmic inclusion bodies (Lewy bodies), found in these patients at autopsy. Biochemically, on postmortem examination, Parkinsonian patients can be shown to have diminished dopamine stores in the principle afferent terminals of the substantia nigra.[3] Decreased levels of homovanillic acid (HVA), a major metabolite of dopamine, are also demonstrated. Thus, Parkinson's disease may be characterized as a disease involving primarily the nigrostriatal dopaminergic system.

During the 1950s, several major breakthroughs occurred which greatly enhanced our understanding of the biochemical changes occurring in Parkinson's disease. Carlsson et al.[4] discovered that dopamine constitutes approximately one-half of brain catecholamine stores. Furthermore, 80% of this dopamine is located in the basal ganglia. The basal ganglia, however, constitutes only about 0.5% of the total brain weight.[5] Not long after this discovery, Hornykiewicz, at the University of Vienna, discovered that some brains, on postmortem examination, had low levels of dopamine, norepinepherine, and serotonin.[6] Upon reviewing the medical histories of these patients, Hornykiewicz discovered that all the patients with low levels of brain biogenic amines had suffered from Parkinson's disease at the time of death. Also, of the biogenic amines, dopamine was the most drastically reduced. Thus, Parkinson's disease became the first example of a disease of the brain correlated with a deficiency of a specific neurotransmitter. Incidentally, this finding led to vigorous attempts to find neurotransmitter deficiency as a basis for schizophrenia, depression, dementia, and other diseases.

Definition

True Parkinson's disease should be distinguished from Parkinsonian syndromes. Essentially, any disease which impairs the function of the caudate and putamen can impair voluntary movement and cause bradykinesia and rigidity. Encephalitis can result in a syndrome clinically indistinguishable from Parkinson's disease.[1,7] Indeed, many of the survivors of the encephalitis lethargica epidemic of 1918 to 1924 suffered signs and symptoms remarkably similar to those of patients with idiopathic Parkinson's disease. Shy–Drager syndrome is prominent among those disease states which can closely mimic Parkinson's disease. This syndrome is associated with central autonomic failure and is often accompanied by nigrostriatal degeneration and Parkinsonian symptoms. Among the other multisystem degenerative diseases which may mimic Parkinson's disease are progressive supranuclear palsy, striatonigral degeneration, and olivopontocerebellar atrophy.[1] While these syndromes often mimic Parkinson's disease clinically, they rarely respond to anti-Parkinsonian medication [primarily L-3,4-dihydroxyphenylalanine (L-DOPA)], thus providing a pharmacologic means of differentiation.

One disease which has recently been linked to Parkinson's disease is Alzheimer's syndrome. Many patients with this latter disease display extrapyramidal movements, bradykinesia, and forgetfulness. Impairment of mentation in patients with Parkinson's disease is usually due to L-DOPA therapy, although it may be part of the disease in a subgroup of patients who demonstrate progressive loss of intellectual function, personality changes, and failing memory.[7] This finding of impaired mentation in Parkinsonian patients may be explained by the fact that parts of the nuclei in the basal ganglia participate in cognitive aspects of behavior.[5] While the motor functions of the basal ganglia are carried out primarily by the putamen, the cognitive functions are thought to be regulated by the caudate nucleus. Segregation of function is consistent with experimental data in primates. For example, bilateral lesions in the dorsolateral prefrontal neocortex produce deficits in performance of tasks measuring spatial memory. On the other hand, lesions in the orbitofrontal neocortex result in impaired performance in direct reversal tasks.[5]

Other syndromes which may be incorrectly diagnosed as idiopathic Parkinson's disease are cases of drug-induced Parkinsonism. Reserpine, phenothiazines, and butyrophenones have been implicated in Parkinsonian syndromes, because of their ability to cause a deficiency of dopamine at postsynaptic striatal receptors. Drug-induced Parkinsonism is commonly seen in institutionalized patients who have been on long-term therapy with anti-psychotic drugs. This syndrome may persist for several weeks after discontinuation of therapy. On the other hand, a Parkinsonian syndrome may follow even a single administration of a drug which antagonizes dopamine. Rivera et al described a case of a healthy 16-year-old patient who underwent a dental procedure under general anesthesia.[8] During the procedure, the patient received 3 ml of intravenous Innovar. The patient's postoperative course was complicated by uncontrollable tremor and cogwheel rigidity. The patient was treated with anti-Parkinsonian medications and her symptoms resolved after approximately 2 weeks.

Medical Therapy

In Parkinson's disease, as in other disease states, there is no single
therapy which is appropriate for all patients. In recent years, there has
been great emphasis on tailoring treatment to the specific needs of each
patient. Patients are usually divided into categories according to the
severity of their disease, i.e., those suffering from early, moderate, and
severe disease. Patients with early disease are usually able to perform
most functions with little difficulty, though with some inconvenience.
Moderate sufferers usually experience some limitation in daily activity
due to the disease. Those with severe disease must limit their daily
activities despite medical therapy. It is useful to refer to the staging
system of Hoehn and Yahr, for Parkinson's patients. (see Table 24.1.).[9]

Generally, patients with early disease can be treated with amantadine
(Symmetrel) or anticholinergic agents (trihexyphenidyl, benztropine,
biperidin, and procyclidine). These agents are particularly useful in
patients in whom tremor is a major problem. However, anticholinergic
therapy is limited because of autonomic side effects, such as urinary
retention and dry mouth.

Undoubtedly, the greatest revolution in the therapy of the Parkinsonian
patient was the introduction of L-DOPA therapy in 1967.[2,7,10] For
patients with moderate disease (stage III of the Hoehn and Yahr
classification), dopamine replacement therapy can provide dramatic relief
in as many as 90% of patients. So effective is L-DOPA therapy in the
Parkinsonian patient that patients who do not respond have probably
been misdiagnosed.

L-DOPA, an aromatic amino acid, easily crosses the blood–brain
barrier. Thus, the rate-limiting step in the synthesis of dopamine and
other catecholamines hydroxylation of L-tyrosine to produce L-DOPA, is
bypassed. The decarboxylation of L-DOPA to produce dopamine
proceeds easily (see Figure 24.1.).

However, because dopamine is a biogenic amine, and because its
presence peripherally results in a number of untoward cardiovascular

TABLE 24.1. Progressive Staging System for Parkinson's Disease

Stage I: Unilateral involvement only
Stage II: Bilateral involvement without impairment of balance
Stage III: Bilateral involvement with some imbalance, impaired righting reflex, mild to
  moderate disability. Patient may still work depending on the type of employment.
Stage IV: Fully developed, severely disabling disease, Patient stands unassisted.
Stage V: Confined to bed or wheelchair.

Reprinted with permission, from Hoehn MM, and Yahr, MD: Parkinsonism: Onset,
Progression, and Mortality. Neurology 17: 433, 1967.

effects, it is now routine to administer L-DOPA with a peripheral decarboxylase inhibitor. This has the dual purpose of increasing the amount of L-DOPA available in the CNS, and decreasing the amount of dopamine in the perpiphery. Commercially prepared drugs are available which combine L-DOPA with carbidopa (Sinemet) or benserazide (Madopar).[7] For example, Sinemet 25/250 contains 250 mg of L-DOPA and 25 mg of carbidopa. However, the problem of maintaining therapeutic levels of dopamine and avoiding drug toxicity are clearly illustrated below (Figure 24.2.).

For patients with moderate to severe disease, the direct-acting dopaminergic agents, such as bromocriptine (Parlodel), are added to the regimen to limit exposure to L-DOPA. This is particularly advantageous as patients tend to develop tolerance to L-DOPA after prolonged therapy. In addition, with time, patients develop adverse CNS effects from L-DOPA, including delirium, dyskinesia, and confusion. On the other hand, bromocriptine itself is not without adverse effects, including dyskinesia, delir-

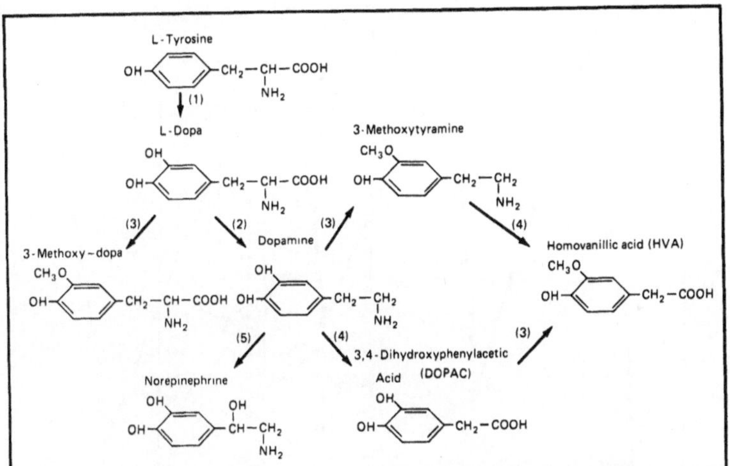

FIGURE 24.1. The biosynthesis and metabolism of catecholamines. (1) Formation of L-dopa from L-tyrosine by tyrosine hydroxylase, the rate-limiting step in catecholamine synthesis. (2) Aromatic L-amino acid decarboxylase converts L-dopa to dopamine. Pyridoxine is a coenzyme for this reaction. (3) Methylation of the hydroxyl group at the 3 position metabolizes L-dopa to 3-methyldopa, dopamine to 3-methoxytyramine, or DOPAC to HVA. Catechol-O-methyltransferase and a methyl-group donor are necessary. (4) Deamination of dopamine by monoamine oxidase to DOPAC, or 3-methoxytyramine to HVA. Norepinephrine is similarly metabolized to dihydroxymandelic acid (not shown). (5) Hydroxylation of dopamine to norepinephrine through the action of dopamine-β-hydroxylase. Reprinted, with permission, from Ngai, S.H. "Parkinsonism, Levodopa, and Anesthesia", Anesthesiology 37:3, 345, 1972.

ium, vasospasm, and edema. For this reason, most experts utilize
bromocriptine in conjunction with L-DOPA therapy.

Some physicians utilize the so-called "drug holiday" for Parkinsonian
patients.[11] Patients are withdrawn from their medications in an inpatient
setting in an attempt to reduce dyskinsia and tolerance. This is one
approach to the "on–off" phenomenon in which abrupt changes from
dyskinesia to akinesia occur in Parkinsonians on long-term L-DOPA
therapy.[12] The cause of the "on-off" phenomenon is not known, but it is
thought to be a result of drug-induced alterations of central dopaminergic
receptor sensitivity.[13] However, the "drug holiday" approach is controversial as it is questionable whether patients derive any true long-term
benefit from such holidays.[14] In addition, these pauses in treatment are
associated with adverse reactions, among these nocturnal myoclonus,
nightmares, and disturbances in the sleep cycle.

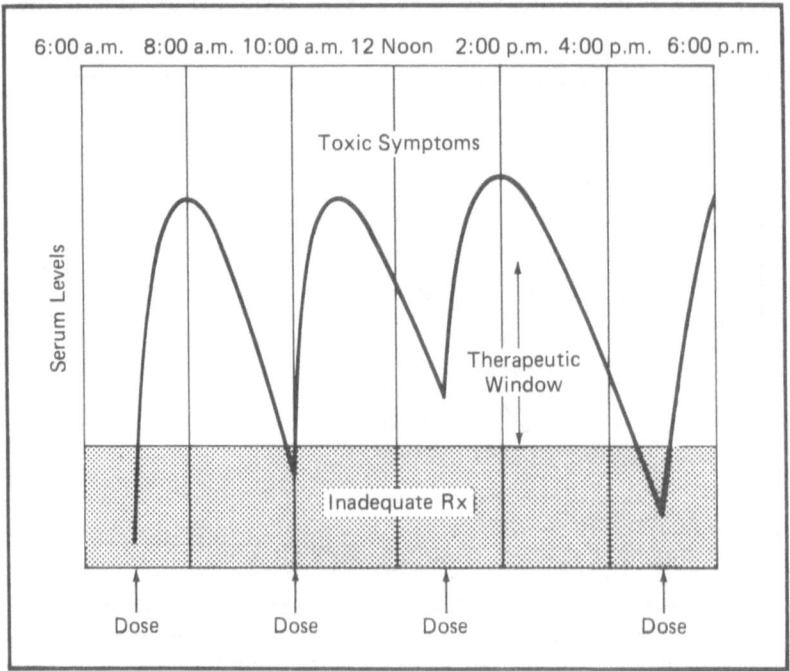

FIGURE 24.2. Symptoms viewed through a therapeutic window. Fluctuations are
the most difficult treatment problems in Parkinson's disease. At peak tissue levels
after a dose, a patient may demonstrate confusion, delirium, and dyskinesia—
symptoms of dopamine excess. Within hours, the same patient may experience
deterioration and freezing up—symptoms of dopamine deficiency. Most of these
effects are pharmacokinetic problems, due to a short half-life and an increasingly
narrow therapeutic window. Reprinted, with permission, from Sudarsky, L.,
"Management of Parkinson's Disease: 1987" in *Resident and Staff Physician*,
March 1987 Vol. 33, No. 3, p. 32.

Surgical Treatment

Medical therapy is limited by adverse drug reactions and the development of tolerance. Previous attempts at ablative procedures have been less than successful. Thus, there is considerable interest in perfecting a surgical treatment for Parkinson's disease.[15,16] In 1979, laboratory trials were begun with experimentally produced deficiencies of dopamine in the caudate nucleus.[17,18] Dopaminergic cells from the substantia nigra of fetal animals were then implanted into the caudate nucleus. The results indicated that, not only was there quantitative improvement in brain dopamine stores in the animals, but there was clinical improvement in the motor deficits. Because of ethical problems inherent in the use of human fetal tissue in transplants, an alternative had to be found for human Parkinson's patients. The chromaffin cells of the human adrenal medulla provide such an alternative as they produce dopamine. Also, these cells have proven to be transplantable in animals.

The first attempts at transplantation of adrenal medullary tissue into the caudate nucleus of human Parkinson's patients occurred in Sweden in 1982.[19] The tissue appeared to survive but the operation did not result in significant improvement in the patients' symptoms. However, the two patients who underwent the procedure were not randomly selected Parkinsonians, but severely afflicted sufferers who had failed to respond to other therapies.

An important advance ocurred in 1987 when Drucker-Colin and Madrazo reported on two patients who successfully received an adrenal tissue implant into the head of the caudate nucleus where it contacts the lateral ventricle.[20] This report was received with great enthusiasm, and a second series of 11 patients was operated.[21] There were two deaths in this group (one patient suffered a myocardial infarction 5 months postoperatively, and one died following a cerebrovascular accident 45 days postoperatively). Among the surviving patients, results were similar to those noted at several other centers. Patients generally showed an initial response, then a relapse. However, after 3 months, most patients improved markedly. At the present time, the procedure is being performed at a number of centers in the US, Europe, and China and while these outcomes are cause for optimism, successful results are not universal. While the initial reports were of transplants accomplished via craniotomy, the procedure has been modified, with the cell implantation performed stereotactically.[22]

Despite early encouraging results, a number of questions remain unanswered with respect to human adrenal implants as a cure for Parkinson's disease. For example, Drucker-Colin et al found no increase in brain levels of dopamine in patients receiving the transplants. This suggests a mechanism other than augmentation of brain dopamine levels to explain the observed clinical improvement. However, they did find that enkephalin levels increased 40-fold postoperatively. Striatal enkephalin neurons regulate release of presynaptic dopamine from striatal dopaminergic terminals. Also, in some cases of Parkinson's disease, striatal met-enkephalin and leu-enkephalin levels are reportedly reduced by 70% and 30%, respectively.[23] A marked increase in CNS enkephalins and endorphins has been reported in patients with Parkinson's disease treated with L-DOPA. This, together with the fact that adrenal chromaffin cells are known to contain high concentrations of opioids, raises speculation that the mechanism involved in the clinical improvements in patients post-adrenal transplant is due not to augmentation of brain dopamine, but activation of the endogenous opioid system.[24]

Anesthetic Considerations

Anesthetic considerations for the patient with Parkinson's disease may be classified, generally, as those directly related to the disease, those related to therapy of the disease, and unrelated factors, although, there is much interaction between the groups.

Parkinson's Disease

Parkinsonian patients present a number of challenging problems to the anesthesiologist which are directly attributable to the disease. Systemic evaluation is indicated.

Respiratory Assessment

The facial rigidity characteristic of Parkinson's disease may make intubation difficult,[25] and a thorough preoperative evaluation of the patient's airway is in order. Diffuse rigidity, particularly of the chest wall musculature, may impair assisted ventilation. Preoperative questioning and the use of pulmonary function testing can alert the anesthesiologist to the presence of restrictive lung disease.

Cardiovascular Assessment

Orthostatic hypotension in the Parkinsonian patient is often a prominent problem, [26] most probably due to an imbalance of excitatory and inhibitory reflexes in the spinal cord.[5] Should the patient report dizziness on sudden position change, modification of anesthetic technique should be considered, including avoidance of the sitting position when placing a regional block. If the surgical procedure requires the lithotomy position, achieving that position should be accomplished slowly with continuous blood pressure monitoring (use of a finger plethysmograph such as the Finapres is an ideal non-invasive monitor in this situation). Frequently, the anesthesiologist encounters the Parkinsonian patient coming to the operating room for an orthopedic procedure after a traumatic fall. A clear history of events immediately preceeding and following the event must be obtained. Did the patient fall because of poor coordination secondary to Parkinson's disease, or did he have a syncopal episode resulting from a dysrhythmia? A rhythm strip from electrocardiographic testing may indicate abnormaities requiring better pharmacologic control of ventricular activity, or even insertion of a pacemaker.

Neurologic assessment

A subgroup of Parkinson's patients suffer from dementia. This may be either due to the presence of coexisting Alzheimer's disease, a manifestation of Parkinson's disease itself, or a result of L-DOPA therapy. In any case, the anesthesiologist should document any abnormalities in the patient's status preoperatively. If the patient is, indeed, mentally impaired, he may be unable to give informed consent for anesthesia and surgery. A psychiatric consultation may be important for documentation. Rigidity often makes ambulation difficult. Falls are not infrequent, and the anesthesiologist should note all injuries (including bruises) preoperatively, lest they later be mistakenly attributed to malpositioning during anesthesia and surgery.

If a regional technique is to be used, the anesthesiologist must ascertain that the patient can tolerate a position necessary for insertion of a subarachnoid or epidural needle without undue pain.

Nutritional Status

As with any chronic disease sufferer, the Parkinsonian is prone to poor nutrition. Based on the patient's overall nutritional status, body weight relative to ideal body weight, serum albumin, hematocrit, and cholesterol, preoperative hyperalimentation may be indicated. Also, if the time since the injury until the patient received help was hours or days, dehydration is likely and the volume status should be corrected prior to induction of anesthesia.

Drug-related considerations

Problems encountered with the use of therapeutic agents for Parkinson's disease are primarily a result of L-DOPA interactions. As mentioned, L-DOPA has been the mainstay of medical therapy since its introduction in 1967. By crossing the blood–brain barrier, L-DOPA bypasses the rate-limiting step in dopamine biosynthesis, the hydroxylation of L-tyrosine. Therapy with L-DOPA results in increased brain levels of dopamine, as well as increased HVA, the primary metabolite of dopamine.

L-DOPA causes adverse effects in up to 90% of treated patients. Among these are nausea, vomiting, and faintness. It was initially felt that nausea in Parkinson's patients was a result of direct irritation of the stomach by L-DOPA. However, studies in dogs revealed that intravenous injection of L-DOPA also caused nausea and vomiting, probably secondary to stimulation of the chemoreceptor trigger zone. Therefore, patients on L-DOPA are at risk for vomiting via a central mechanism, and there are clinical implications for the anesthesiologist. Appropriate precautions must be taken. With a strong history of uncontrolled vomiting, regional anesthesia or a rapid-sequence induction of general anesthesia with cricoid pressure, may be indicated. It may also be prudent to pretreat the patients with antacids before inducing anesthesia.

Psychic disturbances may complicate therapy with L-DOPA. Patients may experience euphoria, depression, or inappropriately aggressive behavior. The anesthesiologist must take note of such behavior when deciding upon an anesthetic technique. A "local standby" approach may be unsuccessful in a patient with a psychic disturbance. If a patient has experienced dysphoria and hallucinations, a "dissociative" technique using ketamine is contraindicated, although this drug has been used with benefit in some patients with Parkinson's disease.

By far the most potentially serious effects of L-DOPA are those related to the cardiovascular system. These adverse effects, notably postural hypotension, dysrhythmias, and hypertension, are of paramount importance to the anesthesiologist. As noted earlier, Parkinsonians suffer from postural hypotension regardless of whether or not treatment is initiated. Treatment with L-DOPA may exacerbate this problem by a number of proposed mechanisms. For example, in experimental animals, the carotid sinus reflex is blunted during infusion of L-DOPA. Because pretreatment with peripheral decarboxylase inhibitors does not prevent L-DOPA-induced postural hypotension, a central mechanism has also been proposed. Another possible mechanism to account for the postural hypotension in patients on L-DOPA is a dopamine-mediated rise in glomerular filtration rate and renal plasma flow.

It is currently accepted practice to continue L-DOPA therapy until the day of surgery, in spite of potential complications resulting from its use. Sudden withdrawal of L-DOPA can result in ventilatory insufficiency due to chest wall rigidity, akinesia, and tremor. Because of the short half-life of L-DOPA (1 1/2 to 2 hours), very little remains in peripheral stores approximately 6 hours after the last dose is given. While the theoretical risk of serious ventricular dysrhythmias exists in a patient on L-DOPA, these are rarely encountered.

Other Considerations

Among the anesthetic considerations not related to Parkinson's disease are those relevant to the middle-aged and elderly patient. Though Parkinson's disease may appear in patients as young as 25, it commonly presents in the 5th decade of life and later. Therefore, patients suffering from Parkinson's disease are in an age group where cardiovascular, cerebrovascular, renal, pulmonary, and genitourinary disease are commonly found. Also, because the number of adults surviving into old age is increasing with better nutrition and medical care, the anesthesiologist can expect to encounter an even greater number of Parkinsonian patients. For this reason, a thorough preparative evaluation and review of systems is in order, with special emphasis on clinical chemistry and electrocardiogram. A thorough understanding of all medication which the patient is receiving is of utmost importance.

Anesthetic Plan

There is no clear choice of anesthetic technique in patients with Parkinson's disease. If the patient is mentally intact with minimal rigidity, a regional technique may be preferable. Immobility, pain, or dementia may dictate use of general anesthesia.

Anesthetic agents which should be avoided in the Parkinsonian due to an anti-dopaminergic effect are the phenothiazines and butyrophenones. As noted earlier, the risk of Parkinson syndrome resulting from the use of droperidol (a butyrophenone) exists in the patient with no prior history of Parkinson's disease. Wiklund and Ngai[27] described a case of rigidity and pulmonary edema in a Parkinsonian on L-DOPA therapy after administration of droperidol and fentanyl (Innovar). It is best to avoid the butyrophenones and phenothiazines and the possibility of exacerbating Parkinsonism.

The use of peripheral decarboxylase inhibitors can decrease, but not prevent, the incidence of untoward sympathomimetic events associated with L-DOPA. Because of a tendency to dysrhythmias in patients on L-DOPA, agents which lower the threshold for rhythm disturbances should be avoided. Halothane should not be used in a patient taking L-DOPA, nor should epinephrine be added to local anesthetics. Some have advocated the avoidance of sympathomimetic agents such as ketamine,[28] but this is somewhat controversial. In fact, one case report sugggests a beneficial effect of ketamine on the symptomatology of Parkinson's disease.[29] This, together with experimental data indicating that ketamine increases dopamine stores in the brains of rats,[30] suggests that more work needs to be done regarding the risk to benefit ratio of ketamine use in the Parkinsonian on L-DOPA.

Recently, some concern has been expressed regarding Parkinsonians' sensitivity to succinylcholine. Specifically, Gravlee[31] described a case of hyperkalemia in a Parkinsonian who had received an intubating dose of succinylcholine. This, however, is generally considered an isolated instance, and is not sufficient cause to abandon the use of succinylcholine in the Parkinsonian patient. For example, Cooperman[32] noted insignificant changes in serum pottassium in Parkinsonians given succinylcholine. In addition, the patient in whom Gravlee described the episode of hyperkalemia had undergone two prior lumbar laminectomies with neurologic sequelae.[33] Thus, hyperkalemia may have occurred as a result of potassium release from denervated muscle, and not as a result of Parkinson's disease.

General anesthesia is probably best managed by administering no or minimal premedication, slowly titrated doses of thiopental or etomidate for induction, muscle relaxation with atracurium, and maintaenance with low dose isoflurane (0.5%) and small boluses of fentanyl (25 μg as indicated) in a nitrous oxide–oxygen mixture. Normocarbia should be maintained. The aim should be to awaken the patient promptly and allow him to ambulate as soon as possible.

References

1. Adams RD, Victor M: Principles of Neurology New York: McGraw-Hill 1985;874–97.
2. Ngai SH: Parkinsonism, levodopa, and anesthesia. Anesthesiology 1972; 37(3):344–51.
3. Hornykiewicz O: Dopamine (3-hydroxytyramine) and function. Pharmacol Rev 1966; 18:925–64.
4. Carlsson A, Lindquist M, Magnusson T, et al: On the presence of 3 hydroxytyramine in brain. Science 1958; 127:471.
5. Cote L, Crutcher MD: Motor functions of the basal ganglia and diseases of transmitter metabolism, in Kandel ER, Schwartz JH (eds): Principles of Neural Science, Elsevier New York: Elsevier, 1985; 523–34.
6. Erlinger H, Hornykiewicz O: Verteilung von Noradrenalin und Dopamin (3-Hydroxytyramine) im Gehirn des Menschen und ihr Verhalten bei Erkrankungen des extrapyridaren Systems. Klin Wochenschr 1960; 38:1236–39.
7. Sudarsky, L: Management of Parkinson's Disease: 1987. Resident Staff Phys 1987; 33(3):29–37.
8. Rivera V, Keichian A, Oliver R: Persistent parkinsonism following neuroleptanalgesia. Anesthesiology 1975; 28(5):635–37.
9. Hoehn MM, Yahr, MD: Parkinsonism: onset, progression and mortality. 1967; Neurology 17:427.
10. Cotzias GC, VanWoert MH, Schiffer LM: Aromatic amino acids and modification of Parkinsonism. N Engl J Med 1967; 276:374–79.

11. Weiner W, Koller WC, Perliks S, et al: Drug holiday and the management of Parkinson's disease. Neurology 1980; 30:1257–61.
12. Markham CH: The on-off side effect of L-dopa, in McDowell F, Barbeare A (ed): Advances in Neurology, Vol. 5 Second Canadian-American Conference on Parkinson's disease. New York: Raven Press 1974;287–395.
13. Pycock CJ, Marsden CD: Central dopaminergic receptor supersensitivity and its relevance to Parkinson's disease. J Neurol Science 1977; 31:113–31.
14. Mayeux R, Stern Y, Mulvey K, et al: Reappraisal of temporary Levodopa withdrawal ("drug holiday") in Parkinson's disease. N Engl J Med 313: 724–28.
15. Gildenberg PL: The present role of stereotactic surgery in the management of Parkinson's disease, Advances in Neurology 1984;40,447–52.
16. Gildenberg PL: The present role of stereotactic surgery in the management of Parkinson's disease, in Hassler RG, Christ JF (eds): Parkinson-Specific Motor and Mental Disorders. Advances in Neurology, Vol. 40. New York: Raven Press 1984; 447–52.
17. Freed WJ: Functional brain tissue transplantation: reversal of lesion-induced rotation by intraventricular substantia nigra and adrenal medulla grafts. Biol. Psychiatry 1983; 18:1205–67.
18. Freed WJ, Cannon-Spoor HE, Wyatt RJ: Embryonic brain grafts in an animal model of Parkinson's disease; Criteria for human application. Appl Neurophysiol 1984; 47:16–22.
19. Backlund EO, Granberg PO, Hanberger B, et al: Transplantation of adrenal medullary tissue to striatum in Parkinsonism. First clinical trials. J Neurosurg 1985; 62:169–73.
20. Madrazo I, Drucker-Colin R, Diaz V, et al: Open microsurgical autograft of adrenal medulla to the right caudate nucleus in two patients with intractable Parkinson's disease. N Engl J Med 1987; 316:831–34.
21. Drucker-Colin R, Madrazo I, Shkurovich M, et al: Open microsurgical autograft of patients with Parkinson's disease. Schmitt Neurological Sciences Symposium. June 30–July 3, 1987, Rochester, NY.
22. Gildenberg PL: Surgical therapy of movement disorders, in Wilkins RH, Rengachary SS (eds): Neurosurgery. New York: McGraw-Hill 1985; 2507–16.
23. Agid Y, Javoy-Agid F: Peptides and Parkinson's disease. Trends Neurosci 1985; 7:30–35.
24. Iacono R, Sandyk, R: Adrenal medullary tissue transplantation in Parkinson's disease. J Neurosug 1988; 68:158.
25. Cullen BF: Anesthesia for patients with Neurologic Disease. ASA Refresher Courses in Anesthesiology 1983; 11:59.
26. Aita JF: Why patients with Parkinson's disease fall. JAMA 1982; 247(4): 515–16.
27. Wiklund RA, Ngai S: Rigidity and pulmonary edema after Innovar in a patient on levodopa therapy: report of a case. Anesthesiology 1971; 35(5):545–47.
28. Ngai SH, Wiklund RA: Levodopa and surgical anesthesia. Neurology 1972; 22:38–42.
29. Hetherington A, Rosenblatt R: Ketamine and paralysis agitans. Anesthesiology 1980; 52(6):527.
30. Glisson SN, EL-Etr AA, Bloor BC: The effects of ketamine upon norepineph-

rine and dopamine levels in rabbit brain parts. Naunyn Schmiedebergs Arch Pharmacol 1976; 295:149–52.

31. Gravlee G: Succinylcholine-induced hyperkalemia in a patient with Parkinson's disease. Anesth Analg 1980; 59(6): 444–46.

32. Cooperman LH: Succinylcholine induced hyperkalemia in neuromuscular disease. JAMA 1970; 213:1867–71.

33. Azar I: The response of patients with neuromuscular disorders to muscle relaxants: a review. Anesthesiology 1984; 61:175–87.

Self-Assessment Questions

Select the single letter response that most correctly answers the question or completes the sentence.

Chapter 1

1. Infrarenal crossclamping of the aorta causes:
   a. 75% increase in renal vascular resistance
   b. 75% decrease in renal vascular resistance
   c. 50% decrease in renal vascular resistance
   d. no change in renal vascular resistance
2. MAC for endotracheal intubation free of coughing and straining is:
   a. 2 × MAC for surgical anesthesia
   b. 3.2 × MAC for surgical anesthesia
   c. 1.3 × MAC for surgical anesthesia
   d. 0.5 × MAC for surgical anesthesia
3. Hypoxic or ischemic events in the spinal cord during infrarenal aortic crossclamping can be recognized by:
   a. intraoperative assessment of foot extension unresponse to stimulation of the lateral peroneal nerve
   b. monitoring of somatosensory evoked potentials
   c. continuous EEG recording
   d. calculation of a large arteriol-venous oxygen difference
4. In a patient with a ruptured aortic aneurysm, anesthesia should be started:
   a. as soon as the patient arrives in the operating room, to prevent psychological trauma
   b. as soon as ECG electrodes and the blood pressure monitor are in place
   c. only after the patient is prepared surgically and draped
   d. after placement of the Swan-Ganz pulmonary artery catheter and intraarterial cannula

5. The most common cause of death following intact abdominal aortic aneurysm repair is:
   a. uncontrolled bleeding intraoperatively or in the immediate post-operative period
   b. disseminated intravascular coagulopathy following massive blood transfusion
   c. myocardial infarction
   d. acute pulmonary embolism

6. Infrarenal crossclamping of the abdominal aorta causes:
   a. increased cardiac output by 15–20%
   b. decreased cardiac output by 15–35%
   c. no significant change
   d. decreased pulmonary resistance by 40%

7. Deleterious effects of unclamping the aorta during AAA repair can best be prevented by:
   a. titrating the infusion of a vasopressor such as phenylephrine hydrochloride (Neo-synephrine®) to maintain the blood pressure near the preoperative level
   b. raising the PCWP to 4–5 mm above the control value by infusion of intravenous fluids before the clamp is released
   c. intravenous administration of ephedrine 10–25mg doses intermittently
   d. norepinephrine infusion to maintain peripheral resistance near normal

8. The chance of rupture of an abdominal aortic aneurysm of 7cm diameter is:
   a. 10% per year
   b. 40% per year
   c. 15% per year
   d. same chance of rupture as an aneurysm of 5cm diameter

9. A patient complains of bounding abdominal pulsations between the umbilicus and xiphoid areas. Thus:
   a. he has an abdominal aortic aneurysm at least 10cm in diameter that is beginning to rupture
   b. he possibly has an aneurysm, but it is impossible to tell the size
   c. it is a sign of nervousness
   d. he probably does not have an aneurysm as pulsations from abdominal aortic aneurysm should be felt between the umbilicus and symphysis pubis

10. Infrarenal crossclamping of the aorta causes:
    a. an increase in venous return from the inferior extremities
    b. no change in venous return
    c. a decrease in venous return from the pelvis but an increase from the inferior extremities
    d. a decrease in venous return both from the pelvis and the inferior extremities

Chapter 2

1. Choose the one incorrect statement below:
   a. Pituitary tumors cause increased hormone secretion.
   b. Pituitary tumors cause decreased hormone secretion.
   c. The gland lies in close proximity to cranial nerve VIII.
   d. Tumors of the pituitary may produce headaches and blindness.
2. The posterior lobe of the pituitary secretes:
   a. antidiuretic hormone (ADH) and growth hormone (GH)
   b. oxytocin and ADH
   c. thyroid-stimulating hormone (TSH) and adrenocorticotropic hormone (ACTH)
   d. follicle-stimulating hormone (FSH) and prolactin
3. Hormone secretion by the pituitary is controlled by all of the following *except:*
   a. neurotransmitters
   b. releasing factors
   c. hypertension
   d. circulating levels of hormone
4. Choose the one correct statement below:
   a. ACTH controls release of cortisol from the adrenals.
   b. Luteinizing hormone (LH) stimulates skeletal development.
   c. FSH is essential for lactation.
   d. GH regulates the synthesis of thyroid hormone.
5. ADH is:
   a. released by the anterior pituitary
   b. an essential factor in the control of fluid balance
   c. the hormone that produces dilute urine concentration
   d. important for its role in the delivery process
6. Panhypopitutitarism results in all of the following *except:*
   a. hypotension
   b. cortisol deficiency
   c. hyperthermia
   d. short stature
7. Cushing's disease is caused by:
   a. tumors of the adrenal gland
   b. excess secretion of ACTH by pituitary microadenomas
   c. ectopic production of ACTH by nonpituitary tumors
   d. longterm treatment with steroids
8. Choose the one incorrect statement below:
   a. Phenothiazine therapy may elevate serum prolactin.
   b. Elevated serum prolactin causes suppression of the menstrual cycle.
   c. Males with elevated prolactin levels report increased libido.
   d. Galactorrhea is found in up to 50% of cases of prolactin-secreting tumors.

9. Acromegaly includes all of the following features *except:*
   a. hypoglycemia
   b. cardiomegaly
   c. coarse facial features
   d. osteoarthritis
10. Perioperative complications of pituitary surgery may include which of the following:
   a. hypertension and dysrhythmias
   b. air embolism
   c. diabetes insipidis
   d. all of the above

Chapter 3

1. HbS differs from HbA in all of the following ways *except:*
   a. it has two hydrophobic areas on its surface when deoxygenated
   b. its beta-6 amino acid is valine
   c. it forms long polymerized chains
   d. small amounts confer resistance to Falciparum malaria
2. The delay seen before onset of HbS gelation can be explained by:
   a. the time needed for the cell to assume a sickled shape
   b. the time needed for synthesis of HbF
   c. the time needed for cell division
   d. the time needed for formation of nucleation sites for polymer generation
3. Sequestration crises are not usually seen in patients beyond the age of 5 years because:
   a. the bone marrow has matured by that age
   b. patients are functionally asplenic beyond that age
   c. the incidence of viral infections has decreased
   d. the MCHC increases after repeated cycles of sickling
4. A 35-year-old SCA patient with pneumonia and a temperature of 102.5°F is receiving I.V. fluids at a rate of 75ml/hr. His urine output is 75ml/hr, with a specific gravity of 1.007. What can we conclude about this patient's fluid status?
   a. he is in neutral fluid balance
   b. severe dehydration is present
   c. a pulmonary artery catheter should be placed to answer the question
   d. the amount of urine excreted does not indicate fluid status
5. The mechanism of action of cytarabine and hydroxyurea may be:
   a. elimination of the mutant HbS stem cell
   b. induction of extramedullary hematopoiesis
   c. induction of secondary erythropoiesis with a predominance of HbF synthesis
   d. a direct effect on HbS, with formation of ketoamine derivatives

6. Drugs that increase membrane permeability inhibit sickling because:
   a. they decrease the intracellular concentration of HbS
   b. they decrease splenic removal of sickled cells
   c. they cause systemic alkalosis
   d. they increase levels of glyceraldehyde
7. Nitrous oxide-narcotic-relaxant techniques are preferred for SCA patients because:
   a. muscle relaxation decreases oxygen consumption
   b. the premise is false; any well-conducted general anesthetic technique is acceptable
   c. use of hepatotoxic volatile anesthetics is avoided
   d. high inspired concentrations of oxygen can be administered
8. The presence of valine in position 6 of the beta chain of HbS allows polymerization because:
   a. it binds less tightly to the heme group
   b. it destroys tactoids,
   c. it is a nonpolar amino acid which can interact with a hydrophobic area on adjacent molecules
   d. its aromatic ring structure leads to resonance stabilization of polymerized HbS
9. With respect to Hb electrophoresis and the sickle cell prep, all of the following are true *except:*
   a. both allow quantitation of the amount of HbS present
   b. electrophoresis depends on differences in mobility of Hb molecules in electric fields, while the sickle cell prep depends on morphologic criteria
   c. the sickle cell prep relies on addition of a reducing agent
   d. the sickle cell prep does not distinguish SCA from sickle trait
10. An SCA patient with signs of right-sided heart failure, right ventricular hypertrophy, and a loud pulmonic component of the second heart sound is likely to have all of the following *except:*
    a. elevated pulmonary artery pressures
    b. occlusion of significant amounts of the pulmonary vascular bed
    c. ECG evidence of right ventricular hypertrophy
    d. a ruptured papillary muscle of the mitral valve

Chapter 4

1. Myocardial O_2 demand is increased by all of the following *except:*
   a. tachycardia
   b. coronary spasm
   c. increased contractility
   d. increased wall tension
2. The best prognostic indicator of short- and longterm survival in patients with CAD is:
   a. ejection fraction

    b. triple-vessel disease

    c. history of congestive heart failure

    d. unstable angina

3. The percentage of CABG candidates who are candidates for PTCA is:

    a. 15%

    b. 10%

    c. 30%

    d. 25%

4. After failed PTCA and the need for emergency CABG, the best intervention to preserve myocardial function is:

    a. dopamine

    b. intravenous nitroglycerin

    c. combination of dopamine and nitroglycerin

    d. intraaortic balloon pump

5. For a 60-year-old man, after failed PTCA for LAD disease, with an ejection fraction of 38% and LVEDP of 22mmHg, the acceptable anesthetic technique includes all of the following *except:*

    a. fentanyl/O_2/vecuronium

    b. sufentanil/O_2/pancuronium

    c. halothane/O_2/pancuronium

    d. fentanyl/O_2/atracurium

6. A normal ECG is present in the following percentage of patients with CAD:

    a. 25–50%

    b. 30–60%

    c. 40–60%

    d. 10–20%

7. After failed PTCA with streptokinase, appropriate placement of central venous access may be performed via all of the following routes *except:*

    a. external jugular vein

    b. subclavian vein

    c. brachial vein

    d. cephalic vein

8. Acute withdrawal of clonidine causes:

    a. myocardial ischemia

    b. arrhythmias

    c. rebound hypertension

    d. myocardial infarction

9. The two-year mortality rate for a 65-year-old woman with triple-vessel disease and an ejection fraction of 48% is:

    a. 20%

    b. 36%

    c. 40%

    d. 25%

10. Significant coronary artery stenosis is present when narrowing of a major coronary artery is:
    a. 70%
    b. 60%
    c. 65%
    d. 50%

Chapter 5

1. Meningomyelocele:
   a. has an incidence of 5–10 per 1000 live births in the United States
   b. has an increased risk of occurring in families who have had a previous child with meningomyelocele
   c. is slightly more common in males and higher socioeconomic populations
   d. has a specific teratogen, polyvinyl chloride, which is associated with an increased incidence of the defect
2. Meningomyelocele is commonly associated with other congenital defects; choose the one correct statement below.
   a. The Chiari II malfunction is rare, occurring in only 25% of patients with meningomyelocele.
   b. Hydrocephalus occurs in almost 99% of patients with meningomyelocele.
   c. Congenital abnormalities such as cardiac defects or diaphragmatic hernias have rarely been reported in association with a meningomyelocele.
   d. Orthopedic malformations are common with meningomyelocele, the most severe of which are kyphosis and scoliosis.
3. Hydrocephalus in patients with meningomyelocele:
   a. often worsens after closure of the back defect
   b. rarely appears if the infant did not have it at birth
   c. commonly causes acute rises in intracranial pressure (ICP) in infants
   d. is a direct cause of decreased intelligence in patients with meningomyelocele
4. Surgery for meningomyelocele:
   a. should not be delayed beyond 48 hours as the infant has an increased risk of developing ventriculitis or sepsis
   b. if completely withheld, does not change the mortality rate of these infants
   c. has the same effect on the recovery of neurologic deficits associated with the lesion whether it is performed early or late
   d. if done on all infants who present with meningomyelocele, will guarantee a high percentage of surviving patients unable to function at all socially

5. Preoperative evaluation of the infant by the anesthesiologist is essential, and must consider all of the following *except:*
   a. Patients with meningomyelocele delivered by cesarean section have less injury than those delivered vaginally.
   b. Infants with high thoracic or cervical lesions may have paralysis of intercostal and abdominal musculature and limited respiratory reserve.
   c. Meningomyelocele infants presenting for surgery rarely have problems with fluid status or temperature control.
   d. Meningomyelocele infants may have stridor, apnea, and gastro-esophageal reflux associated with Chiari II malformations.

6. Effects of atropine, often used as a preoperative medication in infants with meningomyelocele, has the effect of:
   a. increasing vagal tone
   b. increasing lower esophageal sphincter tone
   c. decreasing gastric acidity while increasing gastric fluid volume
   d. decreasing oral and pharyngeal secretions

7. The following statements all apply to temperature control in infants with meningomyelocele *except:*
   a. The central nervous system control of temperature in infants with meningomyelocele is normal.
   b. These infants cannot shiver, and must use brown fat to generate heat.
   c. Paralysis, if present, decreases the metabolic rate and thus the ability to generate heat.
   d. Infants lose heat rapidly because of a high surface area to volume ratio.

8. The following methods of inducing anesthesia in infants with meningomyelocele are all acceptable *except:*
   a. awake intubation with the patient left side down followed by an inhalation induction via the endotracheal tube
   b. an I.V. induction with sodium thiopental followed by a nondepolarizing muscle relaxant to facilitate intubation
   c. intramuscular ketamine followed by establishing an I.V. route and giving succinylcholine to facilitate intubation
   d. an inhalation induction by mask followed by establishing an I.V. route and giving a nondepolarizing muscle relaxant to facilitate intubation

9. Infants with meningomyelocele commonly have problems intra-operatively with all of the following *except:*
   a. significant blood loss requiring transfusion
   b. hypothermia requiring active measures to maintain normal temperature
   c. ventilatory compromise from incorrectly placed thoracic or abdominal bolsters

    d. life-threatening increases in ICP
10. Postoperatively, the infant with meningomyelocele:
    a. will be nursed in the prone position
    b. can always be extubated immediately
    c. has the same risk of apnea postanesthetically as any other infant of similar gestational age
    d. does not need further protection against hypothermia

Chapter 6

1. Which condition is most likely to be associated with poor outcome in a child with tracheoesophageal fistula (TEF)?
    a. birth weight between 1800gm and 2500gm
    b. tetralogy of Fallot
    c. anal atresia
    d. radial limb dysplasia
2. Gastrostomy is indicated initially:
    a. in all patients
    b. only in babies under 2500gm
    c. in critically ill babies under 1800gm
    d. in babies with pure esophageal atresia
3. The most common type of TEF and EA is:
    a. type A
    b. type B
    c. type C
    d. type D
4. Primary definitive repair is performed:
    a. in infants over 1800gm
    b. only when no cardiac anomalies are present
    c. after treatment of aspiration is completed
    d. as an elective procedure after hyperalimentation
5. Preoperatively, during transport and for endotracheal intubation the infant with TEF and EA should be positioned in the:
    a. Trendelenburg position
    b. reverse Trendelenburg position
    c. right lateral decubitus position
    d. left lateral decubitus position
6. The anesthetic plan for the infant with TEF and EA includes:
    a. awake intubation
    b. continuous suctioning of the proximal pouch
    c. intravenous atropine prior to induction
    d. all of the above
7. The most common cardiac lesion associated with TEF and EA is:
    a. ventricular septal defect
    b. pulmonic stenosis

    c. coarctation of the aorta

    d. aortic stenosis

8. The definitive finding for the diagnosis of TEF and EA is:
   a. inability to pass a soft rubber catheter through the nose
   b. demonstration by chest x-ray of a catheter curled in the upper esophagus
   c. large amounts of thick secretions noted at birth
   d. choking with feedings

9. The incidence of TEF and EA is:
   a. 1/3000–1/4000 live births
   b. 1/10,000–1/11,000 live births
   c. 1/1000 live births
   d. 1/8000 live births

10. The percentage of infants with TEF who are premature is approximately:
   a. 50%
   b. 80%
   c. 30%
   d. no association; TEF is related to the sex of the child

Chapter 7

1. Hypotension in burn patients occurs because of:
   a. increased vascular permeability leading to decreased intravascular volume
   b. release of histamine and prostaglandins
   c. loss of skin barrier leading to hypoproteinemia
   d. all of the above

2. Volume replacement:
   a. should be given as rapidly as possible for the first 24 hours of hospitalization after thermal injury
   b. should contain 10% dextrose
   c. may result in generalized edema because of increased vascular permeability
   d. can cause edema that is limited to the burn site

3. Routine therapy for burn patients includes all of the following *except:*
   a. tetanus prophylaxis
   b. full-thickness-wound biopsy to identify organisms prior to clinical evidence of infection
   c. prophylactic intravenous antibiotics
   d. monitoring of antibiotic level after intravenous antibiotics are started

4. Mortality in burn patients is most directly affected by:

    a. age
    b. percent of body surface area affected
    c. inhalation injury
    d. depth of burn
5. A difference between pediatric and adult patients is that:
    a. adults require more glucose during resuscitaton
    b. adults are more likely to have airway obstruction after inhalation injury
    c. adults have higher baseline relative O_2 and metabolic demands, which are increased with large surface burns
    d. adults have more respiratory reserve, and fatigue less rapidly with the increased work associated with respiratory tract injury
6. Carbon monoxide:
    a. is a foul-smelling gas with a high affinity for hemoglobin
    b. inhalation causes a fall in PaO_2
    c. in the blood may cause nausea, dizziness, and headache
    d. can result in coma at concentrations of 5% carboxyhemoglobin
7. Intraoperative management of the burn victim should include all of the following *except:*
    a. warmed intravenous fluids to avoid hypothermia
    b. ready use of surgical placement of intravenous cannulae if there are extensive skin burns
    c. central venous pressure measurements
    d. urinary catheter
8. Anesthetic management of the burn victim should include:
    a. heavy sedation prior to examination of possibly injured airways
    b. avoidance of narcotics because of patient's altered metabolism
    c. avoidance of positive end-expiratory pressure (PEEP) in the presence of airway injury
    d. inflation of endotracheal cuff just enough to prevent a leak
9. In burn patients:
    a. use of succinylcholine should be completely avoided because of risk of hyperkalemia
    b. use of all muscle relaxants should be avoided because of their prolonged action
    c. nondepolarizing muscle relaxants can be safely used up to 25% of the usual dose
    d. reversal of muscle relaxants requires the usual dose
10. All of the following regarding topical antibiotics in burn patients are true *except:*
    a. Topical antibiotics have been found to increase bacterial superinfection.
    b. Mafenide can cause a metabolic acidosis and pain upon application

   c. Silver nitrate often stains skin and clothing.
   d. Silver sulfadiazine has less toxicity and intermediate absorption when compared to other topical agents.

Chapter 8

1. The definitive treatment for paranasal sinusitis related to nasotracheal intubation is:
   a. surgical drainage of the maxillary sinus
   b. instillation of antibiotics through the tube
   c. antibiotic treatment alone
   d. removal of the nasal tube and a course of antibiotics
2. Complement activation in sepsis is associated with:
   a. a diffuse maculopapular rash
   b. peripheral, symmetric polyneuropathy
   c. aggregation of granulocytes
   d. disturbances of GI tract motility
3. The myocardial depression seen in sepsis may be caused by:
   a. a circulating depressant factor
   b. global myocardial ischemia
   c. bacterial invasion of the heart
   d. hypoxic myocardial dysfunction
4. Survivors of human septic shock differ from nonsurvivors in that:
   a. they show less severe metabolic acidosis
   b. their pulmonary compliances remain normal
   c. they show a reversible decrease in ejection fraction
   d. they maintain adequate cerebral perfusion
5. The incidence of sepsis is rising for all the following reasons *except:*
   a. the increased use of invasive procedures
   b. the prevalence of acquired immunodeficiency syndrome
   c. the aging of the patient population
   d. the emergence of multiply resistant bacteria
6. A patient who does not have fever during a bacteremic episode:
   a. has only a minor bacteremia
   b. has high levels of endogenous cortisol
   c. probably has a superficial infection
   d. is at high risk of dying
7. The first step in treating sepsis is:
   a. ventilation with 100% oxygen
   b. starting a norepinephrine infusion
   c. making the diagnosis of sepsis
   d. starting antibiotics
8. Acute acalculous cholecystitis is best diagnosed by:
   a. PIPIDA scintigraphy

  b. clinical criteria alone

  c. percutaneous samples of bile for smear and culture

  d. gallium scan of the abdomen

9. The nutritional support of the septic patient involves all of the following *except:*

  a. 35–40 kcal/kg/day

  b. 1.5–2gm protein/kg/day

  c. 70% of total calories as lipid

  d. not more than 5–6mg carbohydrate/kg/min

10. Corticosteroids in septic shock:

  a. slow the clearance of bacteria from the circulation

  b. may be of use in certain patients if used early

  c. increase serum levels of prostacyclin

  d. reduce the inflammatory response to endotoxin

Chapter 9

1. The most common types of lung tumors are:

  a. hamartomas

  b. benign lesions

  c. adenocarcinomas

  d. squamous cell carcinomas

2. With appropriate staging, the incidence of unnecessary thoracotomy is about:

  a. 40%

  b. 20%

  c. 5%

  d. less than 1%

3. Candidates for surgical resection of lung tumors include patients with:

  a. small-cell carcinomas

  b. extrathoracic metastases

  c. ipsilateral hilar and peribronchial involvement

  d. malignant pleural effusions

4. Lobectomy:

  a. is the treatment of choice for lung carcinoma

  b. can be performed if there is involvement of the mainstem bronchus

  c. has a mortality rate of 10%

  d. is considered in all patients with small-cell carcinoma

5. Which of the following is least useful in treating post-thoracotomy pain?

  a. transcutaneous electrical nerve stimulation (TENS)

  b. epidural opioids

  c. cryoanalgesia

    d. intrapleural local anesthetics

6. Patients with the greatest risk for lung resection include all of the following *except:*
    a. $PaCO_2 > 45$ mmHg
    b. recent myocardial infarction
    c. cor pulmonale
    d. recent coronary artery bypass graft (CABG)

7. Cessation of smoking one week prior to surgery will:
    a. improve pulmonary function studies
    b. precipitate withdrawal
    c. reduce carboxyhemoglobin levels
    d. increase PaO_2

8. Signs of decompensated cor pulmonale include all of the following *except:*
    a. tender liver
    b. râles
    c. peripheral edema
    d. jugular venous distention

9. True statements about intraoperative monitoring include all the following *except:*
    a. An arterial line should be used with double-lumen endobronchial tubes.
    b. Pulmonary diastolic pressures may be substantially elevated above pulmonary wedge pressures with severe lung disease.
    c. Central venous pressure always provides accurate information about left heart filling pressures in patients with pulmonary disease.
    d. A spirometer is useful for determining pulmonary compliance.

10. Correct steps to prevent arterial hypoxemia include all of the following *except:*
    a. maintaining dual lung ventilation as long as possible
    b. using a tidal volume of 10ml/kg during one-lung ventilation
    c. avoiding N_2O during one-lung ventilation
    d. maintaining hypocapnea to maximize hypoxic vasoconstriction

Chapter 10

1. The percentage of cardiac output that travels to the liver is:
    a. 5%
    b. 15%
    c. 25%
    d. 40%

2. The best biochemical index to assess the severity of hepatocellular dysfunction in a patient with chronic liver disease is:
    a. prothrombin time

  b. partial thromboplastin time
  c. Factor VIII level
  d. serum albumin
3. The effect of systemic hypotension on hepatic blood volume is:
  a. an increase
  b. a decrease
  c. no effect
  d. dependent on acid-base balance
4. The cardiovascular system of a patient presenting for hepatic transplantation can typically be characterized by:
  a. extreme instability
  b. decreased pulse pressure
  c. increased systemic vascular resistance
  d. a high cardiac index and wide pulse pressure
5. The thromboelastograph can:
  a. indicate platelet count
  b. pinpoint the cause of bleeding disorders
  c. detect the presence of heparin
  d. differentiate coagulopathy from surgical bleeding
6. The postanhepatic phase of a liver transplant begins with:
  a. application of the vascular clamps to the blood supply of the native liver
  b. removal of the native liver
  c. reperfusion of the donor liver
  d. the onset of the venovenous bypass
7. All of the following factors contribute to ascites formation *except:*
  a. increased plasma colloid oncotic pressure
  b. portal hypertension
  c. impaired water excretion
  d. increased flow of hepatic lymph
8. Advantages of venovenous bypass include all of the following except:
  a. enhancement of cardiovascular stability during the anhepatic phase
  b. decreased intraoperative acidosis
  c. increased venous stasis in the gut
  d. increased time available for the surgical revascularization
9. Deleterious side effects of vasopressin include:
  a. coronary ischemia
  b. thrombocytopenia
  c. decreased portal venous pressure
  d. all of the above
10. Prothrombin time is sensitive to all of the following coagulation factors except:
  a. Factor II

    b. Factor VII
    c. Factor IX
    d. Factor X

Chapter 11

1. Short acting barbiturates administered prior to ECT:
   a. raise the seizure threshold
   b. lower the seizure threshold
   c. have no interactions with antidepressants
   d. have no interactions with phenothiazines
2. Hypertensive patients during ECT may show:
   a. exaggerated pressor response
   b. blunted pressor response
   c. same response as in a normotensive patient
   d. none of the above
3. The most common induction agent used in ECT is:
   a. methohexital
   b. thiopental
   c. diazepam
   d. midazolam
4. Medications that should be discontinued prior to ECT are:
   a. calcium channel blockers
   b. beta-adrenergic blockers
   c. antiarrhythmic agents
   d. MAO inhibitors
5. The anticholinergic premedication of choice in patients on phenothiazines is:
   a. atropine
   b. scopolamine
   c. glycopyrrolate
   d. anticholinergic medication is contraindicated
6. Tricyclic antidepressants:
   a. interfere with intraneuronal metabolism of catecholamines
   b. increase the rate of synthesis of dopaminergic precursors
   c. interfere with neuronal reuptake of norepinephrine
   d. increase intraneuronal metabolism of catecholamines
7. Monoamine oxidase inhibitors:
   a. decrease the rate of synthesis of norepinephrine
   b. need not be discontinued prior to general anesthesia
   c. interfere with intraneuronal enzymatic degradation of catecholamines
   d. decrease neuronal reuptake of norepinephrine
8. Administration of succinylcholine to modify ECT:

a. precedes administration of a short-acting barbiturate
b. follows administration of a short-acting barbiturate
c. requires pretreatment with a non-depolarizing agent
d. is frequently associated with post-fasciculation muscle pain

9. A patient on phenothiazine and tricyclic antidepressant therapy who is scheduled for ECT may have the following response to anesthesia:
   a. severe hypotension
   b. severe hypertension
   c. cardiac arrhythmias
   d. all of the above

10. The proper choice and dosage of muscle relaxant for ECT in a patient on lithium therapy is:
    a. 0.5mg/kg of succinylcholine
    b. a decreased dose of succinylcholine because of anticipated increased sensitivity to the drug
    c. an increased dose of succinylcholine in the range of double the calculated dose
    d. pancuronium 0.1mg/kg

Chapter 12

1. Immersion into the lithotriptor water bath is associated with all of the following changes *except:*
   a. an increase in cardiac output
   b. an increased incidence of dysrhythmias
   c. an initial increase in mean arterial pressure
   d. an increase in central venous pressure

2. Of the 250,000 patients hospitalized each year with renal calculi, the majority:
   a. are admitted for pain control
   b. are black women
   c. have congenital anomalies
   d. have calculi 1cm in size

3. All of the following are factors contributing to stone formation *except:*
   a. paraplegia
   b. dehydration
   c. sex
   d. anemia

4. Shock wave characteristics that make ESWL suitable as a noninvasive treatment include:
   a. its sinusoidal pressure variation
   b. its ability to be generated outside the body
   c. rapid attenuation on encountering biological tissue

    d. its exclusively high-frequency composition

5. All of the following are true of shock waves *except:*
    a. they should preferably pass through fluid-air transition zones
    b. they are focused onto a circular area, located 24cm above the electrode at the second focus
    c. they cause shear and tear forces when encountering a change in acoustic impedance
    d. they are 1000× more powerful than ultrasonic waves

6. Regional anesthesia:
    a. must encompass segments T12–L4, which are the renal tract innervation
    b. allows the patient to assist with his position, thereby decreasing the number of lifting personnel needed
    c. provides inadequate anesthesia
    d. has a shorter preparation time

7. The advantages of general anesthesia include all of the following *except:*
    a. superior postoperative pain relief
    b. greater patient acceptance
    c. ability to allow more precise localization and fixation of the urinary calculus, especially when high-frequency jet ventilation (HFJV) is utilized
    d. greater predictability

8. Dysrhythmias associated with ESWL:
    a. are observed in 80% of all patients
    b. may include premature ventricular contractions as well as supraventricular contractions
    c. may be prevented by maintaining a fast rate with atropine
    d. are prevented by triggering the shock wave to be delivered 20msec after the R wave

9. The hemodynamic changes associated with immersion into a water bath are such that:
    a. a patient with valvular disease is best given regional anesthesia and fluid boluses
    b. a pulmonary artery catheter may be indicated for a patient with ischemic heart disease
    c. a patient with a history of congestive heart failure and a pacemaker should never undergo ESWL
    d. there is very little change in the intrathoracic blood volume

10. The least likely complication associated with the use of ESWL is:
    a. perinephric hematomas
    b. neurologic injury
    c. urosepsis
    d. intractable pain

Chapter 13

1. The most probable cause of early (first trimester) abortion is:
   a. nutritional disorders
   b. infection
   c. fetal genetic abnormalities
   d. cervical incompetence
2. The critical period of organogenesis in gestational days is:
   a. 2–8
   b. 8–15
   c. 13–60
   d. 56–112
3. Which anesthetic agents have been found to be teratogenic in animal studies?
   a. halothane
   b. nitrous oxide
   c. both
   d. neither
4. Which anesthetic agents have been shown to be teratogenic in humans?
   a. halothane
   b. nitrous oxide
   c. both
   d. neither
5. The most important consideration in deciding patient position for cerclage is:
   a. aortocaval compression; therefore, the uterus should be displaced to the left
   b. aspiration prophylaxis; therefore, the patient should be positioned in the head-up position
   c. pressure on the fetal membranes; therefore, the patient should be placed in the Trendelenberg position
   d. uterine perfusion; therefore, the patient should remain in the sitting position
6. Which is the vasopressor of choice during pregnancy?
   a. ephedrine
   b. phenylephrine
   c. epinephrine
   d. methoxamine
7. Which of the following statements about the preoperative assessment is incorrect?
   a. It is important to ask the patient about nutritional status and possible metabolic disorders.
   b. A preoperative chest film should be obtained in all cases.

    c. Appropriate lab evaluation consists of hemoglobin, platelets, and glucose.

    d. One should auscultate for new murmurs and inquire about dyspnea, since the cardiac output begins to rise in the first trimester.

8. Which choice of anesthetic is appropriate for a woman in the 13th week of gestation without significant preoperative findings?
    a. spinal anesthesia at L4–5 with a 25-gauge needle using 6mg hyperbaric tetracaine
    b. epidural anesthesia at L3–4 with 10ml of 3% chloroprocaine
    c. general anesthesia with rapid-sequence-induction endotracheal intubation and maintenance with nitrous oxide and halothane
    d. all of the above

9. For general anesthesia for cerclage, which induction sequence can be recommended for the otherwise healthy patient?
    a. thiamylal-succinylcholine
    b. ketamine-atracurium
    c. midazolam-vecuronium
    d. all of the above

10. Which of the following should be recommended to the gravida requesting the anesthetic method with the least drug exposure to the fetus?
    a. general anesthesia
    b. spinal anesthesia with bupivacaine
    c. epidural anesthesia with lidocaine
    d. spinal anesthesia with tetracaine

Chapter 14

1. Of the following, choose the statement that is true about brain tumors.
    a. Primary tumors occur most often in patients between 30 and 40 years of age.
    b. Lung and breast are the most common primary sites of metastatic intracranial tumors.
    c. They occur most commonly in the posterior fossa.
    d. Glioblastomas have uniformly good prognoses with surgical excision.

2. Of the following, choose the least true statement concerning presenting signs and symptoms of brain tumors.
    a. Altered neuronal excitability may be manifested as generalized seizures.
    b. Characteristically, patients will complain of a headache that worsens with ambulation.

   c. Direct local tissue destruction produces neurologic deficits that are immediately dense and complete.

   d. Classic symptoms of raised ICP include diplopia and an occipital headache on awakening.

3. In monitoring ICP:

   a. subdural pressure monitoring is usually performed over the occipital region

   b. intracranial compliance is best derived using subdural pressure monitoring

   c. ventricular pressure monitoring carries the lowest risk of hemorrhage and infection

   d. the contralateral laterally displaced ventricle is catheterized for ventricular pressure monitoring

4. Cerebral blood flow:

   a. is constant as increased oxygen demand is met solely by increased oxygen extraction

   b. increases linearly at a slope of 2%/mmHg decrease in PaO_2 below a PaO_2 of 80mmHg

   c. is effectively lowered by hyperventilation, and at a $PaCO_2$ of 20mmHg flow is halved

   d. is controlled by autoregulation, which is a neurogenic response dependent on an intact sympathetic nervous system

5. In patients with an intracranial mass the least true statement is:

   a. ECG changes most commonly are tachycardia, prolonged QT interval, large U waves, and T- and ST-wave changes

   b. dexamethasone is routinely given because of the highly stressful nature of a craniotomy

   c. drug-induced sedation may mask decreasing levels of consciousness that may accompany increases in ICP

   d. steroid administration may lead to increases in intravascular volume and hypertension

6. The following is true about venous air embolism (VAE):

   a. VAE is a risk only in the sitting position.

   b. The precordial Doppler is the most sensitive monitor to detect VAE, detecting air at 1ml/kg/min.

   c. Increasing end-tidal nitrogen is a useful means of detecting VAE if a mass spectrometer is used.

   d. A paradoxical air embolus may occur through a probe-patent foramen ovale, which is present in 50% of the population.

7. In considering the effects of anesthetic agents on CBF and ICP:

   a. enflurane produces greater cerebral vasodilatation than halothane

   b. prior hyperventilation is necessary to prevent increased CBF with isoflurane administration

   c. enflurane may cause seizure activity on the EEG in the presence of hypocarbia

    d. N$_2$O effectively decreases CBF but may lead to postoperative pneumocephalus

8. Concerning adjuvants to decrease ICP and provide cerebral protection:
   a. mannitol is not associated with rebound intracranial hypertension
   b. disadvantages of urea include venoirritation, renal reabsorption, and rebound intracranial hypertension
   c. glucose infusion is necessary to provide cerebral energy intraoperatively
   d. phenytoin decreases blood glucose by stimulating insulin secretion

9. Of the following, choose the statement that is true about the intracranial contents.
   a. Tumors with a volume less than 200ml have no effect on ICP.
   b. The critical level of CPP is 25mmHg.
   c. CSF is secreted by arachnoid villi and reabsorbed by the choroid plexus.
   d. Blood in the intracranial vessels constitutes 5% of the intracranial contents.

10. Of the following, choose the statement that is true concerning intracranial dynamics.
   a. Compensation for increased brain bulk is initially via translocation of CSF to the spinal space.
   b. CSF production decreases acutely as ICP increases.
   c. A waves are periods of lowered ICP to improve CPP.
   d. The cardiovascular response to rising ICP is systemic hypotension to decrease CBF and thus reduce ICP.

Chapter 15

1. Normal intraocular pressure (IOP) is:
   a. 10–20mmHg
   b. 3–5mmHg
   c. greater than 25mmHg
   d. zero

2. Intraocular pressure is determined by:
   a. the amount of aqueous humor
   b. choroidal blood volume
   c. the amount of vitreous humor
   d. all of the above

3. Aqueous humor:
   a. is produced mainly in the anterior chamber
   b. is produced mainly via an active secretory process involving carbonic anhydrase

    c. drains through the canal of Schlemm into the circle of Willis

    d. outflow is inhibited by miotic agents

4. All of the following are true *except:*

    a. Coughing can increase IOP 30–40mmHg

    b. IOP increases with respiratory acidosis due to vasodilation.

    c. Hypoxia increases IOP.

    d. A Valsalva maneuver lowers IOP.

5. Succinylcholine, when used alone:

    a. causes a dose-dependent increase in IOP

    b. has never led to a loss of intraocular contents

    c. is the muscle relaxant of choice for a rapid-sequence induction

    d. lowers IOP when used in very high doses

6. All of the following are true *except:*

    a. Inhalation agents diminish IOP.

    b. Free water can lower IOP.

    c. CNS depressants lower IOP.

    d. Miotic agents can lessen IOP.

7. The muscle relaxant that lowers IOP most is:

    a. vecuronium

    b. succinylcholine

    c. curare

    d. gallamine

8. All of the following are true *except:*

    a. Nonpenetrating corneal foreign bodies can be removed under local anesthesia.

    b. Foreign bodies in the anterior chamber are removed via an incision at the corneoscleral limbus.

    c. Metallic foreign bodies can be removed with the aid of a magnet.

    d. It is best to wait until intraocular foreign bodies have become enmeshed in fibrin before removing them.

9. Bucking at the time of extubation can raise IOP and place the surgical closure in jeopardy. Bucking can be safely minimized by all of the following methods *except:*

    a. small dose of succinylcholine

    b. lidocaine 1.5mg/kg intravenously

    c. adequate narcotization

    d. deep extubation despite the presence of a full stomach

10. All children with open eye injuries:

    a. should have preoperative blood work and an intravenous line

    b. should have their parents remain with them if possible, to prevent them from crying

    c. must be separated from their parents before entering the operating room

    d. are absolute emergencies and cannot wait several hours for surgical correction

Chapter 16

1. Factors that affect airway management in patients with maxillofacial trauma include:
   a. presence of airway obstruction
   b. cervical and skull fractures
   c. associated injuries
   d. all of the above

2. Which portion of the mandible is most frequently broken?
   a. the condylar neck
   b. the symphysis
   c. the ramus
   d. the coronoid process

3. After a bilateral mandibular fracture, airway obstruction results from:
   a. laryngeal obstruction
   b. tracheobronchial disruption
   c. obstruction by the maxilla
   d. displacement of the tongue against the posterior pharyngeal wall

4. LeFort I fractures:
   a. never result in airway obstruction
   b. are dental-alveolar fractures
   c. extend through the orbital rim
   d. are the most common of the LeFort injuries

5. All of the following are true of a LeFort II injury *except:*
   a. It can be associated with a fracture of the cribriform plate
   b. It can cause airway obstruction by posterior displacement of the maxilla.
   c. It results in craniofacial dysjunction.
   d. It results in a pyramid-shaped fracture.

6. A LeFort III fracture:
   a. is a pyramidal fracture
   b. causes craniofacial dysjunction
   c. is a dental-alveolar fracture
   d. includes bilateral mandibular (Andy Gump) fractures

7. Airway obstruction from maxillofacial injuries can result from:
   a. blood, teeth, dentures, and bony fragments in the oropharynx
   b. pharyngeal obstruction from bilateral mandibular fractures
   c. posterior displacement of the mobile maxilla
   d. all of the above

8. Tracheostomy is indicated:
   a. in all maxillofacial injuries
   b. as a life-saving maneuver in the emergency room
   c. if concomitant laryngeal or tracheal disruption is present
   d. in the presence of any airway obstruction in patients with maxillary fractures

9. Most repairs of facial lacerations:
   a. are performed under general anesthesia at the time of injury
   b. are done with local anesthesia
   c. do not need to be done in the operating room if sedatives are given
   d. require lidocaine without any epinephrine
10. All of the following techniques can be used to minimize intraoperative blood loss *except:*
    a. reverse Trendelenberg of 15–30°
    b. controlled hypotension
    c. positive end-expiratory pressure
    d. subcutaneous epinephrine

Chapter 17

1. The incidence of hydrocephalus in the pediatric population is:
   a. approximately 1:1000 as a single entity
   b. increased with maternal age
   c. approximately 8:1000 when associated with meningomyelocele
   d. decreasing with improved prenatal care
2. CSF production will increase when:
   a. mean arterial pressure is lowered
   b. mean arterial pressure is raised
   c. high-dose steroids are given
   d. none of the above occurs
3. CSF is absorbed:
   a. via CNS lymphatics
   b. via active pumping of ions across choroidal cells
   c. at the arachnoid villi via vacuoles
   d. across the dura into the epidural space
4. Of the following, the *least* likely to be associated with acute hydrocephalus is:
   a. headache
   b. pituitary abnormalities
   c. nausea/vomiting
   d. coma
5. Which of the following would be a contraindication for shunt placement?
   a. unresectable lesion
   b. history of abdominal surgery
   c. acute ventriculitis
   d. reversible neurologic defects
6. Normal-pressure hydrocephalus is characterized by:
   a. sixth nerve palsy, decreased olfaction, dysphagia
   b. seizures, headaches, vomiting
   c. papilledema, optic atrophy, mental status changes

d. gait disturbances, mental status changes, incontinence in adults
7. Complications particular to VA shunts include:
   a. infection
   b. intestinal obstruction
   c. renal insufficiency
   d. shunt obstruction
8. Induction agents suitable for patients with hydrocephalus include all of the following *except:*
   a. lidocaine
   b. fentanyl
   c. ketamine
   d. thiamylal
9. Maintenance of anesthesia may *best* be accomplished by:
   a. O_2/N_2O/halothane
   b. O_2/N_2O/fentanyl drip
   c. O_2/isoflurane/fentanyl drip
   d. O_2/enflurane/fentanyl drip
10. Prior to extubation, all of the following must be accomplished *except:*
    a. complete removal of the lesion
    b. assessment of patient's ability to maintain his airway
    c. reversal of residual muscle blockade
    d. return of adequate spontaneous ventilation

Chapter 18

1. Ideal qualities of irrigating solutions for TURP include all of the following *except:*
   a. hyposmolar solution
   b. nonhemolytic
   c. electrically inert
   d. nontoxic
2. Approximately what percentage of irrigating solution is absorbed directly into the blood vessels during TURP?
   a. 5%
   b. 97%
   c. 29%
   d. 50%
3. Symptoms of glycine toxicity include:
   a. seizures
   b. diaphoresis
   c. transient blindness
   d. hearing loss
4. The most significant contributory factor in mortality due to bladder perforation is:

a. location of perforation
b. delay of diagnosis
c. type of irrigating solution used
d. age greater than 65 years

5. Complications of TURP include all of the following *except:*
a. hyponatremia
b. circulatory overload with congestive heart failure
c. sepsis
d. hypernatremia

6. The amount of absorption of irrigating fluid is least dependent on:
a. the height of the container of irrigating fluid above the surgical table
b. the length of time of the resection
c. the size of the prostate gland
d. the type of irrigating solution used

7. Hyponatremia is *least* likely to cause:
a. bradycardia
b. widening of the QRS complex
c. tachycardia
d. T-wave inversion

8. Rapid correction of hyponatremia may result in all of the following except:
a. pulmonary edema
b. disseminated intravascular coagulopathy
c. pontine myelinolysis
d. death

9. Distilled water is not used as an irrigating solution today because:
a. it has poor optical qualities
b. it facilitates dispersion of high-frequency current from the resectoscope
c. it causes transient blindness
d. it is extremely hypotonic

10. Coagulopathy after TURP is most probably due to:
a. DIC with secondary fibrinolysis
b. hyponatremia
c. thromboplastin destruction
d. aspirin ingestion

Chapter 19

1. Patients presenting for thyroidectomy are *least* likely to be:
a. euthyroid
b. hypothyroid
c. hyperthyroid
d. in a fluctuating state

2. Thioureylenes act by inhibiting:
   a. iodide uptake
   b. iodination and coupling
   c. peripheral deiodination of T_4
   d. TSH production by anterior pituitary
3. Protein binding of thyroid hormone is inhibited by all of the following *except:*
   a. thiobarbiturates
   b. salicylates
   c. testosterone
   d. estrogens
4. Most of the thyroid nodules diagnosed as "cold" by thyroid scans are:
   a. benign
   b. metastatic disease
   c. malignant
   d. abscesses
5. All of the following symptoms are common in hyperthyroid patients *except:*
   a. increased nervousness
   b. increased perspiration
   c. cold intolerance
   d. palpitations
6. Antithyroid agents can cause:
   a. granulocytopenia
   b. thrombocytopenia
   c. anemia
   d. prolongation of coagulation time
7. The anesthetic method of choice for thyroidectomy is:
   a. local
   b. high spinal
   c. general endotracheal
   d. cervical plexus block
8. The "thyroid storm":
   a. is best prevented
   b. has to be differentiated from malignant hyperthermia
   c. carries a 10% mortality
   d. is characterized by all of the above
9. The recurrent laryngeal nerves:
   a. always lie within the body of the gland
   b. supply only the vocal cords
   c. are most commonly damaged on one side only
   d. provide sensory innervation of the larynx
10. The muscle(s) most sensitive to calcium deficiency is (are):
    a. the diaphragm

b. intrinsic muscles of the larynx
c. the myocardium
d. vascular smooth muscle

Chapter 20

1. Which of the following viruses are herpesviruses?
   a. cytomegalovirus
   b. varicella-zoster virus
   c. Epstein-Barr virus
   d. all of the above
2. What percentage of adults in the United States is seropositive for chickenpox?
   a. 75%
   b. 22%
   c. 96%
   d. 51%
3. Which age group has the highest incidence of mortality when exposed to chickenpox?
   a. <1 year old
   b. 1–10 years old
   c. 10–19 years old
   d. >19 years old
4. The varicella-zoster virus replicates in:
   a. pacinian corpuscles
   b. epithelial derivatives of organ systems
   c. mucoid droplets
   d. intranuclear inclusion bodies
5. The chest x-ray of varicella pneumonitis demonstrates:
   a. perihilar nodular densities
   b. pneumothoraces
   c. pulmonary edema
   d. bronchiectasis
6. Lumbar puncture of patients with varicella-induced meningoen-cephalitis reveals:
   a. increased lymphocytes, PMNs. and granulocytes
   b. increased glucose and protein
   c. varicella-zoster particles
   d. xanthochromia
7. The liver function test that is often elevated in patients with varicella-induced hepatitis is:
   a. prothrombin time
   b. total bilirubin
   c. albumin
   d. SGOT

8. VZ globulin is used in chickenpox for:
   a. curing varicella
   b. stimulating antibody development
   c. attenuating the clinical course
   d. alleviating pulmonary symptoms
9. Acyclovir acts on the VZ virus by:
   a. prevention of viral attachment to cell membranes
   b. inhibiting DNA polymerase
   c. increasing levels of cAMP
   d. immunosuppressing host defenses
10. A patient exposed to chickenpox is infectious during which period?
   a. throughout the course of the disease
   b. 24 hours prior to the appearance of the exanthem
   c. up to 2 weeks after all lesions are crusted
   d. 5 days prior to the development of fever

Chapter 21

1. Factors associated with a poor prognosis in RA patients include:
   a. thrombocytopenia and a hematocrit of more than 35
   b. Caucausian race, age of 50 years, and male sex
   c. combination of hypertension and diabetes
   d. thrombocytosis, vasculitis, and female sex
2. Potential airway management difficulty is most likely with:
   a. sleeping stridor and cricoarytenoid arthritis
   b. visualization of the uvula and dysphagia
   c. TMJ greater than 3cm and a large tongue
   d. edentulous mouth with oral candidiasis
3. Laryngeal abnormalities in the RA patient include:
   a. caudal displacement and rightward deviation
   b. leftward deviation and caudal displacement
   c. leftward rotation and rightward deviation
   d. less mobile vocal cords and leftward deviation
4. Cervical spine involvement in the RA patient includes:
   a. caudad odontoid migration and subluxation at C1–2
   b. subaxial subluxation and atlantoaxial subluxation
   c. atlantoaxial subluxation and tracheal elevation
   d. dizziness with neck movement and a normal TMJ
5. The axial cruciform ligament fixes the odontoid process and includes
   the following ligaments:
   a. transverse and horizontal ligaments
   b. alar ligament and hilar bands
   c. superior and inferior longitudinal bands
   d. intermediate and intramediate ligaments
6. Impending neuropathology in the RA patient is indicated by:

   a. cervical subluxation less than 10%
   b. pain radiating to lumbar spine
   c. inferior migration of the odontoid process
   d. an atlas/odontoid interval greater than 3cm
7. Which of the following systems is *least* likely to be affected by rheumatoid arthritis?
   a. immunologic
   b. hematologic
   c. respiratory
   d. renal
6. Impending neuropathology in the RA patient is indicated by:
   a. cervical subluxation less than 10%
   b. pain radiating to lumbar spine
   c. inferior migration of the odontoid process
   d. an atlas/odontoid interval greater than 3 cm
7. Which of the following systems is *least* likely to be affected by rheumatoid arthritis?
   a. immunologic
   b. hematologic
   c. liver
   d. kidney
8. Preoperative assessment of the patient with severe RA could reveal all *except:*
   a. hypochromic macrocytic anemia
   b. valvular dysfunction or dysrhythmia
   c. temporomandibular dysfunction
   d. renal amyloidosis
9. Medication side effects noted in the RA patient include:
   a. marrow depression and polycythemia
   b. renal dysfunction and rigidity
   c. rigidity and edema
   d. adrenal suppression and marrow suppression
10. The method of intubation *least* desirable in the RA patient is:
    a. fiberoptic
    b. blind nasal
    c. tracheostomy
    d. retrograde

Chapter 22

1. The incidence of cataract disease:
   a. diminishes with increasing age of the population
   b. is significant only in industrialized countries
   c. as shown in the Framingham Study is about 16%
   d. is not expected to alter over the next 30 years

2. Causes of cataracts: Which of the following statements is true?
   a. The most frequent cause of cataracts is congenital problems.
   b. Diabetes insipidus is associated with increased risk of cataracts.
   c. Ultraviolet light has been proved to cause cataracts in humans.
   d. Myotonic dystrophy is associated with increased risk of cataracts.

3. Concerning the pathophysiology of cataracts, which of the following statements is true?
   a. The physiologic changes of aging in the lens are responsible for cataracts.
   b. Exaggeration of normal sclerosis of fibers in the lens nucleus produces a nuclear cataract.
   c. Incipient cataracts show decreased fluid content compared to the normal lens.
   d. Changes in epithelial cells are not important in the development of subcapsular cataracts.

4. Opthalmologic assessment of cataract disease includes all of the following *except:*
   a. assessment of lens opacity
   b. culture and sensitivity of conjunctival fluid
   c. diagnostic ultrasound
   d. electronystagmography

5. Concerning treatment of cataract disease, which of the following is true?
   a. Extracapsular extraction is the most common form of treatment.
   b. Refractive therapy has no role.
   c. Optimal blood glucose control is unlikely to improve vision.
   d. Miotic drugs are of benefit.

6. Regional anesthesia is recommended for all patients *except:*
   a. patients with myotonic dystrophy
   b. patients with NYHA class III angina
   c. patients with severe spasmodic torticollis
   d. patients with history of cerebrovascular accident

7. The most frequent complications of regional anesthesia for eye surgery are:
   a. oculocardiac reflex during performance of the block
   b. minor local problems (ecchymosis)
   c. brain stem anesthesia
   d. intraneural injection

8. Physiologic changes of aging include all of the following *except:*
   a. loss of cellular free water
   b. reduced glomerular filtration rate
   c. increased autonomic end organ responsiveness
   d. elevated plasma epinephrine

9. Which of the following is true concerning peribulbar anesthesia?

a. Local anesthetic is placed as close as possible to the ciliary ganglion.
b. It is preceded by use of mydriatic and local anesthetic eye drops.
c. It does not cause paresis of orbicularis oculi.
d. It has achieved high patient acceptance because of its one-injection technique.

10. The awake patient undergoing eye surgery
   a. requires replacement of the fasting fluid deficit before performance of the block
   b. requires sedation to overcome anxiety
   c. is easily disturbed by extraneous conversation and noise
   d. frequently becomes restless because of the prolonged duration of surgery.

Chapter 23

1. Reduction of hematocrit from a mean of 45.2% to 35% is associated with:
   a. 35% decrease in calf blood flow at rest
   b. 56% increase in calf blood flow at rest
   c. Two fold decrease in peak flow
   d. mean hemoglobin delivery is increased by 40%

2. Fall in the colloid osmotic pressure of the plasma from 25 mm to 20 mmHg is associated with a volume deficit of:
   a. 13 liters
   b. 8 liters
   c. 5 liters
   d. no correlation

3. ST depression on ECG is caused by all of the following except:
   a. left ventricular hypertrophy
   b. digitalis overdose
   c. hyperkalemia
   d. ischemia

4. Thalium redistribution after dipyridamole indicates:
   a. blood collateral coronary circulation
   b. poor coronary perfusion to that segment
   c. improved blood flow to that segment
   d. A Robinhood effect

5. ECG changes due to ischemia are late signs and are preceeded by:
   a. reginal wall motion abnormalities
   b. increase in ventricular compliance
   c. increase in CVP
   d. decrease in lung compliance

6. Earliest consequences of myocardial ischemia include all of the following *except:*

    a. increase in PCWP in the presence of unchanged cardiac output
    b. appearance of prominent AC waves in PCWP
    c. appearance of "V" wave in PCWP
    d. inversion of "T" waves on the ECG
7. Coexisting risk factors in mortality of patients with chronic leg ischemia are all of the following except:
    a. smoking
    b. diabetes
    c. hypertension
    d. thyrotoxicosis
8. Atherosclerosis has last predilection for which vessels?
    a. coronary arteries
    b. axillary and brachial arteries
    c. carotid arteries and intracranial cerebral vessels
    d. aorta and arterial supply to the kidneys and lower legs
9. The elderly heart demonstrates all of the following *except:*
    a. increase in resistance to B-adrenergic blockade
    b. marked reduction of the tachycardic response to atropine
    c. marked increase in sensitivity to isoproterenol
    d. less flexibility as a biological pump
10. Mortality in claudicants after 10 years in comparison to the general population is:
    a. three times that of the general population
    b. about the same
    c. 80% that of general population
    d. at least 10 times higher

Chapter 24

1. Parkinson's disease results from a deficiency of dopamine in the
    a. third ventricle
    b. pons
    c. thalamus
    d. basal ganglia
2. Surgical implantation of adrenal tissue into the brain of a Parkinsonian will most likely
    a. increase dopamine stores in the substantia nigra
    b. increase secretion of epinephrine via a feedback mechanism to the adrenal medulla
    c. increase striatal levels of enkephalins
    d. decrease urinary homovanilic acid (HVA) levels
3. True statements regarding postural hypotension in the Parkinsonian are:
    a. postural hypotension may exist in the untreated Parkinsonian and in the patient treated with L-DOPA

b. Postural hypotension in the Parkinsonian may improve with age.

c. The mechanism for postural hypotension in the Parkinsonian has been elucidated

d. Postural hypotension can be treated effectively by increasing the morning dose of L-DOPA.

4. The rate-limiting step in dopamine synthesis is:
   a. Decarboxylation of L-DOPA to dopamine
   b. Deamination of dopamine to HVA
   c. Hydroxylation of L-tyrosine to L-dopa
   d. Methylation of L-DOPA to 3-methoxydopa

5. Which of the following agents may cause a Parkinsonian patient to decompensate?
   a. Ketamine
   b. Diazepam
   c. Haloperidol
   d. Sufentanil

6. Each of the following statements is true except
   a. Parkinsonian patients who are not optimally managed may suffer some degree of restrictive lung disease
   b. Hyperkalemia is a significant problem when succinylcholine is administered to the Parkinsonian patient.
   c. Parkinsonian patients may suffer altered mentation as a result of their disease or treatment.
   d. Poor nutrition may complicate the routine management of Parkinsonians.

7. Which of the following has helped reduce the incidence of untoward cardiovascular effects in patients maintained on L-DOPA?
   a. the routine use of β-blockers in these patients
   b. the use of selective MAO-B inhibitors
   c. the use of reserpine in these patients
   d. the use of peripheral decarboxylase inhibitors

8. Which of the following best explains the association between Parkinson's disease and dementia?
   a. a linked gene governing inheritance of Parkinson's and Alzheimer's disease
   b. segregation of function in the caudate nucleus
   c. degeneration of the frontal cortex
   d. Lewy Bodies can be found in the ventral thalamus and motor cortex on the postmortem exam of Parkinsonians.

9. Which represents the best rationale for the use of bromocriptine in Parkinsonian patients?
   a. Bromocriptine and L-DOPA enter the CNS to be converted to dopamine.
   b. The use of bromocriptine allows patients to better tolerate untoward effects of L-DOPA.

    c. Bromocriptine allows clinicians to use smaller doses of L-DOPA, thereby delaying the onset of tolerance.

    d. Bromocriptine has been shown to reverse the pathological changes in the brains of Parkinsonians.

10. Which statements are true regarding anesthetic management of Parkinsonians?

    a. They may suffer from a number of system disorders other than Parkinson's.

    b. They may be at higher risk of aspiration of gastric contents due to a central action of L-DOPA.

    c. They may present airway management problems due to facial rigidity.

    d. All of the above.

Answers to Self-Assessment Questions

Chapter 1	Chapter 2	Chapter 3	Chapter 4
1. a	1. c	1. a	1. b
2. c	2. b	2. d	2. a
3. b	3. c	3. b	3. d
4. c	4. a	4. d	4. d
5. c	5. b	5. c	5. c
6. b	6. c	6. a	6. a
7. b	7. b	7. b	7. b
8. b	8. c	8. c	8. c
9. a	9. a	9. a	9. b
10. d	10. d	10. d	10. a

Chapter 5	Chapter 6	Chapter 7	Chapter 8
1. b	1. b	1. d	1. d
2. d	2. c	2. c	2. c
3. a	3. c	3. c	3. a
4. c	4. a	4. c	4. c
5. c	5. b	5. d	5. b
6. d	6. d	6. c	6. d
7. a	7. a	7. b	7. c
8. c	8. b	8. d	8. a
9. d	9. a	9. d	9. c
10. a	10. c	10. a	10. b

Chapter 9	Chapter 10	Chapter 11	Chapter 12
1. d	1. c	1. a	1. c
2. b	2. d	2. a	2. a
3. c	3. b	3. a	3. d
4. a	4. d	4. d	4. b
5. a	5. d	5. c	5. a
6. d	6. c	6. c	6. b
7. c	7. a	7. c	7. a

8. b	8. c	8. b	8. b
9. c	9. a	9. d	9. b
10. d	10. c	10. b	10. d

Chapter 13	*Chapter 14*	*Chapter 15*	*Chapter 16*
1. c	1. b	1. a	1. d
2. c	2. c	2. d	2. a
3. c	3. d	3. b	3. d
4. d	4. c	4. d	4. b
5. c	5. b	5. a	5. c
6. a	6. c	6. b	6. b
7. b	7. c	7. c	7. d
8. d	8. b	8. d	8. c
9. a	9. d	9. d	9. b
10. d	10. a	10. b	10. c

Chapter 17	*Chapter 18*	*Chapter 19*	*Chapter 20*
1. a	1. a	1. b	1. d
2. b	2. c	2. b	2. c
3. c	3. c	3. d	3. d
4. b	4. b	4. a	4. b
5. c	5. d	5. c	5. a
6. d	6. d	6. a	6. a
7. c	7. c	7. c	7. d
8. c	8. b	8. d	8. c
9. c	9. d	9. c	9. b
10. a	10. a	10. b	10. b

Chapter 21	*Chapter 22*	*Chapter 23*	*Chapter 24*
1. d	1. c	1. b	1. d
2. a	2. d	2. c	2. c
3. d	3. b	3. c	3. a
4. b	4. d	4. b	4. c
5. c	5. a	5. a	5. c
6. d	6. c	6. d	6. b
7. c	7. b	7. d	7. d
8. a	8. c	8. b	8. b
9. d	9. b	9. c	9. c
10. b	10. c	10. a	10. d

Index